Pulmonary Diseases

Guest Editor

ALI I. MUSANI, MD

MEDICAL CLINICS
OF NORTH AMERICA

www.medical.theclinics.com

November 2011 • Volume 95 • Number 6

SAUNDERS an imprint of ELSEVIER, Inc.

W.B. SAUNDERS COMPANY
A Division of Elsevier Inc.

1600 John F. Kennedy Boulevard • Suite 1800 • Philadelphia, Pennsylvania 19103-2899

http://www.theclinics.com

MEDICAL CLINICS OF NORTH AMERICA Volume 95, Number 6
November 2011 ISSN 0025-7125, ISBN-13: 978-1-4557-2370-6

Editor: Rachel Glover
Developmental Editor: Donald Mumford

Medical Clinics of North America (ISSN 0025-7125) is published bimonthly by Elsevier Inc., 360 Park Avenue South, New York, NY 10010-1710. Months of issue are January, March, May, July, September, and November. Periodicals postage paid at New York, NY, and additional mailing offices. Subscription prices are USD 218 per year for US individuals, USD 404 per year for US institutions, USD 110 per year for US students, USD 277 per year for Canadian individuals, USD 525 per year for Canadian institutions, USD 173 per year for Canadian students, USD 336 per year for international individuals, USD 525 per year for international institutions and USD 173 per year for international students. To receive student/resident rate, orders must be accompanied by name of affiliated institution, date of term, and the *signature* of program/residency coordinator on institution letterhead. Orders will be billed at individual rate until proof of status is received. Foreign air speed delivery is included in all *Clinics* subscription prices. All prices are subject to change without notice. **POSTMASTER:** Send address changes to *Medical Clinics of North America*, Elsevier Health Sciences Division, Subscription Customer Service, 3251 Riverport Lane, Maryland Heights, MO 63043. **Customer Service: Telephone: 1-800-654-2452** (U.S. and Canada); **1-314-447-8871** (outside U.S. and Canada). **Fax: 1-314-447-8029.** E-mail: **journalscustomerservice-usa@elsevier.com** (for print support); **journalsonlinesupport-usa@ elsevier.com** (for online support).

Reprints. For copies of 100 or more of articles in this publication, please contact the Commercial Reprints Department, Elsevier Inc., 360 Park Avenue South, New York, NY 10010-1710. Tel.: 212-633-3812; Fax: 212-462-1935; E-mail: reprints@elsevier.com.

Medical Clinics of North America is also published in Spanish by McGraw-Hill Interamericana Editores S. A., P.O. Box 5-237, 06500 Mexico, D.F., Mexico.

Medical Clinics of North America is covered in *MEDLINE/PubMed (Index Medicus), Current Contents, ASCA, Excerpta Medica, Science Citation Index,* and *ISI/BIOMED.*

Printed in the United States of America.

GOAL STATEMENT

The goal of *Medical Clinics of North America* is to keep practicing physicians up to date with current clinical practice by providing timely articles reviewing the state of the art in patient care.

ACCREDITATION

The *Medical Clinics of North America* is planned and implemented in accordance with the Essential Areas and Policies of the Accreditation Council for Continuing Medical Education (ACCME) through the joint sponsorship of the University of Virginia School of Medicine and Elsevier. The University of Virginia School of Medicine is accredited by the ACCME to provide continuing medical education for physicians.

The University of Virginia School of Medicine designates this enduring material activity for a maximum of 15 *AMA PRA Category 1 Credit*(s)™ for each issue, 90 credits per year. Physicians should only claim credit commensurate with the extent of their participation in the activity.

The American Medical Association has determined that physicians not licensed in the US who participate in this CME enduring material activity are eligible for a maximum of 15 *AMA PRA Category 1 Credit*(s)™ for each issue, 90 credits per year.

Credit can be earned by reading the text material, taking the CME examination online at http://www.theclinics.com/home/cme, and completing the evaluation. After taking the test, you will be required to review any and all incorrect answers. Following completion of the test and evaluation, your credit will be awarded and you may print your certificate.

FACULTY DISCLOSURE/CONFLICT OF INTEREST

The University of Virginia School of Medicine, as an ACCME accredited provider, endorses and strives to comply with the Accreditation Council for Continuing Medical Education (ACCME) Standards of Commercial Support, Commonwealth of Virginia statutes, University of Virginia policies and procedures, and associated federal and private regulations and guidelines on the need for disclosure and monitoring of proprietary and financial interests that may affect the scientific integrity and balance of content delivered in continuing medical education activities under our auspices.

The University of Virginia School of Medicine requires that all CME activities accredited through this institution be developed independently and be scientifically rigorous, balanced and objective in the presentation/discussion of its content, theories and practices. All authors/editors participating in an accredited CME activity are expected to disclose to the readers relevant financial relationships with commercial entities occurring within the past 12 months (such as grants or research support, employee, consultant, stock holder, member of speakers bureau, etc.). The University of Virginia School of Medicine will employ appropriate mechanisms to resolve potential conflicts of interest to maintain the standards of fair and balanced education to the reader. Questions about specific strategies can be directed to the Office of Continuing Medical Education, University of Virginia School of Medicine, Charlottesville, Virginia. The faculty and staff of the University of Virginia Office of Continuing Medical Education have no financial affiliations to disclose.

The authors/editors listed below have identified no professional or financial affiliations for themselves or their spouse/ partner:

Esam H. Alhamad, MD, FCCP; Todd M. Bull, MD; Brendan Carolan, MD; Laurie L. Carr, MD; Ahmad Chebbo, MD; Gregory P. Cosgrove, MD, FCCP; James I. Finigan, MD; Rachel Glover, (Acquisitions Editor); David Hsia, MD; James M. Hunt, MD; Shirley F. Jones, MD, FCCP; Steve Lommatzsch, MD; Girish B. Nair, MD; Amy L. Olson, MD, MSPH; Evans R. Fernández Pérez, MD, MS; Amer Tfaili, MD; and Andrew Wolf, MD (Test Author).

The authors/editors listed below identified the following professional or financial affiliations for themselves or their spouse/ partner:

Ron Balkissoon, MD, DIH, MSc, FRCP(C) is on the Speakers' Bureau and Advisory Board for Astra Zeneca and GSK, and is on the Speakers' Bureau for Novartis, Genentech, and Forest Labs.

Stephen K. Frankel, MD is employed by the National Jewish Health, and is an Investigator (Gov) for the National Institutes of Health.

Nabeel Hamzeh, MD, FCCP receives research support from Centocor.

Jeffrey A. Kern, MD is an industry funded research/investigator for Cepheid, Inc, is a patent holder with Genentech, owns stock in Abbot Labs and Bristol Myers Squibb, amd is employed by Cleveland VAMC.

Richard W. Light, MD is a consultant, and is on the Speakers' Bureau and Advisory Board for Care Fusion.

Barry Make, MD is on the Advisory Board for Boehringer Ingelheim, Forest, AstraZeneca, MedImmune, Pfizer, Merck, Breathe, Novartis, and Abbott; is on the Speakers' Bureau for GSK and Boehringer Ingelheim; and, trains personnel and educates speakers for Forest.

Ali I. Musani, MD, FCCP is a consultant for Olympus USA, Cardinal health (Carefusion), and Super Dimension Inc, and receives research funding from Allegro Inc, Spiration Inc, and Boston Scientific (Asthmatics).

Michael S. Niederman, MD is a consultant and is on the Advisory Board for Pfizer, Merck, and Johnson and Johnson, and receives research funding from Novartis.

Rodolfo M. Pascual, MD is a consultant for Astra-Zeneca, is a consultant and an industry funded research/investigator for Actelion, and is on the Advisory Board for United Therapeutics and Gilead.

Stephen P. Peters, MD, PhD is on the Advisory Board for AstraZeneca, Aerocrine, Airsonett AB, Delmedica, GSK, Merck, and TEVA; has Editorial Activities with Resp Med, Resp Research, and J. Allergy; participates on the Speakers' Bureau for Merck, CME Programs for the American Thoracic Society, American Academy of Allergy, Asthma & Immunology, American College of Allergy, Asthma & Immunology, and Integrity Continuing Education; is a member of a Wake Forest University Climical Trails Group sponsored by Actelion, Amgen, Astra-Zeneca, Boehringer-Ingelheim, Centocor, Cephalon, Genentech, GSK, Medimmune, and Sanofi-Aventis; and participates in clinical trails and humans studies in asthma and COPD under the auspices of the NIH.

Disclosure of Discussion of Non-FDA Approved Uses for Pharmaceutical Products and/or Medical Devices

The University of Virginia School of Medicine, as an ACCME provider, requires that all faculty presenters identify and disclose any off-label uses for pharmaceutical and medical device products. The University of Virginia School of Medicine recommends that each physician fully review all the available data on new products or procedures prior to clinical use.

TO ENROLL

To enroll in the Medical Clinics of North America Continuing Medical Education program, call customer service at 1-800-654-2452 or visit us online at http://www.theclinics.com/home/cme. The CME program is available to subscribers for an additional fee of USD 228.

RELATED INTEREST

Clinics in Chest Medicine, December 2011 (Volume 34, Issue 4)
Respiratory Tract Infections: Advances in Diagnosis, Management and Prevention
Michael S. Niederman, MD, *Guest Editor*

VISIT US ONLINE!
Access your subscription at:
www.theclinics.com

Contributors

GUEST EDITOR

ALI I. MUSANI, MD, FCCP, FACP
Associate Professor of Medicine and Pediatrics, Director, Interventional Pulmonology Program, National Jewish Health; Associate Professor of Medicine, University of Colorado, Denver, Colorado

AUTHORS

ESAM H. ALHAMAD, MD, FCCP, FACP
Assistant Professor of Medicine, Division of Pulmonary Medicine, College of Medicine, King Saud University, Riyadh, Kingdom of Saudi Arabia

RON BALKISSOON, MD, DIH, MSc, FRCP(C)
National Jewish Health, Denver, Colorado

TODD M. BULL, MD
Division of Pulmonary Sciences and Critical Care Medicine, University of Colorado Denver, Aurora, Colorado

BRENDAN CAROLAN, MD
National Jewish Health, Denver, Colorado

LAURIE L. CARR, MD
Assistant Professor of Medicine, Division of Oncology, National Jewish Health, Denver, Colorado

AHMAD CHEBBO, MD
Division of Pulmonary, Critical Care and Sleep Medicine, Department of Internal Medicine, Scott and White Healthcare/Texas A&M Health Science Center, Temple, Texas

GREGORY P. COSGROVE, MD, FCCP
Assistant Professor of Medicine, Interstitial Lung Disease Program, National Jewish Health, Denver, Colorado

JAMES H. FINIGAN, MD
Assistant Professor of Medicine, Division of Oncology, National Jewish Health, Denver, Colorado

STEPHEN K. FRANKEL, MD
Associate Professor of Medicine, Interstitial Lung Disease Program, Autoimmune Lung Center, National Jewish Health, Denver; Division of Pulmonary Sciences & Critical Care Medicine, University of Colorado Denver, Aurora, Colorado

NABEEL HAMZEH, MD, FCCP
Assistant Professor, Division of Environmental and Occupational Health Sciences, National Jewish Health, Denver, Colorado

DAVID HSIA, MD
Division of Respiratory and Critical Care Physiology and Medicine, Harbor–University of California, Los Angeles Medical Center, Torrance, California

JAMES M. HUNT, MD
Division of Pulmonary Sciences and Critical Care Medicine, University of Colorado Denver, Aurora, Colorado

SHIRLEY F. JONES, MD, FCCP, FAASM
Division of Pulmonary, Critical Care and Sleep Medicine, Department of Internal Medicine, Scott and White Healthcare/Texas A&M Health Science Center, Temple, Texas

JEFFREY A. KERN, MD
Director of Lung Cancer Center, Professor, Division of Oncology, National Jewish Health, Denver, Colorado

RICHARD W. LIGHT, MD
Professor of Medicine, Division of Allergy, Pulmonary & Critical Care, Vanderbilty University Medical Center, Nashville, Tennessee

STEVE LOMMATZSCH, MD
National Jewish Health, Denver, Colorado

BARRY MAKE, MD
National Jewish Health, Denver, Colorado

ALI I. MUSANI, MD, FCCP, FACP
Associate Professor of Medicine and Pediatrics, Director, Interventional Pulmonology Program, National Jewish Health; Associate Professor of Medicine, University of Colorado, Denver, Colorado

GIRISH B. NAIR, MD
Fellow, Pulmonary and Critical Care Medicine, Winthrop-University Hospital, Mineola, New York

MICHAEL S. NIEDERMAN, MD
Chairman, Department of Medicine, Winthrop-University Hospital, Mineola; Professor and Vice-Chairman, Department of Medicine, SUNY at Stony Brook, Stony Brook, New York

AMY L. OLSON, MD, MSPH
Assistant Professor of Medicine, Interstitial Lung Disease Program, Autoimmune Lung Center, National Jewish Health, Denver; Division of Pulmonary Sciences & Critical Care Medicine, University of Colorado Denver, Aurora, Colorado

RODOLFO M. PASCUAL, MD
Assistant Professor of Internal Medicine, and Translational Science, Section on Pulmonary, Critical Care, Allergy & Immunologic Diseases, Department of Internal Medicine, Center for Genomics and Personalized Medicine Research, Wake Forest University School of Medicine, Winston-Salem, North Carolina

EVANS R. FERNÁNDEZ PÉREZ, MD, MS
Assistant Professor of Medicine, Interstitial Lung Disease Program, Autoimmune Lung Center, National Jewish Health, Denver, Colorado

STEPHEN P. PETERS, MD, PhD
Professor of Internal Medicine, Pediatrics, and Translational Science, Section on Pulmonary, Critical Care, Allergy & Immunologic Diseases, Department of Internal Medicine, Center for Genomics and Personalized Medicine Research, Wake Forest University School of Medicine, Winston-Salem, North Carolina

AMER TFAILI, MD
Division of Pulmonary, Critical Care and Sleep Medicine, Department of Internal Medicine, Scott and White Healthcare/Texas A&M Health Science Center, Temple, Texas

Contents

bronchoscopy, therapeutic modalities for central airway obstructions, pleural interventions, and novel therapies for asthma and chronic obstructive pulmonary disease. This article is an introduction to pertinent interventions within the context of the diseases encountered by the trained interventional pulmonologist.

and most clinicians periodically encounter patients with one or more of the eosinophilic lung diseases and need to understand how to recognize, diagnose, and manage these diseases. This review focuses on the clinical features, general diagnostic workup, and management of the eosinophilic lung diseases.

Preface

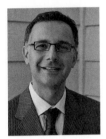

Ali I. Musani, MD, FCCP
Guest Editor

Pulmonary medicine is arguably one of the most complex and exciting disciplines in medicine. It overlaps with critical care medicine, sleep medicine, infectious diseases, and thoracic surgery, making it one of the largest contributors to the field of medicine.

Within the field of pulmonary medicine, technological and biomedical advances continue to yield new treatments for some of the most common and deadly diseases. The subspecialty of interventional pulmonology, for example, has revolutionized the diagnosis and staging of lung cancer and now shows promise in treating asthma and emphysema. Identification of clinically significant genetic mutations in lung cancer has led to targeted chemotherapeutic agents that expand treatment options and prolong survival. In community-acquired pneumonia, increasingly complex patients, new pathogens, and drug-resistant organisms pose continuing challenges, which may be met with new patient assessment tools, including biomarkers. Advances in molecular phenotyping have shed light on the pathogenesis and treatment of hypereosinophilic syndrome. As an understanding of these heterogeneous diseases unfolds, we may anticipate further advances in our ability to impact disease course and progression.

In this issue of *Medical Clinics of North America*, we are fortunate to have contributors who are experts in their fields, and who have spearheaded progress in their respective subspecialties. I am profoundly grateful to them for their dedication and efforts in creating this evidence-based, state-of-the-art edition.

I sincerely hope that the comprehensive and succinct articles in this issue will enhance the knowledge of general practitioners and subspecialists alike, with the ultimate, shared goal of creating better outcomes for our patients.

Ali I. Musani, MD, FCCP
Interventional Pulmonology Program
National Jewish Health
University of Colorado
J 225, Molly Blank, 1400 Jackson Street
Denver, CO 80206, USA

E-mail address:
Musani@njhealth.org

Med Clin N Am 95 (2011) xiii
doi:10.1016/j.mcna.2011.10.001
0025-7125/11/$ – see front matter © 2011 Elsevier Inc. All rights reserved.

Evaluation and Treatment of Patients with Non–Small Cell Lung Cancer

Laurie L. Carr, MD[a],*, James H. Finigan, MD[b], Jeffrey A. Kern, MD[c]

KEYWORDS

• Lung cancer • Treatment • Staging • Molecular testing

This article reviews the current diagnosis and treatment of patients with lung cancer, focusing on the role of the internist in lung cancer screening, staging, and follow-up. Historically, lung cancer is associated with high mortality rates and little effective therapy. Because this disease predominantly affects those of advanced age with significant comorbidities, treatment can be difficult to deliver safely with manageable adverse effects. All these factors can lead to a sense of futility among clinicians and patients when discussing lung cancer therapy. However, in the last several years, novel therapies have emerged to make lung cancer therapy better tolerated and more effective, even among those with significant comorbidities. Advances in surgical and radiation techniques, as well as the introduction of better-tolerated cytotoxic chemotherapy and targeted agents, have made lung cancer therapy tenable for many more patients. In addition, advances in lung cancer screening using low-dose computed tomography (CT) scans have demonstrated a benefit in lung cancer mortality for the first time and will make the early detection of lung cancer an active part of the management plan of high-risk individuals. Thus, although the morbidity and mortality of lung cancer remain high, novel approaches to screening and therapy have begun to make a significant impact on the burden of this disease.

The authors have nothing to disclose.

[a] Division of Oncology, National Jewish Health, 1400 Jackson Street, J-326a, Denver, CO 80206, USA

[b] Division of Oncology, National Jewish Health, 1400 Jackson Street, K-736a, Denver, CO 80206, USA

[c] Division of Oncology, National Jewish Health, 1400 Jackson Street, J-213, Denver, CO 80206, USA

* Corresponding author.

E-mail address: carrl@njhealth.org

Med Clin N Am 95 (2011) 1041–1054

doi:10.1016/j.mcna.2011.08.001

0025-7125/11/$ – see front matter © 2011 Elsevier Inc. All rights reserved.

medical.theclinics.com

EPIDEMIOLOGY

More men and women in the United States die of lung cancer than any other form of cancer.[1] Although more women are diagnosed with breast cancer each year, nearly twice as many women die of lung cancer than breast cancer. One reason for the high mortality rate of lung cancer is the advanced stage at diagnosis.[2] For example, only 16% of new lung cancer cases are diagnosed with localized disease that is potentially curable compared with 61.2% of breast cancer cases and 39.8% of colon cancer cases. This is one of the main reasons that the 5-year overall survival rate of lung cancer is only 15% compared with 89.1% for breast cancer and 65.2% for colon cancer. Not only is the 5-year survival rate for lung cancer low, it has also remained relatively unchanged since 1977 (12.3%). Currently, small cell lung cancer (SCLC) constitutes approximately 13% of newly diagnosed lung cancer cases; non–small cell lung cancer (NSCLC), which includes squamous cell carcinoma, adenocarcinoma, and large cell carcinoma, makes up most of the remaining cases (85.3%). Over time, there has been a change in the type of lung cancer diagnosed. In the late 1980s, adenocarcinoma became the most common histologic lung cancer type diagnosed in the United Sates, overtaking squamous cell carcinoma.[3] The change in the histology of NSCLC is attributed to changes in cigarette design introduced in the late 1950s. The introduction of filter-tip cigarettes and blended tobacco allowed for deeper inhalation and delivery of tobacco carcinogens more distally to the bronchoalveolar junction where adenocarcinomas often arise.

Lung cancer is a growing health problem on a global level because the prevalence of tobacco smoking in developing countries has steadily increased. The most recent global statistics provided by the World Health Organization for 2008 report an incidence of more than 1.6 million cases of lung cancer. Globally, more than 1.3 million men and women died of lung cancer in 2008, making lung cancer the leading cause of cancer death worldwide. The number of deaths attributed to lung cancer is expected to continue to increase up to 2030 because of smoking trends in developing countries in the past several decades.[4] In 2009, 57% of the adult male population of China and India smoked. The use of solid fuels for cooking and heating in poorly ventilated living spaces contributes to the risk of lung cancer, predominantly in low-income homes in Asia. Several studies of never-smoking women in China demonstrated an increased risk of lung cancer associated with the use of indoor coal burning for cooking.[5]

In the United States, cigarette smoking remains the most important risk factor for lung cancer. The lung cancer mortality rate for a nonsmoking man is 11.9/100,000 person-years; that rate increases to 224.3/100,000 person-years for a man who has smoked a pack per day for 20 years.[3] Trends for lung cancer occurrence follow cigarette-smoking trends with approximately a 20-year lag. The most recent data (2009) provided by the Centers for Disease Control document that 20.6% of US adults currently smoke (smoked >100 cigarettes in their lifetime, now smoke every or some days). Although smoking rates have decreased since 1997 (24.7%), they have remained unchanged in the past several years.

Former smokers in the United States also make up a significant part of the population at just more than 20%. Unfortunately, even after smoking cessation, the risk of lung cancer remains high for many years, although it does slowly decrease. When compared with a never smoker, the risk of lung cancer for an individual who smoked a pack per day remains nearly sevenfold higher even 10 years after quitting.[6] The risk decreases with longer cessation intervals and lower amounts of former smoking. For those with high levels of previous exposure, the risk remains increased for more than

20 years. Today, more than 40% of new lung cancer cases are diagnosed in patients who are former smokers.

Approximately 15% of all lung cancers are diagnosed in those who have never smoked.[7] Analysis of 2 large American Cancer Society Cancer Prevention Study cohorts, CPS-I (1959–1972) and CPS-II (1982–2000), revealed that the rate of lung cancer death between nonsmoking women and men is the same and that the total rate of lung cancer among never smokers has not increased with time.[7] Certainly, other risk factors, such as environmental tobacco smoke (ETS), radon gas exposure, and occupational exposures, contribute to the incidence of lung cancer in this population. Multiple studies have analyzed the association between ETS and lung cancer. A comprehensive meta-analysis performed in 1997 estimated an excess risk of lung cancer for never smokers married to smoking spouses at 23% (95% CI 13%–43%), accounting for 3000 to 5000 lung cancer deaths annually in the United States.[8] Radon gas exposure was originally shown to be associated with lung cancer through analysis of uranium miners. A recent analysis in North America demonstrated a significant risk associated with increased levels of indoor radon gas (10% increased risk per 100 Bq/m^3 increase in radon exposure).[9] The occupational exposure to asbestos, arsenic, and silica has consistently been reported to increase the risk of lung cancer among never smokers.[10–12] Each of these occupational exposures has a positive relationship between duration of exposure and cumulative exposure to lung cancer risk. Other agents implicated in case-control studies include pesticides, metal dust and fumes, and organic solvents.[13] Although not an occupational exposure, previous treatment with radiation to the chest for medical purposes has also been shown to increase future lung cancer diagnoses.[14] A cohort study of patients with Hodgkin disease who received greater than 9 Gy of thoracic radiation therapy demonstrated an increased risk of future lung cancer versus those patients who did not receive thoracic radiation.

PATHOPHYSIOLOGY

Advances in molecular biology have enabled the search for novel molecular abnormalities in lung cancer that provide insights into tumorigenesis as well as potential therapeutic targets. The identification of driver mutations, those mutations that drive neoplastic transformation and contribute to tumor progression, has provided at least 2 clinically important targets to date. Epidermal growth factor receptor (EGFR) is a member of the human epidermal growth factor receptor (HER) family, a group of 4 transmembrane tyrosine kinase receptors expressed on epithelial cells of many organs, including the lung. In response to ligand binding, EGFR (HER1) forms a homodimer with another EGFR molecule or heterodimerizes with a different HER family receptor (HER 2, 3, or 4). This leads to tyrosine phosphorylation on the EGFR intracellular domain and activation of EGFR's kinase activity, resulting in phosphorylation of target proteins and initiation of downstream signaling. Normal functions of EGFR include epithelial growth and differentiation, cell-cell adhesion, and cell migration.[15]

Many NSCLCs harbor at least one EGFR mutation. Most EGFR mutations are in the tyrosine kinase domain and result in EGFR activation and unregulated signaling.[16,17] The discovery of these mutations forms the basis for the use of the EGFR tyrosine kinase inhibitors (TKI) erlotinib and gefitinib as a treatment for lung cancer. The presence of EGFR mutations strongly predicts a response to TKI therapy. One pooled analysis of 3 studies demonstrated a response rate to TKI treatment of 81% in mutation-positive cancers compared with less than 10% in mutation-negative cancers.[18] Given the poor response of mutation-negative cancers, therapy selection based on molecular characteristics is superior to using standard clinical criteria.

However, further analyses have revealed growing complexity and certain EGFR mutations are associated with resistance to TKI treatment. In addition, over time, almost all TKI responsive lung cancers acquire secondary mutations rendering them resistant to further treatment and relapse is inevitable.[19]

Certain clinical characteristics are associated with EGFR mutation-positive lung cancer. Mutation-positive cancers are almost exclusively NSCLC, specifically adenocarcinoma.[16] EGFR mutations have been reported in 10% to 15% of Western and 25% to 30% of Asian patients with lung cancer. EGFR mutations are significantly more common in women and nonsmokers. Mutation status is not associated with tumor stage and some studies suggest a survival benefit in patients with EGFR-mutated lung cancer, regardless of treatment.[20] Currently, our practice is to test all adenocarcinomas of the lung for the presence of an EGFR mutation. Use of a TKI as first-line therapy is reserved for those with mutation-positive tumors. However, TKI therapy can be used as third-line or fourth-line therapy in mutation-negative cancers.

Another clinically relevant molecular subset of NSCLC are those that are driven by the newly discovered echinoderm microtubule-associated protein-like 4 (EML4) and anaplastic lymphoma kinase (ALK) translocation.[21] The EML4-ALK translocation in NSCLC leads to the constitutive activation of the ALK kinase domain and promotes cell growth and survival. This translocation is found in approximately 2% to 5% of NSCLC, most commonly seen in never smokers or light smokers with adenocarcinomas. It is rarely found in tumors that harbor activating mutations in EGFR. As discussed later, a novel TKI, crizotinib, has been developed to target ALK mutations.

Genome-wide studies of multiple lung cancers have revealed other recurring mutations within additional signaling pathways that could provide additional targets and may account for most NSCLC cases. A recently reported study of 1000 cases of adenocarcinoma revealed that 60% of the tumors contained 1 of 10 individual driver mutations that were analyzed (**Fig. 1**).[22]

SCREENING

Although currently there are no accepted recommendations for lung cancer screening, the recent publication of the results of the National Lung Screening Trial (NLST) has the potential to change our approach to lung cancer screening. Based on previous observational studies demonstrating that low-dose helical CT scans increased the detection of early-stage lung cancer,[23] the NLST is the first large randomized lung cancer

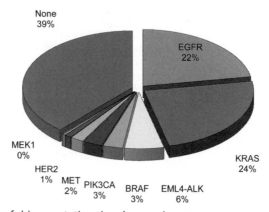

Fig. 1. Frequency of driver mutations in adenocarcinoma.

screening trial to decrease lung cancer mortality.[24] From 2002 to 2004, the NLST randomized more than 50,000 subjects (aged 55–74 years who had a history of cigarette smoking of at least 30 pack-years and were either actively smoking or had quit within the past 15 years) to low-dose helical CT scan or chest radiograph with a baseline imaging study and annual studies for 2 additional years. The study demonstrated a relative reduction in lung cancer mortality of 20.0% ($P = .004$) after a median 6.5 years of follow-up. The authors estimate that 7 million Americans would currently meet the eligibility criteria used for this study. Although this study is a major step forward in the efforts to find an effective lung cancer screening tool, many questions remain unanswered. There were many false-positive findings. More than 23% of the low-dose helical CT scans had a false-positive result, leading to concerns of expense and morbidity associated with unnecessary diagnostic procedures in follow-up. The NLST reported that the rate of complications from diagnostic procedures for nodule evaluation was low (1.4%) with only 0.06% leading to a major complication. However, the cost-effectiveness of CT screening is yet to be analyzed. In addition, the number of lung cancer diagnoses remained stable at each round of imaging, leading to the question of whether screening should continue longer than 2 years. Although the dose of radiation with these scans is reduced (1.5 mSv, approximately one-third the dose of a conventional chest CT), there is concern regarding the risk of repeated radiation exposure. The use of additional predictors for lung cancer risk, such as serum biomarkers, could potentially improve the risk assessment for a given individual (beyond age and smoking history) to focus on those who will benefit the most from CT screening.

WORK-UP

Although NSCLC can be asymptomatic and incidentally found on chest imaging performed for other reasons, often patients present with nonspecific pulmonary symptoms. For those at increased risk (significant smoking history, age >55 years, and family history of lung cancer), there are several signs/symptoms that necessitate a closer evaluation for lung cancer. New or worsening cough, dyspnea, and chest wall pain are often manifestations of a lung tumor, although they are also common complaints in nonmalignant disease. However, when these symptoms are accompanied by hemoptysis, weight loss, or progressive fatigue in a high-risk patient, consideration of lung cancer should be included in the work-up. Patients may present with signs and symptoms of postobstructive pneumonitis, including cough, fever, and increased sputum production. Therefore, it is important that high-risk patients who present with a consolidation thought to be caused by infection are evaluated following treatment to ensure that the consolidation has cleared. If imaging and clinical evaluation are concerning for lung cancer, assessment of underlying comorbidities, including pulmonary function, is important when considering further diagnostic procedures and treatment.

The initial evaluation of a patient with chest imaging suspicious for lung cancer centers on obtaining tissue for pathologic evaluation. The safest and least invasive procedure should be chosen based on radiographic evidence that ideally could provide not only a tissue diagnosis but also staging information. The approach chosen must be balanced by obtaining sufficient material to enable the pathologist to make a histologic determination, including enough tissue for immunohistochemistry (IHC) and molecular testing, if needed.[25] For example, testing pleural effusions for malignant cells can establish an advanced stage, but often leads to insufficient tissue for molecular testing and the patient requires an additional biopsy procedure. If a patient has radiologic evidence of a solitary site of metastatic disease, attempts should be made to sample that site to provide a diagnosis and have pathologic confirmation of advanced disease. For patients with evidence of extensive metastatic disease, if the metastatic site is not safe or easily amenable to biopsy, it is often most efficient to sample the primary lung lesion. Bronchoscopy can be used in the diagnosis and local staging of both central and peripheral lesions. Standard bronchoscopy has a low yield for diagnosis of peripheral lesions less than 2 cm in size, with a 28% to 30% diagnostic accuracy.[26] However, emerging technology in interventional pulmonary techniques now allows for navigational bronchoscopy with an increased ability to sample small peripheral lesions with a diagnostic yield of 70%[27] and should be considered before referring the patient for a transthoracic approach.[28] In addition, the use of endobronchial ultrasound-guided transbronchial needle aspiration (EBUS-TBNA) allows for sampling of mediastinal and hilar lymph nodes. EBUS-TBNA can be used to confirm suspicious findings on CT and positron emission tomography (PET) scans. Coupling EBUS-TBNA with esophageal ultrasound techniques allows noninvasive access to almost all nodal stations important to the staging evaluation. CT-guided transthoracic needle aspiration (TTNA) can be used to sample peripheral lesions, with a diagnostic yield for malignancy of 85% to 90%. The amount of nondiagnostic procedures, as well as complications with pneumothorax, increases with more centrally located tumors.[29] For a small peripheral lung lesion that is highly suspicious for lung cancer (spiculated, increasing in size, PET avid, and so forth), often a surgical resection provides both diagnosis and treatment.

STAGING

Accurate staging of newly diagnosed lung cancer provides information regarding prognosis and risk of disease recurrence. This information is necessary to develop the appropriate therapeutic plan for each patient and provide patients with the necessary information to determine risk versus benefit of therapy. Staging is based on an algorithm that encompasses primary tumor size and invasion, nodal involvement, and the identification of metastases. The current staging algorithm for lung cancer was revised in 2009 and published in *TNM Classification of Malignant Tumors*, 7th edition (**Table 1**).[30] Initial clinical staging involves a CT of the chest that includes the adrenal glands to determine tumor size, invasion, and local and regional nodal status. The addition of an fluorodeoxyglucose (FDG)-PET scan to evaluate for metastatic disease and further assess possible involvement of the mediastinal lymph nodes has been proven to prevent futile thoracotomies.[31] The specificity and sensitivity for mediastinal lymph node involvement, when assessed by CT scan, are 69% and 71%, respectively.[32] These are increased to 86% and 85% when PET/CT is added. EBUS with TBNA of suspected lymph nodes can be used to confirm suspicious hilar and mediastinal lymph nodes that are positive on imaging studies. However, mediastinoscopy should be used to confirm a negative EBUS evaluation for those tumors at high risk for nodal involvement (based on size and central location). Magnetic resonance imaging (MRI) of the brain is recommended for stage II and III disease before initiating aggressive local therapy. This should also be considered for stage I disease when the primary tumor is a centrally located adenocarcinoma.[33]

TREATMENT

The treatment for lung cancer is determined by stage, patient preference, comorbidities, and overall performance status (**Table 2**). Treatment planning should include presentation and discussion at a multidisciplinary tumor board with review of

Table 1
Staging of NSCLC

T (Primary Tumor)	
T1 (T1a/T1b)	Tumor ≤3 cm in greatest dimension, surrounded by lung or visceral pleura, without evidence of invasion more proximal than the lobar bronchus
T2 (T2a/T2b)	Tumor >3 cm but ≤7 cm or tumor with any of the following: involves main bronchus, ≥2 cm distal to the carina, invades visceral pleura, associated with atelectasis or obstructive pneumonitis that extends to the hilar region but does not involve the entire lung
T3	Tumor >7 cm or one that involves any of the following: chest wall, diaphragm, phrenic nerve, mediastinal pleura, parietal pericardium, or tumor in the main bronchus <2 cm from the carina, or atelectasis/obstructive pneumonitis of the entire lung, or separate nodule(s) in the same lobe
T4	Tumor that invades: mediastinum, heart, great vessels, trachea, recurrent laryngeal nerve, esophagus, vertebral body, carina, or separate nodule(s) in an ipsilateral lobe
N (Regional Lymph Nodes)	
N0	No regional lymph node metastasis
N1	Metastasis in ipsilateral peribronchial and/or ipsilateral hilar lymph nodes and intrapulmonary lymph nodes, including involvement by direct extension
N2	Metastasis in ipsilateral mediastinal and/or subcarinal lymph node(s)
N3	Metastasis in contralateral mediastinal, contralateral hilar, ipsilateral or contralateral scalene, or supraclavicular lymph node(s)
M (Distant Metastasis)	
M0	No distant metastasis
M1 (M1a/M1b)	Distant metastasis
TNM Stage Grouping	
Stage I	IA (T1a, or T1b, N0, M0) IB (T2a, N0, M0)
Stage II	IIA (T1a, or T1b, or T2b, N1, M0 or T2b, N0, M0) IIB (T2b, N1, M0 or T3, N0, M0)
Stage III	IIIA (T3 or T4, N1, M0 or T4, N0, M0 or T1–3, N2, M0) IIIB (T1–4, N3,M0 or T4, N2, M0)
Stage IV	T1–4, N0–3, M1

From AJCC. AJCC cancer staging manual. 7th edition. New York: Springer; 2009; with permission.

pathology and staging.[35] The recommended therapy for stage I disease is surgical resection, with stereotactic body radiation therapy (SBRT) reserved for those who are medically inoperable. Stage II disease is also treated with surgery followed by adjuvant chemotherapy to prevent disease recurrence. Stage IIIA disease has multiple treatment options determined by the extent of regional (nodal) involvement. Stage IIIA disease is often treated with concurrent chemotherapy and radiation, adding surgical resection (trimodality therapy) for those who are medically fit and have responded well to initial concurrent therapy. Stage IIIB disease is not amenable to surgical resection and is therefore treated with concurrent chemotherapy and radiation only. Metastatic disease is treated with systemic therapy, chemotherapy, and/or molecular targeted agents, with radiation used for palliation of painful lesions or brain metastasis.

Table 2 Treatment of NSCLC by stage				
	Stage I (IA/IB)	Stage II (IIA/IIB)	Stage III (IIIA/IIIB)	Stage IV
Percentage at diagnosis[2,a]	15%	Regional: 22%		56%
Treatment	Surgical resection or SBRT (medically inoperable)	Surgical resection and adjuvant chemotherapy	IIIA: Concurrent chemo/ radiation or trimodality therapy IIIB: Concurrent chemo/ radiation	Palliative systemic therapy (chemotherapy or erlotinib)
5-year survival[34]	73%/58%	46%/36%	24%/9%	13%

[a] 7% are unknown (unstaged at diagnosis).

SURGERY FOR EARLY-STAGE LUNG CANCER

The Lung Cancer Study Group has published the only randomized study to date comparing lobectomy with sublobar resection for stage I (T1N0M0) NSCLC.[36] This study determined that the rate of local recurrence among those treated with sublobar resection was significantly higher than those with a lobectomy. Although survival was better for the lobectomy group, this did not reach statistical significance. Because of these results, lobectomy is considered the appropriate surgery for stage I NSCLC, whereas sublobar resections are considered a reasonable approach for those with compromised pulmonary function. More recent studies, predominantly retrospective analyses have determined that tumors 2 cm in size or less have similar outcomes with either surgical approach.[37] Tumors comprised entirely of adenocarcinoma in situ (formerly bronchioloalveolar carcinoma) and less than 2 cm in size have a 100% cure rate with surgical resection. These tumors appear as pure ground-glass opacities on chest CT and can be resected with a sublobar approach.[38] A national clinical research study, CALGB-140503, is currently randomizing patients with peripheral NSCLC less than or equal to 2 cm in size to lobectomy versus sublobar resection to determine if this less invasive approach provides appropriate local control.

Video-assisted thoracoscopic surgery (VATS), a recent advance in the surgical treatment of patients with early-stage lung cancer, has improved the adverse events associated with surgical resection without compromising treatment outcomes.[39] A secondary analysis of data from the American College of Surgeons Oncology Group compared outcomes from those who underwent either video-assisted thoracoscopic or open lobectomy for early-stage lung cancer.[40,41] Those undergoing VATS had shorter operating time, fewer postoperative complications, and shorter hospital stays despite having similar rates of negative surgical margins and lymph nodes dissected. VATS is now considered a preferred approach to lung cancer resection for those patients without contraindications.[33]

RADIATION THERAPY FOR LUNG CANCER

Radiation therapy can be used to treat lung cancer in multiple settings. It can be given concurrently with chemotherapy as definitive treatment for stage III disease that is not amenable to surgery, as adjuvant therapy for positive resection margins identified postoperatively or nodal fields at high risk for relapse, and in selective fields for palliation of advanced disease. Recently, new techniques have made radiation as a single modality more effective for early-stage disease in medically inoperable patients. A general term for this new approach is SBRT. In this approach, highly focused beams of ionizing radiation are delivered to the target with high precision. The entire treatment is given over 5 or fewer sessions with the use of image-guided intensive radiation dosing as opposed to weeks of therapy required for a full course of standard external beam radiotherapy. A phase II study published in 2010 reported on patients with medically inoperable T1-T2 N0 NSCLC treated with SBRT.[42] For the 55 patients who were evaluable, the 3-year primary tumor control rate was 97.6% (95% CI 84.3%–99.7%). The rate of overall survival at 3 years was 55.8% (95% CI 41.6%–67.9%). This is a significant improvement over previous reports of external beam radiation for inoperable, early-stage NSCLC that described 2-year overall survival of only 39%.[43] The adverse event rate was low (~17%), with acceptable levels of pulmonary toxicity in this group of patients with significant lung disease (2% with grade 3 [severe but not life-threatening] pneumonitis, 3% with grade 3 reduction in pulmonary function tests).[44] The most disappointing finding in this trial was the rate of disseminated recurrence at 3 years (22.1%), suggesting occult metastatic disease at the time of therapy that cannot be controlled by local therapy. Although randomized studies are yet to be reported using SBRT, the data are promising and studies are currently underway to determine the appropriate dose and if SBRT can be safely used for more centrally located tumors. This modality shows promise to improve the outcomes of those with significant comorbidities and limited surgical options.

SYSTEMIC THERAPY FOR NSCLC
Molecular Targeted Therapy

As described above, several driver mutations have been identified in subsets of patients with NSCLC and have become therapeutic targets for advanced disease. The presence of driver mutations allows targeting of mutant proteins that are only present in the lung cancer, avoiding systemic toxicity seen in nontargeted therapy. Currently, an oral TKI, erlotinib, is US Food and Drug Administration (FDA)-approved drug targeting a driver mutation in lung cancer, mutant EGFR, additional TKIs and monoclonal antibodies are in clinical trials. Erlotinib received FDA approval based on an improvement in overall survival seen in a randomized phase III trial of erlotinib versus best supportive care in heavily pretreated patients with NSCLC.[45] The identification of specific activating mutations within EGFR that predict for disease response to EGFR inhibitors has made routine genetic testing feasible.[46] Multiple randomized clinical trials have demonstrated that patients with activating mutations within EGFR have significant improvement in disease response with decreased toxicity when treated with erlotinib, compared with traditional chemotherapy, as first-line therapy.[47] As a result of these findings, it is recommended that all patients with newly diagnosed advanced adenocarcinoma of the lung have their cancer tested for EGFR activating mutations and be treated with erlotinib if a mutation is identified.[48] The most common toxicities seen with EGFR inhibitors are acneform type rash, diarrhea, and a small risk of interstitial lung disease (<1% in white patients). Patients treated with EGFR TKIs develop drug resistance on average about 1 year after treatment.[47] Mechanisms of resistance are being studied to provide future targeted therapy in this setting.

The EML4-ALK translocation is another driver mutation discovered in approximately 5% to 7% of NSCLC, again predominantly found in adenocarcinomas. A recently reported nonrandomized clinical trial of crizotinib, a TKI that targets the ALK kinase domain, demonstrated encouraging rates of disease control (90%) in patients with advanced lung cancer with EML4-ALK translocations.[49] Crizotinib is currently being studied in phase III clinical trials as first-line therapy for these patients. The FDA has recently approved crizotinib for treatment of lung cancer patients with EML4-ALK translocations, making it the second TKI approved for use in treatment of advanced lung cancer.

The monoclonal antibody bevacizumab, which targets the vascular endothelial growth factor (VEGF), is approved for first-line treatment of NSCLC when combined with cytotoxic chemotherapy. VEGF is not mutated in NSCLC, and this therapy, although molecularly targeted, is not specific to the tumor. A large randomized phase III study published in 2006 demonstrated an improvement in overall survival (hazard ratio 0.79 P = .003) for those patients who received bevacizumab in addition to chemotherapy for advanced NSCLC.[50] Because of the high risk of life-threatening hemoptysis seen in early clinical trials, patients with squamous cell lung cancer or a history of hemoptysis were excluded from this study. As an antiangiogenesis agent, bevacizumab has several unique adverse effects, including hemoptysis, hypertension, and proteinuria.[51] When carefully used in patients with advanced lung cancer, bevacizumab is a novel targeted agent that can improve the survival of those with advanced disease.

Systemic Chemotherapy

Cytotoxic chemotherapy continues to play an important role in the treatment of lung cancer and remains the recommended first-line therapy for those with metastatic disease without activating mutations in EGFR and for all patients on progression as second-line therapy. In metastatic lung cancer, the goals of chemotherapy are to improve the duration of survival and to palliate the symptoms of disease. Standard first-line therapy is a platinum-based drug (cisplatin or carboplatin) combined with a second agent. Chemotherapy has been demonstrated to improve survival in the elderly ($\geq$70 years) with advanced disease to the same extent as those who are young.[52] Although there is an increase in side effects, particularly cytopenias, advanced age is not a contraindication to chemotherapy. The decision to use chemotherapy in the setting of incurable disease is based on patient preference, comorbidities, and performance status, and requires an ongoing dialog between the patient and physician throughout the disease course.

Chemotherapy is also indicated as concurrent therapy with radiation for those with stage III disease and as adjuvant therapy following definitive surgery in high-risk stage I to III disease (see **Table 2**). By definition the use of chemotherapy in the adjuvant setting is to prevent the recurrence of disease following potentially curative surgery. Although adjuvant chemotherapy has been commonly used for other solid tumors, such as colorectal and breast cancer, for several decades, its use in NSCLC is more recent. A meta-analysis of patients treated with cisplatin-based chemotherapy in the adjuvant setting demonstrated a 5.4% improvement in absolute survival at 5 years.[53] This benefit was seen in those with stage II to III disease and good performance status. Currently, 4 cycles of adjuvant chemotherapy initiated approximately 4 to 8 weeks after surgery is the standard of care for patients after surgery.

SURVIVORSHIP

The follow-up care of those with a history of lung cancer focuses on surveillance for disease recurrence and second primary cancers, monitoring for sequelae of lung cancer therapy, and ongoing smoking cessation. Following potentially curative therapy for lung cancer, patients should undergo a thorough history and examination with a contrasted CT of the chest every 4 to 6 months for 2 years, then annually.[35] Attention should also be paid to the high risk of second primary cancers in this population, particularly head and neck cancer, as well as routine screening for colorectal, breast, and prostate cancer. Ongoing discussions of smoking cessation with referral to counseling for those who continue to smoke are recommended for all lung cancer survivors. Sequelae of lung cancer therapy, including a decline in lung function for those with surgical resection or thoracic radiation, and renal insufficiency, hearing loss, and peripheral neuropathy for those who received cisplatin-based chemotherapy, are commonly seen and may require medical intervention. Although survivorship care is often provided by a medical oncologist, commonly patients turn to their primary care physicians for follow-up.

SUMMARY

Lung cancer continues to cause significant morbidity and mortality in the US population. Although the 5-year survival for this disease has not changed substantially in several decades, several important recent advances have been made that may finally begin to change this dismal statistic. A focus on diagnosing disease at an early stage through the use of low-dose helical CT scan screening, more effective treatment options for those with early-stage disease who are medically inoperable, the adoption of adjuvant chemotherapy through community practice, and the introduction of molecularly targeted therapy to improve survival for those with advanced disease all contribute to changing the outlook for those with lung cancer. Further advances in lung cancer are anticipated in the near future with novel therapeutics currently undergoing evaluation in clinical trials and several lung cancer screening trials nearing completion. Internists play an important role in recognizing those at risk, instituting screening when possible, encouraging the elderly and those with comorbidity to explore what therapy may be available, providing palliative care for those with incurable disease, and ensuring that survivors of lung cancer have appropriate follow-up for the sequelae of lung cancer treatment and disease recurrence.

ACKNOWLEDGMENTS

The authors wish to acknowledge Midge Neel for her assistance with editing and article preparation.

REFERENCES

1. United States Cancer Statistics: 1999-2007 Incidence and mortality web-based report. US Cancer Statistics Working Group 2010; Available at: http://www.cdc.gov/uscs. Accessed July 25, 2011.
2. SEER cancer statistics review 1975-2008. 2011. Available at: http://www.cancer.gov. Accessed July 25, 2011.
3. Thun MJ, Lally CA, Flannery JT, et al. Cigarette smoking and changes in the histopathology of lung cancer. J Natl Cancer Inst 1997;89(21):1580–6.
4. WHO report on the global tobacco epidemic. Geneva: World Health Organization; 2008.
5. Lan Q, He X, Shen M, et al. Variation in lung cancer risk by smoky coal subtype in Xuanwei, China. Int J Cancer 2008;123:2164–9.
6. Hrubec A, McLaughlin JK. Former cigarette smoking and mortality among U.S. veterans: a 26 year follow-up, 1954-1980. Bethesda (MD): US Government Printing Office; 1997. p. 501–30.

7. Thun M, Henley SL, Burns D, et al. Lung cancer death rates in lifelong nonsmokers. J Natl Cancer Inst 2006;98:691–9.

8. Hackshaw A, Law MR, Wald NJ. The accumulated evidence on lung cancer and environmental tobacco smoke. BMJ 1997;315:980–8.

9. Krewski D, Lubin JH, Zielinski JM, et al. Residential radon and risk of lung cancer. a combined analysis of 7 North American case-control studies. Epidemiology 2005;16:137–45.

10. Jarup L, Pershagen G. Arsenic exposure, smoking, and lung cancer in smelter workers - a case-control study. Am J Epidemiol 1991;134(6):545–51.

11. Cassidy A, Mannetje A, van Tongeren M, et al. Occupational exposure to crystalline silica and risk of lung cancer. A multicenter case-control study in Europe. Epidemiology 2007;18(1):36–43.

12. Berry G, Newhouse ML, Turok M. Combined effect of asbestos exposure and smoking on mortality from lung cancer in factory workers. Lancet 2003; 300(7775):476–9.

13. Pohlabeln H, Boffetta P, Ahrens W, et al. Occupational risks for lung cancer among nonsmokers. Epidemiology 2000;11(5):532–8.

14. van Leeuwen F, Klokman WJ, Stovall M, et al. Roles of radiotherapy and smoking in lung cancer following Hodgkin's disease. J Natl Cancer Inst 1995;87:1530–7.

15. Jorissen RN, Walker F, Pouliot N, et al. Epidermal growth factor receptor: mechanisms of activation and signalling. Exp Cell Res 2003;284(1):31–53.

16. Shigematsu H, Lin L, Takahashi T, et al. Clinical and biological features associated with epidermal growth factor receptor gene mutations in lung cancers. J Natl Cancer Inst 2005;97(5):339–46.

17. Sharma SV, Bell DW, Settleman J, et al. Epidermal growth factor receptor mutations in lung cancer. Nat Rev Cancer 2007;7(3):169–81.

18. Pao W, Girard N. EGF receptor gene mutations are common in lung cancers from "never smokers" and are associated with sensitivity of tumors to gefitinib and erlotinib. Proc Natl Acad Sci U S A 2004;101(36):13306–11.

19. Nguyen KS, Kobayashi S, Costa DB. Acquired resistance to epidermal growth factor receptor tyrosine kinase inhibitors in non-small-cell lung cancers dependent on the epidermal growth factor receptor pathway. Clin Lung Cancer 2009; 10(4):281–9.

20. Cooper WA, O'Toole S, Boyer M, et al. What's new in non-small cell lung cancer for pathologists: the importance of accurate subtyping, EGFR mutations and ALK rearrangements. Pathology 2011;43(2):103–15.

21. Soda M, Young LC, Enomoto M, et al. Identification of the transforming EML4-ALK fusion gene in non-small-cell lung cancer. Nature 2007;448:561–6.

22. Kris MG, Johnson DJ, Kwiatkowski DJ, et al. Identification of driver mutations in tumor specimens from 1,000 patients with lung adenocarcinoma: the NCI's Lung Cancer Mutation Consortium (LCMC). J Clin Oncol 2011;29(Suppl): [abstract CRA7506] 477s.

23. Henschke C, Yankelevitz DF, McCauley A, et al. Survival of patients with stage I lung cancer detected on CT screening. N Engl J Med 2006;355:1763–71.

24. Aberle D, Adams AM, Berg CD, et al. Reduced lung-cancer mortality with low-dose computed tomographic screening. N Engl J Med 2011;365(5): 395–409.

25. Travis WD, Brambilla E, Noguchi M, et al. International Association for the Study of Lung Cancer/American Thoracic Society/European Respiratory Society international multidisciplinary classification of lung adenocarcinoma. J Thorac Oncol 2011;6(2):244–85.

26. Mazzone P, Jain P, Arroliga AC, et al. Bronchoscopy and needle biopsy techniques for diagnosis and staging of lung cancer. Clin Chest Med 2002;23(1):137–58, ix.

27. Wilson D, Bartlett RJ. Improved diagnostic yield of bronchoscopy in a community practice. combination of electromagnetic navigation system and rapid on-site evaluation. J Bronchol 2007;14(4):227–32.

28. Rivera MP, Mehta AC. Initial diagnosis of lung cancer. ACCP evidence-based clinical practice guidelines (2nd edition). Chest 2007;132(Suppl 3):131S–48S.

29. Yung RC. Tissue diagnosis of suspected lung cancer. selecting between bronchoscopy, transthoracic needle aspiration, and resectional biopsy. Respir Care Clin N Am 2003;9(1):51–76.

30. AJCC. AJCC cancer staging manual. 7th edition. New York: Springer; 2009.

31. Fischer B, Lassen U, Mortensen J, et al. Preoperative staging of lung cancer with combined PET-CT. N Engl J Med 2009;361(1):32–9.

32. Yang W, et al. Value of PET/CT versus enhanced CT for locoregional lymph nodes in non-small cell lung cancer. Lung Cancer 2008;61(1):35–43.

33. Jazieh AR, Bamefleh H, Demirkazik A, et al. Modification and implementation of NCCN guidelines on non-small cell lung cancer in the Middle East and North Africa region. J Natl Compr Canc Netw 2010;8(Suppl 3):S16–21.

34. Goldstraw P, Crowley J, Chansky K, et al. The IASLC Lung Cancer Staging Project: proposals for the revision of the TNM stage groupings in the forthcoming (seventh) edition of the TNM Classification of malignant tumours. J Thorac Oncol 2007;2(8):706–14.

35. Ettinger DS, Johnson B. Non-small cell lung cancer. J Natl Compr Canc Netw 2010;8(7):740–801.

36. Ginsberg RJ, Rubinstein LV. Randomized trial of lobectomy versus limited resection for T1 N0 non-small cell lung cancer. Lung Cancer Study Group. Ann Thorac Surg 1995;60(3):615–22 [discussion: 622–3].

37. Okada M, Yoshikawa K, Hatta T, et al. Is segmentectomy with lymph node assessment an alternative to lobectomy for non-small cell lung cancer of 2 cm or smaller? Ann Thorac Surg 2001;71(3):956–60 [discussion: 961].

38. Rami-Porta R, Tsuboi M. Sublobar resection for lung cancer. Eur Respir J 2009; 33(2):426–35.

39. Yan TD, Black D, Bannon PG, et al. Systematic review and meta-analysis of randomized and nonrandomized trials on safety and efficacy of video-assisted thoracic surgery lobectomy for early-stage non-small-cell lung cancer. J Clin Oncol 2009;27(15):2553–62.

40. Scott WJ, Allen MS, Darling G, et al. Video-assisted thoracic surgery versus open lobectomy for lung cancer: a secondary analysis of data from the American College of Surgeons Oncology Group Z0030 randomized clinical trial. J Thorac Cardiovasc Surg 2010;139(4):976–81 [discussion: 981–3].

41. Whitson BA, Whitson BA, Andrade RS, et al. Video-assisted thoracoscopic surgery is more favorable than thoracotomy for resection of clinical stage I non-small cell lung cancer. Ann Thorac Surg 2007;83(6):1965–70.

42. Timmerman R, Paulus R, Galvin J, et al. Stereotactic body radiation therapy for inoperable early stage lung cancer. JAMA 2010;303(11):1070–6.

43. Sibley GS. Radiotherapy for patients with medically inoperable Stage I nonsmall cell lung carcinoma: smaller volumes and higher doses–a review. Cancer 1998; 82(3):433–8.

44. Trotti A, Colevas AD, Setser A, et al. CTCAE v3.0: development of a comprehensive grading system for the adverse effects of cancer treatment. Semin Radiat Oncol 2003;13(3):176–81.

45. Shepherd FA, Rodrigues Pereira J, Ciuleanu T, et al. Erlotinib in previously treated non-small-cell lung cancer. N Engl J Med 2005;353(2):123–32.

46. Lynch TJ, Bell DW, Sordella R, et al. Activating mutations in the epidermal growth factor receptor underlying responsiveness of non-small-cell lung cancer to gefitinib. N Engl J Med 2004;350(21):2129–39.

47. Maemondo M, Inoue A, Kobayashi K, et al. Gefitinib or chemotherapy for non-small-cell lung cancer with mutated EGFR. N Engl J Med 2010;362(25):2380–8.

48. Azzoli CG, Baker S, Temin S, et al. ASCO Clinical Practice Guideline update on chemotherapy for stage IV non-small- cell lung cancer. J Clin Oncol 2009; 27(36):6251–66.

49. Kwak EL, Bang YL, Camidge DR, et al. Anaplastic lymphoma kinase inhibition in non-small-cell lung cancer. N Engl J Med 2010;363(18):1693–703.

50. Sandler A, Gray R, Perry MC, et al. Paclitaxel-carboplatin alone or with bevacizumab for non-small-cell lung cancer. N Engl J Med 2006;355(24):2542–50.

51. Crino L, Dansin E, Garrido P, et al. Safety and efficacy of first-line bevacizumab-based therapy in advanced non- squamous non-small-cell lung cancer (SAiL, M019390). a phase 4 study. Lancet 2010;11(8):733–40.

52. Davidoff AJ, Tang M, Seal B, et al. Chemotherapy and survival benefit in elderly patients with advanced non-small- cell lung cancer. J Clin Oncol 2010;28(13): 2191–7.

53. Pignon JP, Tribodet H, Scagliotti GV, et al. Lung adjuvant cisplatin evaluation. a pooled analysis by the LACE Collaborative Group. J Clin Oncol 2008;26(21): 3552–9.

Pleural Effusions

Richard W. Light, MD

KEYWORDS

- Pleura • Pleural effusion • Empyema • Parapneumonic effusion
- Malignant pleural effusion

Approximately 1.5 million people develop a pleural effusion in the United States each year.[1] There are many different causes of pleural effusions (**Box 1**). When a patient is seen who has a pleural effusion, efforts should be made to find the cause of the effusion so that appropriate treatment can be instituted. In this article an approach to the diagnosis of pleural effusions is suggested and the diagnosis and management of the most common causes of pleural effusion are discussed.

SEPARATION OF EXUDATES FROM TRANSUDATES

One of the main reasons to do a thoracentesis in a patient with an undiagnosed pleural effusion is to determine whether the patient has a transudative or an exudative pleural effusion. The reason to make this differentiation is that the existence of a transudative pleural effusion indicates that systemic factors such as heart failure or cirrhosis are responsible for the effusion, whereas the existence of an exudative effusion indicates that local factors are responsible for the effusion. If the patient has a transudative effusion, the systemic abnormality can be treated and no attention need be diverted to the pleura. Alternatively, if an exudative effusion is present investigations need to be directed toward the pleura to find out the cause of the local problem.

For the past several decades, the principal manner by which transudates and exudates are identified is with the Light criteria.[2] According to the Light criteria, an exudative effusion is present if one or more of the following conditions are met: (1) pleural fluid protein/serum protein level greater than 0.5, (2) pleural fluid lactic acid dehydrogenase (LDH)/serum LDH level greater than 0.6, or (3) pleural fluid LDH level greater than two-thirds the upper normal limit for serum LDH.

The primary problem with the Light criteria is that they identify 15% to 20% of transudative effusions as exudative effusions. This situation is particularly likely if the patient has been receiving diuretics before the thoracentesis.[3] If the patient has CHF or cirrhosis but the pleural fluid meets exudative criteria by a small amount, then the difference between the serum protein and the pleural fluid protein should

Financial Disclosures: I am a consultant and am on the speaking bureau for Care Fusion, which makes the PleurX catheter.
Division of Allergy/Pulmonary/Critical Care, Vanderbilty University Medical Center, 1161 21st Avenue South, Nashville, TN 37232, USA
E-mail address: rlight98@yahoo.com

| Box 1 |
| Differential diagnoses of pleural effusion |

1. Transudative pleural effusions
    a. Congestive heart failure (CHF)
    b. Cirrhosis
    c. Nephrotic syndrome
    d. Superior vena caval obstruction
    e. Fontan procedure
    f. Urinothorax
    g. Peritoneal dialysis
    h. Glomerulonephritis
    i. Myxedema
    j. Cerebrospinal fluid leak to pleura
    k. Hypoalbuminemia
2. Exudative pleural effusions
    a. Neoplastic diseases
        i. Metastatic disease
        ii. Mesothelioma
        iii. Body cavity lymphoma
        iv. Pyothorax-associated lymphoma
    b. Infectious diseases
        i. Bacterial infections
        ii. Tuberculosis
        iii. Fungal infections
        iv. Parasitic infections
        v. Viral infections
    c. Pulmonary embolization
    d. Gastrointestinal disease
        i. Pancreatic disease
        ii. Subphrenic abscess
        iii. Intrahepatic abscess
        iv. Intrasplenic abscess
        v. Esophageal perforation
        vi. Postabdominal surgery
        vii. Diaphragmatic hernia
        viii. Endoscopic variceal sclerosis
        ix. Postliver transplant
    e. Heart diseases
        i. Postcoronary artery bypass graft (post-CABG) surgery
        ii. Postcardiac injury (Dressler) syndrome

      iii. Pericardial disease

      iv. Pulmonary vein stenosis postcatheter ablation of atrial fibrillation

  f. Obstetric and gynecologic disease

      i. Ovarian hyperstimulation syndrome

      ii. Fetal pleural effusion

      iii. Postpartum pleural effusion

      iv. Meigs syndrome

      v. Endometriosis

  g. Collagen vascular diseases

      i. Rheumatoid pleuritis

      ii. Systemic lupus erythematosus

      iii. Drug-induced lupus

      iv. Immunoblastic lymphadenopathy

      v. Sjögren syndrome

      vi. Familial Mediterranean fever

      vii. Churg-Strauss syndrome

      viii. Wegener granulomatosis

  h. Drug-induced pleural disease

      i. Nitrofurantoin

      ii. Dantrolene

      iii. Methysergide

      iv. Ergot drugs

      v. Amiodarone

      vi. Interleukin 2

      vii. Procarbazine

      viii. Methotrexate

      ix. Clozapine

  i. Miscellaneous diseases and conditions

      i. Asbestos exposure

      ii. Postlung transplant

      iii. Postbone marrow transplant

      iv. Yellow nail syndrome

      v. Sarcoidosis

      vi. Uremia

      vii. Trapped lung

      viii. Therapeutic radiation exposure

      ix. Drowning

      x. Amyloidosis

      xi. Milk of calcium pleural effusion

      xii. Electrical burns

xiii. Extramedullary hematopoiesis

xiv. Rupture of mediastinal cyst

xv. Acute respiratory distress syndrome

xvi. Whipple disease

xvii. Iatrogenic pleural effusions

j. Hemothorax

k. Chylothorax

l. Pseudochylothorax

be measured. If this difference is greater than 3.1 gm/dL, then the patient in all probability has a transudative pleural effusion.[4]

CHF is by far the leading cause of transudative pleural effusions. In recent years it has been shown that levels of N-terminal probrain natriuretic peptide (NT-proBNP) are increased in the pleural fluid and serum of patients with CHF.[5] Levels more than 1500 pg/mL in either the serum or the pleural fluid are virtually diagnostic of CHF.[5] The levels of NT-proBNP are virtually identical in the pleural fluid and the serum.[6] It has been shown that the pleural fluid BNP levels are less accurate than the pleural fluid NT-proBNP in identifying patients with CHF, although a BNP level of 115 pg/mL does identify most patients with CHF.[7]

Routine Tests on Pleural Fluid

In addition to measuring the protein and LDH levels in the pleural fluid to differentiate transudates and exudates, the following tests are recommended on the pleural fluid[8]: description of the fluid; cell count and differential; glucose; pH particularly if the patient has a parapneumonic effusion; cytology; smears and cultures for bacteria, mycobacteria, and fungi; and adenosine deaminase (ADA) if tuberculous pleuritis is in the differential.

The appearance of the pleural fluid should always be noted. If it is very cloudy or milky, then it should be centrifuged. A clear supernatant indicates that the cloudiness is caused by cells or debris and the patient probably has an empyema. If cloudiness persists after centrifugation, the cloudiness is caused by a high lipid level in the pleural fluid and the patient has a chylothorax or a pseudochylothorax. If the fluid looks very bloody, a hematocrit should be obtained on the pleural fluid. A hemothorax is present if the pleural hematocrit exceeds 50% of the peripheral hematocrit.

Most transudates have a nucleated cell count less than 1000/mm^3, whereas most exudates have a nucleated cell count more than 1000/mm^3. The cell count in empyemas is frequently low because the sediment is caused by debris and dead cells. The cells in the pleural space are classified as neutrophils, small lymphocytes, other mononuclear cells, and eosinophils.[1] The presence of predominantly neutrophils indicates that the pleural process is acute. If the presumptive diagnosis is a parapneumonic effusion and there are not predominantly neutrophils in the pleural fluid, an alternate diagnosis should be sought. The presence of predominantly small lymphocytes in the pleural fluid suggests pleural tuberculosis, malignancy, or a post-CABG surgery pleural effusion. Eosinophilic pleural effusions have more than 10% eosinophils and are most commonly idiopathic or caused by malignancy.[9,10]

A low pleural fluid glucose (<60 mg/dL) indicates that the pleural effusion is probably caused by 1 of the following 4 entities: complicated parapneumonic effusion, malignant pleural effusion, tuberculous pleural effusion, and rheumatoid pleural effusion. Other rare causes of low glucose effusions are hemothorax, paragonimiasis, Churg-Strauss syndrome, and occasionally lupus pleuritis. If a patient has a parapneumonic effusion, the pleural fluid pH should be measured because the lower the pH, the more likely the patient is to require surgery for the effusion.[11] To be clinically useful, the pH must be measured with a blood gas machine; pH meter and indicator strips are not sufficiently accurate.[12]

If there is any suspicion that the patient has a malignancy, a cytologic examination on the pleural fluid is indicated. If the patient has malignancy, the cytology is diagnostic in about 65%. The cytology is more likely to be positive with adenocarcinoma than with squamous cell carcinoma, Hodgkin disease, or lymphoma.

If bacterial infection is suspected as a cause of the pleural effusion, bacterial smears and cultures of the pleural fluid should be obtained. It has been shown that using blood culture bottles inoculated at the bedside increases the number of positive cultures by about 50%.[13] In like manner if tuberculous pleuritis is suspected, use of a BACTEC (BD Franklin Lakes, NJ, USA) system with bedside inoculation provides higher yields and faster results than do conventional methods.[1] If tuberculous pleuritis is suspected, a pleural fluid ADA level should be obtained. Pleural fluid ADA levels more than 40 U/L in a patient with predominantly lymphocytes in their pleural fluid are virtually diagnostic of tuberculous pleuritis.[14]

Approach to Patient with No Diagnosis After a Thoracentesis

When one considers the diseases most likely to cause pleural effusions (**Table 1**), this provides some guidance as to how to proceed. The first procedure that is recommended is a computed tomography (CT) angiogram. Not only does the CT angiogram show whether or not a pulmonary embolus (the fourth leading cause of a pleural effusion) is present, it also identifies the presence of pulmonary infiltrates, pleural masses, or mediastinal lymphadenopathy, providing clues to the cause of the pleural effusion.

Observation

If the CT angiogram is not diagnostic of pulmonary embolism and if there are no other abnormalities in the parenchyma, pleura, or mediastinum, observation is probably the

Table 1
Estimated annual incidence of various causes of pleural effusions in the United States

CHF	500,000
Parapneumonic effusion	300,000
Malignant pleural effusion	200,000
Lung	60,000
Breast	50,000
Lymphoma	40,000
Other	60,000
Pulmonary embolization	150,000
Viral disease	100,000
Cirrhosis with ascites	50,000
Post-CABG surgery	50,000
Gastrointestinal disease	25,000
Tuberculosis	2500

best course of action if the patient is improving. It is estimated (see **Table 1**) that 100,000 cases of pleural effusions each year are caused by viral illnesses. Pleural effusions caused by viral illnesses are self-limited, and invasive procedures such as bronchoscopy or thoracoscopy do not establish the diagnosis.

Needle Biopsy of Pleura

If the patient has a pleural mass or pleural thickening, consideration should be given to performing a CT-guided cutting needle biopsy of the abnormal area.[15] The CT-guided cutting needle biopsy provides a significantly higher diagnostic yield than does the blind needle biopsy of the pleura.[15] In the past blind needle biopsy of the pleural was frequently performed primarily to establish the diagnosis of tuberculous pleuritis or malignancy. However, for the following reasons needle biopsy is rarely indicated if thoracoscopy is readily available. The diagnosis of tuberculous pleuritis is more easily established by showing a pleural fluid ADA more than 40 U/L. Moreover, if the pleural fluid cytology is negative and the patient has malignancy, blind needle biopsy is diagnostic of malignancy in only about 20% of cases.[16]

Bronchoscopy

If the patient has a parenchymal lesion, a massive pleural effusion or hemoptysis, bronchoscopy should be performed. However, if none of these abnormalities is present, then bronchoscopy is not indicated because in this situation it is rarely diagnostic.[17] If the mediastinum is shifted toward the side of the effusion, bronchoscopy is also indicated because this finding is suggestive of an obstructed bronchus.

Thoracoscopy

Thoracoscopy establishes the diagnosis of either malignancy or tuberculosis in nearly 100% of cases.[18] Thoracoscopy should be performed only when less invasive procedures are nondiagnostic. In patients with undiagnosed pleural effusions, 4 characteristics are suggestive that the patient has a malignant pleural effusion, namely, (1) a symptomatic period of more than a month, (2) absence of fever, (3) blood-tinged or bloody pleural fluid, or (4) CT findings suggestive of malignancy (pulmonary or pleural masses, pulmonary atelectasis, or lymphadenopathy).[19] In 1 study of 93 patients with negative cytology who were referred for thoracoscopy, 28 had all 4 criteria and all had malignancy, whereas 21 had at most 1 criterion and none had malignancy.[19] If thoracoscopy is performed for an undiagnosed pleural effusion, a procedure should be performed to create a pleurodesis at the time of the thoracoscopy.

DISEASES THAT MOST COMMONLY CAUSE PLEURAL EFFUSION

In the sections that follow, the diseases that most commonly cause pleural effusions are discussed.

CHF

CHF is responsible for more pleural effusions than any other disease entity. In most cases the origin of the pleural fluid is fluid in the interstitial spaces of the lung resulting from an increased wedge pressure.[20] However, patients with right heart failure may also develop a pleural effusion.[21] The pleural effusion is usually bilateral, but if unilateral it is more commonly on the right.[22]

The diagnosis is usually suggested by the clinical picture of CHF. Initially a thoracentesis is indicated only if the patient has pleuritic chest pain, is febrile, or if the effusions are greatly disparate in size. If the effusion persists after treatment of the CHF is initiated, a thoracentesis can be performed. The pleural fluid is a transudate by definition, but if diuretics have been administered to the patient, the pleural fluid may meet the Light exudative criteria, as discussed earlier. That the fluid is caused by CHF may be established by showing an NT-proBNP level more than 1500 pg/mL or a serum-pleural fluid protein gradient more than 3.1 g/dL. If the effusion is large and the patient is dyspneic, a therapeutic thoracentesis frequently relieves the dyspnea.

Cirrhosis

The other main cause of a transudative pleural effusion is cirrhosis with ascites. The predominant mechanism leading to a pleural effusion in a patient with cirrhosis and ascites is the movement of ascitic fluid through a diaphragmatic defect into the pleural space.[23] At times, the ascites may not be apparent clinically. The initial management of the pleural effusion associated with cirrhosis and ascites should be directed toward treatment of the ascites with a low-salt diet and diuretics. If this strategy is ineffective, then liver transplantation is the best option. If liver transplantation is not feasible, the next best treatment is implantation of a transjugular intrahepatic portosystemic shunt (TIPS).[24] If neither TIPS nor liver transplantation is feasible, the best alternative is probably videothoracoscopy with closure of the diaphragmatic defects and pleurodesis, but this approach is associated with significant morbidity and mortality.[25]

Parapneumonic Effusions and Empyema

A parapneumonic effusion is any pleural effusion associated with bacterial pneumonia, lung abscess, or bronchiectasis. Approximately 1 million individuals are hospitalized each year with pneumonia and because approximately 40% have a pleural effusion, parapneumonic effusion is one of the most common pleural effusions. Parapneumonic effusions that require tube thoracostomy or that are culture positive are designated complicated parapneumonic effusions. If the pleural fluid is pus, an empyema is present.

All patients with parapneumonic effusion should be treated with antibiotics. For patients with severe community-acquired pneumonia in whom *Pseudomonas* is not suspected, the recommended agents are a β-lactam plus either an advance macrolide or a respiratory fluoroquinolone. If a *Pseudomonas* infection is suspect, an anti-*Pseudomonas* antibiotic such as piperacillin, piperacillin-tazobactam, imipenem, meropenem, or cefepime should be included.[26] Because anaerobic bacteria cause many parapneumonic effusions, anaerobic coverage with either clindamycin or metronidazole is recommended.[27] If the patient has a health care-associated pneumonia, vancomycin should be administered because many of these are caused by methicillin-resistant *Staphylococcus aureus*.[28]

When a patient with pneumonia is evaluated, the possibility of a parapneumonic effusion should be considered. If the diaphragms are not visible throughout their lengths on both the posteroanterior and lateral chest radiograph, the possibility of a parapneumonic effusion should be evaluated with ultrasound, chest CT scan, or lateral decubitus chest radiographs. If the thickness of the fluid is greater than 20 mm, a thoracentesis should be performed.[29] Initially it was recommended that all effusions more than 10 mm thick be sampled,[30] but it now seems that only effusions more than 20 mm thick need be sampled because almost all effusions smaller than this resolve with only antibiotics.[29]

It is recommended that the initial thoracentesis be a therapeutic thoracentesis.[1] The reasoning behind this recommendation is that if a patient has a needle in their chest, it is prudent to take all the fluid out. If the fluid does not return, one need not worry about the pleural effusion. Alternative approaches are to insert a small chest tube or perform a diagnostic thoracentesis. There are no controlled studies comparing the efficacy of these 3 approaches. The purpose of the thoracentesis is to determine whether the pleural fluid has those characteristics associated with a bad prognosis, namely a positive Gram stain or culture, a pH level less than 7.20, a glucose level less than 60 mg/dL, an LDH level greater than 3 times the upper limit of normal or the presence of pus. The yield with bacterial cultures is increased if the pleural fluid is inoculated directly into blood culture bottles at the bedside.[13] If the differential cell count does not show predominantly neutrophils, an alternative diagnosis should be sought.[1]

If the pleural fluid cannot be completely removed with the therapeutic thoracentesis or there are bad prognostic factors present, a chest tube should be inserted. Small chest tubes (<14 F) seem to be as effective as large chest tubes and are recommended because they are less painful.[31] If the pleural fluid is not completely removed by the small chest tube, the pleural fluid is probably loculated. The loculations are created by fibrin bands that result from the intense pleural inflammation. Many papers have been written attesting to the effectiveness of fibrinolytics such as streptokinase, urokinase, or tissue plasminogen activator (tPA) in facilitating drainage of loculated pleural effusions. However, these positive studies were mostly uncontrolled. In the largest study ever performed, 454 patients in a multicenter, double-blind randomized study received streptokinase 250,000 IU or saline, both in a total volume of 30 mL, twice a day for a total of 3 days.[32] There was no difference in the number of patients requiring additional therapy or the length of hospitalization in the 2 groups. Moreover, subgroup analysis was unable to show any group that appeared to benefit from the streptokinase.[32]

The same group conducted a second study in which they compared the efficacy of 10 mg tPA, 4 mg DNase (Pulmozyme), saline, and the combination of 10 mg tPA and 4 mg DNase[33] in a double-blind, randomized multicenter study of 210 patients. The primary end point for this study was the reduction in the percentage of the hemithorax occupied by the pleural fluid. The results were as follows: tPA 15.1%, saline 17%, DNase 17.1%, and tPA plus DNase 29.7%. The results with the combination were significantly better than the results with the other 3 regimens.[33] It is recommended that to treat a patient with a loculated parapneumonic effusion with fibrinolytics, the combination of 10 mg tPA plus 4 mg DNase be used.

The primary alternative approach to fibrinolytics for loculated parapneumonic effusions is video-assisted thoracic surgery (VATS) with the breakdown of adhesions, the optimal placement of chest tubes, and possibly decortication. Most patients who undergo VATS need no additional therapy. When 4 studies in the late 1990s are combined, VATS was the definitive procedure in 77% of the patients. After VATS, the median time for chest tube drainage was 5.3 to 12.3 days, the median hospital stay ranged from 5.3 to 12.3 days, and the overall mortality was 3%.[34–37] There have been no randomized studies comparing VATS with the combination of tPA and DNase in the treatment of loculated parapneumonic effusion. If VATS is available and the patient is a surgical candidate, then VATS is the preferred procedure.

When a pleural infection is present, the pleural space must be eradicated before the infection can be cured. At times a rind of fibrous tissue forms on the visceral pleura that prevents the underlying lung from expanding and eliminating the pleural space. In such a situation, the fibrous tissue must be removed from the visceral pleura through a process called decortication. Decortication can frequently be performed at the time of VATS, but on occasion an open thoracotomy must be performed to remove all the fibrous tissue and allow the underlying lung to expand. If the patient does not have uncontrolled pleural sepsis and there is fibrous tissue covering the visceral pleura, the patient need not go to surgery because the fibrous tissue usually resolves with time.

MALIGNANT PLEURAL EFFUSION

Malignant pleural effusions are the second most common exudative pleural effusion (see **Table 1**). Pleural effusions associated with neoplasms arise through at least 5 different mechanisms: (1) the pleural surfaces may be involved by the tumor, which leads to increased permeability of the pleural membranes, possibly because of vascular endothelial growth factor[38]; (2) the neoplasm may obstruct the lymphatics or veins draining the pleural space, leading to the accumulation of pleural fluid; (3) an endobronchial tumor may completely obstruct a bronchus, leading to atelectasis and a pleural effusion from the decreased pleural pressure; (4) a pneumonia distal to a partially obstructed bronchus may lead to a parapneumonic effusion; and (5) the malignancy may disrupt the thoracic duct, leading to a chylothorax.

When a pleural effusion is present in a patient with malignancy, one should attempt to determine the cause of pleural effusion with these 5 causes in mind. The pleural effusion may be caused by a different disease such as CHF, pulmonary embolism, or pneumonia.

The possibility of a malignant pleural effusion should be considered in all patients with undiagnosed exudative pleural effusions. The diagnosis is established by showing malignant cells in the pleural space. The easiest way to establish the diagnosis of a malignant pleural effusion is via cytology of the pleural fluid, as described earlier. If the cause remains undiagnosed after a cytologic examination, the most efficient way to make the diagnosis is with thoracoscopy or with a cutting needle biopsy of the pleura, as described earlier.

The initial step in the management of a malignant pleural effusion is to attempt to identify the site of the primary tumor to decide whether to administer systemic chemotherapy. Approximately 75% of pleural malignancies are caused by lung cancer, breast cancer, or leukemia. To identify the site of the primary, the following studies are indicated: CT scan of the chest looking for a lung primary, mediastinal lymphadenopathy suggestive of a lymphoma, and mammography looking for a breast primary. If these studies are not informative, additional studies should be based on the patient's symptoms and the results of the physical examination.

The prognosis of patients with malignant pleural effusions is grave, with a median life expectancy of 4 to 5 months. The presence of the malignant pleural effusion indicates that the malignancy is disseminated and is not curable with surgery. The aim of therapy for the pleural effusion is to provide the patient with the highest possible quality of life with a minimal amount of hospitalization.

The primary symptom caused by the pleural effusion is dyspnea. Maneuvers designed to remove or prevent the accumulation of pleural fluid are indicated only if the patient's quality of life is reduced by dyspnea and the dyspnea is relieved with a therapeutic thoracentesis. The 2 main treatments for the fluid accumulation with malignant effusions are the implantation of an indwelling catheter and the intrapleural injection of a sclerosing agent to produce a pleurodesis.

The indwelling pleural catheter most commonly used is a 15.5-Fr silicone rubber catheter (PleurX catheter, CareFusion, Waukegan, IL, USA) that can be inserted on an outpatient basis[39,40] by pulmonologists, interventional radiologists, or surgeons. The catheter is tunneled and has a valve on the distal end that prevents fluid or air from passing in either direction through the catheter unless the catheter is accessed with a matching drainage line. The pleural fluid is drained at 24-hour to 48-hour intervals by inserting the access tip of the drainage line into the valve of the catheter and then draining the fluid via an external tube into vacuum bottles.[39]

The indwelling pleural catheter is effective in managing malignant pleural effusions.[41] In 1 retrospective analysis of 250 tunneled pleural catheter insertions in 223 patients at a single center, symptom control was compete in 39% and partial in another 50%.[42] No additional procedure was necessary in 90%.[42] A spontaneous pleurodesis occurs in about 50% of patients who receive the indwelling catheter. In 1 study 173 of 295 catheters (58.6%) were removed because the fluid drainage had become less than 50 mL/d at a mean of 29.4 days after catheter insertion.[43] Reaccumulation of fluid that produced dyspnea occurred in only 5 of the 173 patients (2.9%). The biggest advantage of the indwelling pleural catheter is that it can be inserted as an outpatient. Adverse effects events associated with the indwelling catheter include pleural infection (2.8%) (which can be managed with intravenous antibiotics, leaving the catheter in place), catheter blockage (which can be managed with the instillation of a fibrinolytic into the catheter or replacement of the catheter), and chest pain with the removal of fluid (which can be minimized by draining the fluid more slowly).[44]

The primary alternative to insertion of an indwelling pleural catheter is to inject an irritant into the pleural space, which can create an intense inflammatory response, leading to fusion of the visceral and parietal pleural.[1] Many different agents have been used as pleurodesing agents, but doxycycline 500 mg is the agent I recommend. The only 2 agents approved by the US Food and Drug Administration are talc and bleomycin. Talc is the agent most commonly used,[45] but it is not recommended because it causes fatal acute respiratory distress syndrome (ARDS) in more than 1% of patients.[46] ARDS seems to be related to talc with small particle size, and talc should never be used if the size of the talc particles is not known.[1] Another reason that talc is not recommended is that in the biggest randomized controlled study ever performed for pleurodesis, talc administered either as a slurry or insufflated at thoracoscopy was not particularly effective.[46]

The following is the procedure recommended for pleurodesis. A chest tube (9–14 Fr) is inserted and the pleurodesing agent is injected as soon as the lung is completely expanded. Before the agent is injected, the patient should undergo conscious sedation with systemic medications such as lorazepam or midazolam, because the procedure can be painful. Doxycycline 500 mg in 50 mL saline is injected through the chest tube into the pleural space and then the tube is clamped for the next 1 to 2 hours. The chest tube is then unclamped and negative pressure is applied until the drainage becomes less than 150 mL/d. The chest tube is then removed. Pleurodesis performed in this manner is effective in obliterating the pleural space and controlling the effusion about 80% of the time. The disadvantage of this procedure is that the patient has to remain hospitalized for a median of about 5 days. If patients remain dyspneic after either insertion of the indwelling catheter or pleurodesis, the dyspnea can be treated with opiates, which are titrated just as they are for pain.

PLEURAL EFFUSION CAUSED BY PULMONARY EMBOLISM

Pulmonary embolism is the fourth leading cause of pleural effusions. Approximately 20% to 40% of patients with pulmonary embolism have a pleural effusion.[47] The presence of pleuritic chest pain in a patient with a pleural effusion is suggestive of pulmonary embolus. More than 75% of patients with pleural effusions secondary to pulmonary emboli have pleuritic chest pain.[47]

The pleural effusions secondary to pulmonary emboli are usually unilateral and occupy less than one-third of the hemithorax.[48] Approximately 20% of pleural effusions secondary to pulmonary emboli are loculated, and loculation is more common if the diagnosis is delayed more than 10 days after symptoms develop.[48] There is not a good correlation between the side of the embolus and the side of the effusion.[48] The pleural fluid with pulmonary embolism is almost always exudative.[48,49]

The diagnosis of pulmonary embolism should be considered in every patient with an undiagnosed exudative pleural effusion. If the patient has a high probability of pulmonary embolism (see article on pulmonary embolism by Hunt and Bull elsewhere in this issue), the patient should be immediately started on low-molecular-weight heparin or unfractionated heparin, and a test for pulmonary embolism should be performed before a thoracentesis is attempted. The serum D-dimer level should be measured in patients with a low probability of pulmonary embolism. If the D-dimer level is normal, the diagnosis of pulmonary embolism is virtually ruled out. If the D-dimer level is increased, another test must be performed to confirm the diagnosis of pulmonary embolism.[49] The treatment of patients with pulmonary embolism and pleural effusion is the same as the treatment of patients with pulmonary emboli without pleural effusion. If the effusion increases in size with treatment, a diagnostic thoracentesis should be performed to rule out pleural infection or hemothorax.

PLEURAL EFFUSIONS CAUSED BY VIRAL DISEASES

It is estimated that viral infections are responsible for 100,000 pleural effusions annually in the United States (see **Table 1**). However, the diagnosis of a viral pleural effusion is rarely established because it depends on showing an increase in antibodies to the virus. The importance of viral pleural effusions is that they are self-limited. Accordingly, if a patient with an undiagnosed exudative effusion is improving, no additional diagnostic procedures are indicated.

PLEURAL EFFUSIONS CAUSED BY TUBERCULOSIS

In some parts of the world, tuberculous pleural effusions are the most common pleural effusions, but they are relatively uncommon in the United States (see **Table 1**). However, if a patient has tuberculous pleuritis, it is important to establish the diagnosis because if the patient is not treated, the effusion spontaneously resolves, but the patient has a high likelihood of subsequently developing pulmonary or extrapulmonary tuberculosis.[50]

The diagnosis of tuberculous pleuritis should be suspected in any patient with an undiagnosed exudative pleural effusion.[14] Patients with tuberculous pleuritis usually have a subacute illness characterized by cough, pleuritic chest pain, and fever. The pleural fluid with tuberculous pleuritis is an exudate that usually has predominantly small lymphocytes and often has a protein level more than 5 gm/dL. The diagnosis is established by showing a pleural fluid ADA level more than 40 IU/L in a lymphocytic pleural effusion.[14] In equivocal cases, needle biopsy or thoracoscopy may be necessary to establish the diagnosis. Cultures of pleural fluid are positive in less than 20% of patients with tuberculous pleuritis. The treatment of tuberculous pleuritis is the same as the treatment of pulmonary tuberculosis.

PLEURAL EFFUSIONS AFTER CABG

Almost all patients after CABG develop a pleural effusion, and approximately 10% develop a pleural effusion that occupies more than 25% of the hemithorax.[51] The primary symptom of patients with pleural effusions after CABG is dyspnea. Chest pain and fever are distinctly uncommon. The pleural effusions that occur after

CABG can be divided into those that occur within the first 30 days and those that occur after the first 30 days.[52] The pleural fluid in both instances is an exudate. The early effusions are frequently bloody and many contain more than 10% eosinophils. The late effusions are not bloody and contain mostly small lymphocytes.[53]

Patients who are dyspneic from a pleural effusion after CABG should undergo a therapeutic thoracentesis. Patients who are febrile or have pleuritic chest pain should also undergo a thoracentesis to rule out pleural infection. When a thoracentesis is performed in a patient with an effusion after CABG, studies should be performed to rule out CHF, chylothorax, and pleural infection. The possibility of pulmonary embolus should always be considered.[52] Most patients with a pleural effusion after CABG are cured with 1 to 3 therapeutic thoracenteses.[50] There is no evidence that the administration of diuretics or antiinflammatory agents are effective in the management of post-CABG effusion.[52]

PLEURAL EFFUSIONS CAUSED BY SYSTEMIC LUPUS ERYTHEMATOSUS

Pleural effusions occur in approximately 40% of patients with systemic lupus erythematosus.[1] The effusions are frequently bilateral but may be unilateral and change from 1 side to the other. Pericardial effusions are frequently present concomitantly with the pleural effusion. The pleural fluid is typically a serous exudate with normal pH and glucose levels and an LDH level less than 2 times the upper limit of normal.[54] The diagnosis of lupus pleuritis is established by using the diagnostic criteria published by the American Rheumatism Association. Patients with lupus pleuritis should be treated with oral prednisone, 80 mg every other day, with rapid tapering once the symptoms are controlled.

PLEURAL EFFUSIONS CAUSED BY RHEUMATOID DISEASE

Pleural effusions occur in approximately 4% of patients with rheumatoid pleuritis. Most rheumatoid pleural effusions occur in men and most patients have subcutaneous rheumatoid nodules. The effusion is usually small to moderate in size and only occasionally produces symptoms. The pleural fluid with rheumatoid pleuritis is distinctive, with a glucose level less than 30 mg/dL, an LDH level more than 2 times the upper limit of normal, and a pH level less than 7.20.[54] It is not clear that any medical therapy exerts a positive influence on the course of rheumatoid pleuritis.

PLEURAL EFFUSIONS CAUSED BY GASTROINTESTINAL DISEASE

Many different gastrointestinal diseases can have an associated pleural effusion, and it is beyond the scope of this article to discuss them all in detail. Patients with acute pancreatitis frequently have an associated pleural effusion, and at times chest symptoms dominate the clinical picture. The diagnosis is established by showing a high pleural fluid amylase level. Patients with pancreatic pseudocysts may have a large pleural effusion caused by a sinus tract from the pseudocyst into the mediastinum and then into the pleural space. Chest symptoms almost always dominate in this situation and the diagnosis is made by showing a high pleural fluid amylase level.[55]

Esophageal perforation is a diagnosis that should be considered in every critically ill patient with a pleural effusion because if the diagnosis is not made within several days, mortality approaches 100%. Most patients with an esophageal perforation have either a pleural effusion or a hydropneumothorax. The pleural fluid with esophageal perforation is distinctive, with a high amylase level (salivary type), a low pH level, a low glucose level, and a high LDH level. At times food particles may be seen in the pleural fluid. The treatment is surgical repair of the perforation.

The diagnosis of intra-abdominal abscess should be considered in patients with pleural effusions containing predominantly neutrophils but without pulmonary infiltrates. The abscess can be subphrenic, intrahepatic, intrapancreatic, or intrasplenic. The diagnosis is made with abdominal CT scan and the treatment is drainage of the abscess.[1]

PLEURAL EFFUSIONS CAUSED BY DRUG REACTIONS

The possibility that an undiagnosed pleural effusion is caused by a drug reaction should be considered. The primary drugs responsible for pleural effusions include nitrofurantoin, dantrolene, ergot alkaloids, amiodarone, interleukin 2, procarbazine, methotrexate, and clozapine. The pleural effusions associated with the administration of drugs are frequently eosinophilic.

CHYLOTHORAX AND PSEUDOCHYLOTHORAX

When pleural fluid is found to be milky or opaque, the patient either has a high lipid pleural effusion or an empyema. If the fluid is centrifuged, the supernatant remains milky or opaque only if the patient has a high lipid pleural effusion. Chylothorax and pseudochylothorax are the 2 effusions with high lipid levels. A chylothorax occurs when the thoracic duct is disrupted and chyle accumulates in the pleural space. With chylothorax, the pleural fluid triglyceride levels usually exceed 110 mg/dL. The treatment of chylothorax is the implantation of a pleuroperitoneal shunt, thoracic duct ligation, or the percutaneous transabdominal thoracic duct blockage.[56]

The high lipid levels in a pseudochylothorax are caused by the accumulation of cholesterol or lecithin-globulin complexes in long-standing (>5 years) pleural effusions.[57] Most patients with pseudochylothorax have either rheumatoid pleuritis or have been treated in the past with an artificial pneumothorax for tuberculosis. If the patient is dyspneic from the pleural effusion and if the underlying lung is believed to be functional, a decortication should be considered.[57]

OTHER CAUSES OF PLEURAL EFFUSIONS

There are many other causes of pleural effusions (see **Box 1**), which are not discussed in this article because of space considerations. The reader is referred to Refs[1,58] for additional information.

REFERENCES

1. Light RW. Pleural diseases. 5h edition. Baltimore (MD): Lippincott Williams & Wilkins; 2007.
2. Light RW, MacGregor MI, Luchsinger PC, et al. Pleural effusions: the diagnostic separation of transudates and exudates. Ann Intern Med 1972;77:507–14.
3. Romero-Candeira S, Fernandez C, Martin C, et al. Influence of diuretics on the concentration of proteins and other components of pleural transudates in patients with heart failure. Am J Med 2001;110:681–6.
4. Romero-Candeira S, Hernandez L, Romero-Brufao S, et al. Is it meaningful to use biochemical parameters to discriminate between transudative and exudative pleural effusions? Chest 2002;122:1524–9.

5. Porcel JM, Vives M, Cao G, et al. Measurement of pro-brain natriuretic peptide in pleural fluid for the diagnosis of pleural effusions due to heart failure. Am J Med 2004;15(116):417–20.

6. Kolditz M, Halank M, Schiemanck S, et al. High diagnostic accuracy of NT-proBNP for cardiac origin of pleural effusions. Eur Respir J 2006;28:144–50.

7. Porcel JM, Martínez-Alonso M, Cao G, et al. Biomarkers of heart failure in pleural fluid. Chest 2009;136:671–7.

8. Light RW. Pleural effusion. N Engl J Med 2002;346:1971–7.

9. Kalomenidis I, Light RW. Eosinophilic pleural effusions. Curr Opin Pulm Med 2003;9:254–60.

10. Krenke R, Nasilowski J, Korczynski P, et al. Incidence and etiology of eosinophilic pleural effusion. Eur Respir J 2009;34:1111–7.

11. Colice GL, Curtis A, Deslauriers J, et al. Medical and surgical treatment of parapneumonic effusions: an evidence-based guideline. Chest 2000;118:1158–71.

12. Cheng D-S, Rodriguez RM, Rogers J, et al. Comparison of pleural fluid pH values obtained using blood gas machine, pH meter, and pH indicator strip. Chest 1998; 114:1368–72.

13. Menzies SM, Rahman NM, Wrightson JM, et al. Blood culture bottle culture of pleural fluid in pleural infection. Thorax 2011;66(8):658–62.

14. Light RW. Update on tuberculous pleural effusion. Respirology 2010;15:451–8.

15. Maskell N, Gleeson FV, Davies RJ. Standard pleural biopsy versus CT-guided cutting-needle biopsy for diagnosis of malignant disease in pleural effusions: a randomised controlled trial. Lancet 2003;361:1326–30.

16. Prakash UR, Reiman HM. Comparison of needle biopsy with cytologic analysis for the evaluation of pleural effusion: analysis of 414 cases. Mayo Clin Proc 1985;60:158–64.

17. Chang S-C, Perng RP. The role of fiberoptic bronchoscopy in evaluating the causes of pleural effusions. Arch Intern Med 1989;149:855–7.

18. Diacon AH, Van de Wal BW, Wyser C, et al. Diagnostic tools in tuberculous pleurisy: a direct comparative study. Eur Respir J 2003;22:589–91.

19. Ferrer J, Roldan J, Teixidor J, et al. Predictors of pleural malignancy in patients with pleural effusion undergoing thoracoscopy. Chest 2005;127:1017–22.

20. Wiener-Kronish JP, Matthay MA, Callen PW, et al. Relationship of pleural effusions of pulmonary hemodynamics in patients with congestive heart failure. Am Rev Respir Dis 1985;132:1253–6.

21. Tang KJ, Robbins IM, Light RW. Incidence of pleural effusions in idiopathic and familial pulmonary arterial hypertension patients. Chest 2009;136:688–93.

22. Kataoka H, Takada S. The role of thoracic ultrasonography for evaluation of patients with decompensated chronic heart failure. J Am Coll Cardiol 2000;35:1638–46.

23. Alonso JC. Pleural effusion in liver disease. Semin Respir Crit Care Med 2010;31: 698–705.

24. Rossle M, Ochs A, Gulberg V, et al. A comparison of paracentesis and transjugular intrahepatic portosystemic shunting in patients with ascites. N Engl J Med 2000;342:1701–7.

25. Milanez de Campos JR, Filho LOA, Werebe EC, et al. Thoracoscopy and talc poudrage in the management of hepatic hydrothorax. Chest 2000;118:137.

26. Mandell LA, Barltett JG, Dowell SF, et al. Update of practice guidelines for the management of community-acquired pneumonia in immunocompetent adults. Clin Infect Dis 2003;37:1405–33.

27. Rahman NM, Chapman SJ, Davies RJ. The approach to the patient with a parapneumonic effusion. Clin Chest Med 2006;27:253–66.

28. Davies CW, Gleeson FV, Davies RJ. BTS guidelines for the management of pleural infection. Thorax 2003;58(Suppl 2):II18–28.
29. Skouras V, Awdankiewicz A, Light RW. What size parapneumonic effusions should be sampled? Thorax 2010;65:91.
30. Light RW, Girard WM, Jenkinson SG, et al. Parapneumonic effusions. Am J Med 1980;69:507–11.
31. Rahman NM, Maskell NA, Davies CW, et al. The relationship between chest tube size and clinical outcome in pleural infection. Chest 2010;137:536–43.
32. Maskell NA, Davies CW, Nunn AJ, et al. U.K. controlled trial of intrapleural streptokinase for pleural infection. N Engl J Med 2005;352:865–74.
33. Rahman NM, Maskell N, Davies CW, et al. Primary result of the 2nd multi-centre intrapleural sepsis (MIST2) trial; randomized trial of intrapleural tPA and DNAse in pleural infection. N Engl J Med 2011;365:518–26.
34. Landreneau RJ, Keenan RJ, Hazelrigg SR, et al. Thoracoscopy for empyema and hemothorax. Chest 1995;109:18–24.
35. Cassina PC, Hauser M, Hillejan L, et al. Video-assisted thoracoscopy in the treatment of pleural empyema: stage-based management and outcome. J Thorac Cardiovasc Surg 1999;117:234–8.
36. Lawrence DR, Ohri SK, Moxon RE, et al. Thoracoscopic debridement of empyema thoracis. Ann Thorac Surg 1997;64:1448–50.
37. Striffeler H, Gugger M, Im Hof V, et al. Video-assisted thoracoscopic surgery for fibrinopurulent pleural empyema in 67 patients. Ann Thorac Surg 1998;65: 319–23.
38. Cheng C-S, Rodriguez RM, Perkett EA, et al. Vascular endothelial growth factor in pleural fluid. Chest 1999;115:760–5.
39. Putnam JB Jr, Light RW, Rodriguez RM, et al. A randomized comparison of indwelling pleural catheter and doxycycline pleurodesis in the management of malignant pleural effusions. Cancer 1999;86:1992–9.
40. Tremblay A, Robbins S, Berthiaume L, et al. Natural history of asymptomatic pleural effusions in lung cancer patients. J Bronchol 2007;14:98–100.
41. Van Meter ME, McKee KY, Kohlwes RJ. Efficacy and safety of tunneled pleural catheters in adults with malignant pleural effusions: a systematic review. J Gen Intern Med 2010;26:70–6.
42. Tremblay A, Michaud G. Single-center experience with 250 tunnelled pleural catheter insertions for malignant pleural effusion. Chest 2006;129:362–8.
43. Warren WH, Kim AW, Liptay MJ. Identification of clinical factors predicting PleurX catheter removal in patients treated for malignant pleural effusion. Eur J Cardiothorac Surg 2008;33:89–94.
44. Chee A, Tremblay A. The use of tunneled pleural catheters in the treatment of pleural effusions. Curr Opin Pulm Med 2011;17:237–41.
45. Lee YC, Baumann MH, Maskell NA, et al. Pleurodesis practice for malignant pleural effusions in five English-speaking countries: survey of pulmonologists. Chest 2003;124:2229–38.
46. Dresler CM, Olak J, Herndon JE 2nd, et al. Phase III intergroup study of talc poudrage vs talc slurry sclerosis for malignant pleural effusion. Chest 2005;127:909–15.
47. Stein PD, Terrin ML, Hales CA, et al. Clinical, laboratory, roentgenographic, and electrocardiographic findings in patients with acute pulmonary embolism and no pre-existing cardiac or pulmonary disease. Chest 1991;100:598–603.
48. Porcel JM, Madronero AB, Pardina M, et al. Analysis of pleural effusions in acute pulmonary embolism: radiological and pleural fluid data from 230 patients. Respirology 2007;12:234–9.

49. Light RW. Pleural effusion in pulmonary embolism. Semin Respir Crit Care Med 2010;31(6):716–22.
50. Patiala J. Initial tuberculous pleuritis in the Finnish Armed Forces in 1939–1945 with special reference to eventual post pleuritic tuberculosis. Acta Tuberc Scand 1954;36(Suppl):1–57.
51. Light RW, Rogers JT, Moyers JP, et al. Prevalence and clinical course of pleural effusions after coronary artery and cardiac surgery. Am J Respir Crit Care Med 2002;166:1563–6.
52. Light RW. Pleural effusions after coronary artery bypass graft surgery. Curr Opin Pulm Med 2002;8:308–11.
53. Sadikot RT, Rogers JT, Cheng DS, et al. Pleural fluid characteristics of patients with symptomatic pleural effusion post coronary artery bypass surgery. Arch Intern Med 2000;160:2665–8.
54. Halla JT, Schronhenloher RE, Volanakis JE. Immune complexes and other laboratory features of pleural effusions. Ann Intern Med 1980;92:748–52.
55. Ali T, Srinivasan N, Le V, et al. Pancreaticopleural fistula. Pancreas 2009;38: e26–31.
56. Itkin M, Kucharczuk JC, Kwak A, et al. Nonoperative thoracic duct embolization for traumatic thoracic duct leak: experience in 109 patients. J Thorac Cardiovasc Surg 2010;139:584–9.
57. Hillerdal G. Effusions from lymphatic disruptions. In: Light RW, Lee YC, editors. Textbook of pleural diseases. 2nd edition. London: Hodder Arnold; 2008. p. 389–96.
58. Light RW, Lee YC, editors. Textbook of pleural diseases. 2nd edition. London: Hodder Arnold; 2008.

Interstitial Lung Disease: The Initial Approach

Esam H. Alhamad, MD, FCCP[a],*, Gregory P. Cosgrove, MD, FCCP[b]

KEYWORDS

- Idiopathic pulmonary fibrosis
- High-resolution computed tomography
- Pulmonary hypertension • Gastroesophageal reflux disease

Interstitial lung disease (ILD) is a heterogeneous group of disorders with variable etiology, clinical presentation, radiographic pattern, and histologic appearance that diffusely affects the lung parenchyma. Although ILD comprises more than 100 distinct entities, idiopathic pulmonary fibrosis (IPF), connective tissue disease (CTD)-associated ILD, sarcoidosis, and hypersensitivity pneumonitis (HP) account for the majority of ILD cases. In 2002, The American Thoracic Society and European Respiratory Society provided a consensus classification of idiopathic interstitial pneumonia that includes 7 entities: IPF, nonspecific interstitial pneumonia (NSIP), cryptogenic organizing pneumonia, acute interstitial pneumonia, respiratory bronchiolitis, desquamative interstitial pneumonia (DIP), and lymphocytic interstitial pneumonia (LIP).[1] However, significant progress in the understanding of idiopathic interstitial pneumonia has been made since these criteria were established, and the current consensus view is that respiratory bronchiolitis and DIP are strongly related to cigarette smoke exposure.[2,3] The diagnostic accuracy of high-resolution computed tomography (HRCT) for patients with a usual interstitial pneumonia (UIP) radiographic pattern has been validated. Acceptance of this view is reflected in recently published international guidelines on the diagnosis and management of IPF, which indicate that IPF can be accurately diagnosed by HRCT in the absence of a surgical lung biopsy when a radiographic UIP pattern is present.[4] This review highlights the importance of a meticulous patient history and clinical examination, and the role of laboratory testing, physiologic studies, and radiographic evaluation in narrowing differential diagnoses. The authors also briefly address the value of bronchoscopic and surgical lung biopsy when ILD is

---

Conflict of Interest: The authors have nothing to disclose.
[a] Division of Pulmonary Medicine, College of Medicine, King Saud University, 38, PO Box 2925, Riyadh 11461, KS, USA
[b] Interstitial Lung Disease Program, National Jewish Health, 1400 Jackson Street, A551, Denver, CO 80206, USA
* Corresponding author.
E-mail address: esamalhamad@yahoo.com

Med Clin N Am 95 (2011) 1071–1093
doi:10.1016/j.mcna.2011.08.008
0025-7125/11/$ – see front matter © 2011 Elsevier Inc. All rights reserved.

encountered. In addition, the importance of recognizing common comorbidities associated with ILD is discussed, and the importance of integrating a multidisciplinary approach into clinical practice is underscored.

CLINICAL FEATURES
History

A detailed, thorough history plays a pivotal role in the initial evaluation of patients when ILD is suspected. Among the important information to be gathered from patients as part of a careful systemic review are identification of past medical illness with systemic manifestations, all therapeutic drug use or recreational drug abuse, social history, detailed occupational and environmental exposures, and family history. As such, using patient history helps in limiting the differential diagnosis (**Box 1**) (**Fig. 1**) and guiding physician requests for appropriate investigations.

Patients commonly present with long-standing (months or years) dyspnea, initially with exertion, but which may have progressed to the point where the patient becomes dyspneic at rest. However, when dyspnea has occurred over days to weeks in the absence of infection, one needs to consider cryptogenic organizing pneumonia, acute eosinophilic pneumonia, HP, drug-induced toxicity, vasculitis, and acute interstitial pneumonia. Dry cough is frequently noted in patients with ILD. However, it is a nonspecific finding; when cough is highly productive, special attention should be paid to other diagnoses, such as bronchoalveolar cell carcinoma, bronchiectasis, and gastroesophageal reflux disease (GERD) with the possibility of occult aspiration. Wheezing and hemoptysis are relatively uncommon, and their presence may suggest airway involvement or diffuse alveolar hemorrhage, respectively. Pleurisy, commonly occurring in patients with systemic lupus erythematosus (SLE), can be associated with severe intractable cough, occasionally leading to rib injuries. Fever, fatigue, and weight loss are nonspecific symptoms; however, when weight loss is significant, it raises the possibility of lung cancer–associated ILD. Arthralgias, joint swelling, Raynaud phenomenon, photosensitivity, morning stiffness, dry mouth or dry eyes, dysphagia, skin changes, oral ulceration, and muscle weakness are common symptoms in patients with CTD-associated ILD.

Demographic information, such as gender, age, and smoking status, are important. For example, sarcoidosis[5,6] and CTD[7–9] are more commonly observed in females, whereas IPF is more frequently reported in males.[10,11] However, despite these differences, gender cannot differentiate between various forms of ILDs except lymphangioleiomyomatosis (LAM), which occurs exclusively in women.[12]

Although ILD can present at any age, important inferences can be drawn with respect to age in the context of specific disorders. Sarcoidosis, CTD, NSIP, pulmonary Langerhans cell histiocytosis (PLCH), and familial idiopathic interstitial pneumonias are more often reported among individuals younger than 50 years, whereas the majority of patients with IPF are older than 60. Smoking history provides important clues in cases where associations between smoking and ILDs are well documented, including respiratory bronchiolitis–associated ILD, DIP, PLCH, and pulmonary hemorrhage secondary to Goodpasture syndrome. Family history may identify patients with hereditary forms of ILDs, including familial idiopathic interstitial pneumonias, Hermansky-Pudlak syndrome, tuberous sclerosis complex–associated LAM, Gaucher disease, hypocalciuric hypercalcemia, neurofibromatosis, and Niemann-Pick disease.[13,14]

A wide range of drugs is known to cause lung injury, including chemotherapeutic agents (bleomycin, cyclophosphamide, methotrexate); antibiotics (nitrofurantoin, sulfasalazine); and anti-inflammatory (penicillamine, nonsteroidal anti-inflammatory agents), cardiovascular (amiodarone, procainamide, statins), and recreational (cocaine, heroin, methadone) drugs.[15–17] Diagnosing drug-induced lung injuries can be very challenging for clinicians because of significant variability in clinical presentation and because the presence of coexisting lung diseases may delay the diagnosis. However, a careful review of drug history can provide a great deal of information that helps in narrowing the differential diagnosis and may prevent a fatal outcome.

A thorough assessment of occupational and environmental exposure as well as a consideration of hobbies is important in patients presenting with ILD. Among the common types of occupational-associated ILDs are those that involve exposure to asbestos, silica, beryllium, cobalt, copper sulfate, or isocyanates.[18] In addition, clinicians should carefully evaluate potential fungal, bacterial, and animal protein exposures, which can be potential causes for the development of HP. Because continuous low-grade exposure to these offending substances may progress to diffuse lung fibrosis, detailed assessment and early recognition are important from both a diagnostic and therapeutic perspective. Several occupations, including farming, hairdressing, bird raising, and stone cutting/polishing, as well as exposure to certain occupational hazards such as livestock and/or various dusts (eg, vegetable, animal, metal), were found to be significantly associated with IPF in a case-control study, highlighting the importance of a detailed assessment of occupational and environmental exposures.[19] The significance of the exposures remains unclear as they pertain to the pathogenesis of IPF, but are certainly important for the development of HP.

Physical Examination

Although ILD patients share similar physical findings, careful identification of subtle signs may provide clues to the underlying etiology and provide additional information about comorbidities associated with ILDs.

Bilateral basilar mid-late, end-inspiratory crackles are commonly described in almost all types of ILDs, although they are less frequently present in sarcoidosis.[5,20] However, the absence of crackles does not rule out ILD, particularly in the presence of extrapulmonary signs (**Table 1**).

Pulmonary hypertension is frequently seen in patients with CTD-associated ILD,[21–25] notably in scleroderma, polymyositis, mixed connective tissue disease, and occasionally rheumatoid arthritis, sarcoidosis,[26–28] and IPF.[29,30] Physical signs suggestive of pulmonary hypertension include increased jugular "a" and "v" waves, left parasternal lift, accentuated pulmonary component of the second heart sound, right ventricular S4, diastolic murmur of pulmonary regurgitation, holosytolic murmur of tricuspid regurgitation, and hepatojugular reflux indicating high central venous pressure.[31] Digital clubbing is nonspecific and can be seen in any type of ILD. Arthritis is associated with CTD or sarcoidosis. Subcutaneous calcinosis, Raynaud phenomenon, sclerodactyly, and telangiectasias are characteristic features of systemic sclerosis. Systemic muscle weakness, heliotrope rash, and Gottron papules are features of polymyositis/dermatomyositis. Skin involvement associated with ILD can occur in sarcoidosis, CTD, amyloidosis, PLCH, tuberous sclerosis, and neurofibromatosis. Ocular and salivary gland involvement suggests sarcoidosis or Sjögren syndrome. Uveitis may be associated with sarcoidosis, SLE, or Wegener granulomatosis. Thyroid enlargement raises the possibility of drug reaction (amiodarone) or PLCH. The presence of ILD with lymphadenopathy raises the possibility of sarcoidosis, CTD, PLCH, and drug reaction (methotrexate). Hepatomegaly may be associated with sarcoidosis, CTD, PLCH, LIP, drugs, and amyloidosis. Splenomegaly has been described in sarcoidosis, SLE, PLCH, LIP, amyloidosis, Gaucher disease, and Niemann-Pick disease. Central nervous manifestations may be seen in sarcoidosis, antineutrophil

Box 1
Differential diagnoses to consider in patients presenting with interstitial lung disease

Idiopathic Interstitial Pneumonia

    Idiopathic pulmonary fibrosis

    Nonspecific interstitial pneumonia

    Cryptogenic organizing pneumonia

    Acute interstitial pneumonia

    Lymphocytic interstitial pneumonia

Connective Tissue Disease

    Rheumatoid arthritis

    Systemic sclerosis

    Systemic lupus erythematosus

    Polymyositis/dermatomyositis

    Mixed connective tissue disease

    Undifferentiated connective tissue disease

    Sjögren syndrome

    Ankylosing spondylitis

Smoke Related

    Respiratory bronchiolitis

    Desquamative interstitial pneumonia

    Pulmonary Langerhans cell histiocytosis

Vasculitis

    Wegener granulomatosis

    Churg-Strauss syndrome

    Goodpasture syndrome

    Microscopic polyangitis

    Behçet disease

Granulomatous disease

    Sarcoidosis

Environmental/Occupational

    Hypersensitivity pneumonitis

      Exposure to: animal, bacterial fungal, chemical

    Pneumoconiosis

      Exposure to: asbestos, silica, beryllium, aluminum, coal, cobalt

Drug induced

    Chemotherapeutic agents (cyclophosphamide, methotrexate, bleomycin)

    Biological drug (anti–tumor necrosis factor α: etanercept, infliximab)

    Antibiotics (sulfasalazine)

    Cardiovascular medication (amiodarone)

    Anti-inflammatory (penicillamine, gold)

> Illicit drugs (cocaine, heroin)
>
> Other (oil nose drops)
>
> Inherited
>
> Familial idiopathic interstitial pneumonia
>
> Hermansky-Pudlak syndrome
>
> Tuberous sclerosis
>
> Neurofibromatosis
>
> Niemann-Pick disease
>
> Gaucher disease
>
> Hypocalciuric hypercalcemia
>
> Others
>
> Lymphangioleiomyomatosis
>
> Eosinophilic pneumonia
>
> Amyloidosis
>
> Alveolar proteinosis

cytoplasmic antibody (ANCA)-positive vasculitis, PLCH, or tuberous sclerosis. Coexistence of ILD with oculocutaneous albinism suggests the diagnosis of Hermansky-Pudlak syndrome.

Laboratory Testing

Routine blood tests are nonspecific, but the initial evaluation should include a complete blood count with a full differential, electrolytes panel, serum urea nitrogen, creatinine, calcium, liver function tests, and erythrocyte sedimentation rate. Serologic tests, including those for antinuclear antibody (ANA) and rheumatoid factor (RF), are routine general screens when CTD is suspected or when patients present with acute interstitial pneumonia. However, low titers of circulating ANA and/or RF have been described in patients with IPF.[4] More importantly, negative ANA and RF test results do not exclude CTD-associated ILD, even in the absence of extrathoracic features. It is well established that the lungs may be the primary site of initial clinical symptoms in CTDs, antedating the systemic manifestations by several years (**Figs. 2** and **3**). As such, specific serum markers, including anticyclic citrullinated peptide (anti-CCP) for rheumatoid arthritis, anti–SS-A/Ro and anti–SS-B/La for Sjögren syndrome, anti–double-stranded DNA (dsDNA) and anti-Smith (Sm) for SLE, antiscleroderma (Scl-70) and anticentromere for systemic sclerosis, antiribonucleoprotein (RNP) for mixed CTD, antipolymyositis/scleroderma (PM/Scl) for overlap syndrome, and anti-tRNA synthetase (eg, Jo-1, PL-7, PL-12) for antisynthetase syndrome, may be warranted in patients presenting with interstitial pneumonia.[32] Human immune deficiency virus (HIV) tests should be conducted when LIP or NSIP is clinically suspected. In patients presenting with symptoms or signs suggestive of vasculitis or diffuse alveolar hemorrhage, antineutrophil cytoplasmic antibody, antiglomerular basement membrane antibody, and urine sediment should be determined.

The presence in serum of precipitating antibodies (usually IgG but possibly IgM or IgA) against the offending antigens may be identified in patients with HP. However, these antibodies are nonspecific because they can be detected among exposed

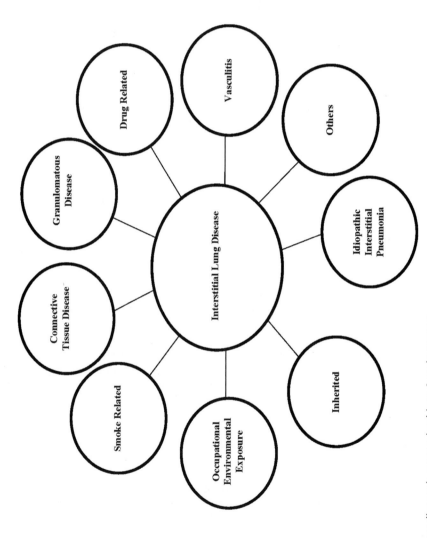

Fig. 1. Interstitial lung disease is categorized into 9 main groups.

Table 1
Extrapulmonary manifestations that can be associated with interstitial lung disease

Features	Possible Diagnosis
Skin lesions	Connective tissue disease, sarcoidosis, Wegener granulomatosis, Churg-Strauss syndrome, amyloidosis, Behçet disease, pulmonary Langerhans cell histiocytosis, tuberous sclerosis, neurofibromatosis, drug induced
Eye lesions	Connective tissue disease, sarcoidosis, Wegener granulomatosis, Behçet disease
Salivary/parotid gland enlargement	Sarcoidosis, Sjögren syndrome, Wegener granulomatosis
Thyroid enlargement	Drug induced (amiodarone), pulmonary Langerhans cell histiocytosis
Lymph node enlargement	Sarcoidosis, connective tissue disease, pulmonary Langerhans cell histiocytosis, amyloidosis, drug induced
Liver enlargement	Sarcoidosis, connective tissue disease, pulmonary Langerhans cell histiocytosis, amyloidosis, drug induced
Spleen enlargement	Sarcoidosis, connective tissue disease, Wegener granulomatosis, pulmonary Langerhans cell histiocytosis, amyloidosis, Gaucher disease, Niemann-Pick disease
Muscle involvement	Connective tissue disease, sarcoidosis
Joint involvement	Connective tissue disease, sarcoidosis, Behçet disease, Wegener granulomatosis
Central nervous system involvement	Connective tissue disease, sarcoidosis, Wegener granulomatosis, Churg-Strauss syndrome

individuals without clinical symptoms.[33,34] More importantly, the precipitating antibodies can be negative in more than 50% of patients with chronic HP.[35] In a multicenter study including a cohort of 199 patients with HP and 462 with other ILDs, investigators identified 6 clinical predictors of HP[36]: (1) exposure to a known offending antigen, (2) positive precipitating antibodies to the offending antigen, (3) recurrent episodes of symptoms, (4) inspiratory crackles, (5) symptoms occurring 4 to 8 hours after exposure to an offending antigen, and (6) weight loss. When all 6 predictors were present, the probability of HP was 98%. Of interest, the best single predictor was positive exposure to a known offending antigen (odds ratio 38.8), highlighting the importance of a thorough history in establishing potential environmental and occupational exposure in any patient with ILD.

Physiologic Testing

Most ILDs share common physiologic aberrations that prevent pulmonary function tests (PFTs) from differentiating between various types of ILDs; thus, these tests need to be performed in conjunction with clinical, radiological, and/or histologic assessments. Nevertheless, PFTs are important in aiding in differential diagnosis, establishing disease severity, and monitoring disease progression and response to therapy. PFTs should include spirometry, lung volumes, and diffusing capacity for carbon monoxide (DLCO). A restrictive ventilatory defect with decreased DLCO is a common physiologic pattern among patients with ILDs. However, purely obstructive, mixed obstructive-restrictive, or (rarely) normal patterns may also be observed.[37] When obstructive findings are detected in patients with ILDs, the differential diagnoses include sarcoidosis, HP, respiratory bronchiolitis-associated ILD (RB-ILD),

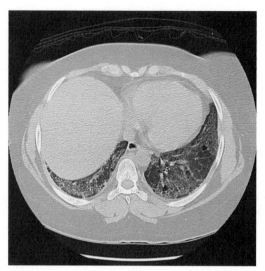

Fig. 2. Connective tissue disease (CTD)–associated usual interstitial pneumonia (UIP) in a 33-year-old woman, without extrathoracic signs or symptoms of CTD, with a high titer of antinuclear antibodies (1:2560) and UIP confirmed by surgical lung biopsy. High-resolution computed tomographic (HRCT) scan demonstrates the predominant pattern of ground-glass opacities associated with traction bronchiectasis, interlobular septal thickening, fine reticulation, and honeycombing.

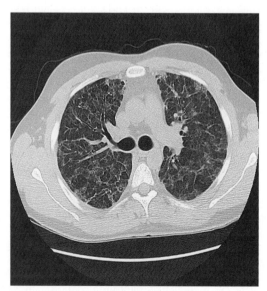

Fig. 3. Organizing pneumonia secondary to CTD in a 27-year-old man, without extrathoracic signs or symptoms of rheumatoid arthritis, with positive finding of anticyclic citrullinated peptide (anti-CPP) and histologically verified organizing pneumonia. HRCT demonstrates diffuse patchy ground-glass opacities with interlobular and intralobular thickening intervening with normal lung tissues, producing a "crazy-paving" appearance.

emphysema, PLCH, and LAM. Decreased DLCO with relatively normal spirometry and lung volumes suggests pulmonary vascular involvement related to CTD, chronic recurrent pulmonary emboli, or idiopathic pulmonary hypertension. When respiratory muscle weakness is suspected (eg, sarcoidosis, polymyositis), quantifiable objective measurements of muscle weakness can be obtained by measuring maximal inspiratory and expiratory pressures.

Over the past decade, the 6-minute walk test (6MWT) has become a popular tool for assessing functional status in patients with cardiopulmonary diseases because it is simple, inexpensive, reproducible, and well received by patients, as it mimics the effort required for daily physical activity. Measuring distance and oxygen desaturation during the 6MWT has been shown to predict the prognoses of patients with various pulmonary and nonpulmonary diseases; it has also become a surrogate measure of efficacy among various forms of ILD in therapeutic drug trials. In IPF, a walking distance less than 350 m and oxygen saturation of 88% or less during the walking test is associated with reduced survival.[38,39] Studies using the 6MWT in sarcoidosis have demonstrated a correlation between 6-minute walk distance and pulmonary function parameters, oxygen saturation, dyspnea, and St. George's Respiratory Questionnaire.[40–42] In systemic sclerosis, the 6-minute walk distance is reduced in 30% of patients.[43] However, exercise limitation is frequently noted in sarcoidosis, systemic sclerosis, and other CTDs because of the involvement of skin, lung, joint, heart, muscles, and nerves as well as pain, fatigue, and corticosteroid use—all of which can affect walking distance. As such, the utility of the 6MWT as a surrogate marker in this group of ILDs is less clear and remains to be determined in future studies.

Radiographic Evaluation

Chest radiography is an important first-line investigational tool when parenchymal pathology is suspected. However, abnormalities are nonspecific; moreover, parenchymal patterns are difficult to characterize and sometimes can be normal with histologically proven infiltrative lung disease.[44,45] HRCT provides essential information for evaluating various ILDs, allowing clinicians to narrow the differential diagnosis and offering guidance for the appropriate lung biopsy site, when needed; HRCT information can also be important in predicting mortality. Classifying HRCT findings into patterns (ground glass, cystic, nodular, and reticular opacities, and consolidation), distributions (upper, central, lower, and peripheral), and associated findings (traction bronchiectasis, mediastinal lymphadenopathy, septal thickening, air trapping, and pleural involvement) has helped clinicians significantly in narrowing the differential diagnosis (**Figs. 2–10**).[46] Several studies[47–51] have shown that the diagnostic accuracy of IPF ranges from 71% to 100% when HRCT findings are typical of UIP (ie, subpleural, basal predominance, presence of reticular abnormality, and honeycombing [cyst] with or without traction bronchiectasis; see **Fig. 4**). Based on these findings, a confident diagnosis of IPF can be made in the absence of a surgical lung biopsy when the characteristic findings of UIP are present on the HRCT imaging.[4] However, it is important that identifying a UIP pattern does not necessarily imply IPF, but can also be seen in other disorders including CTD, chronic HP, and pneumoconiosis (see **Fig. 5**).[4] For other types of interstitial lung disorders, HRCT has been shown to yield a correct diagnosis of 83% for sarcoidosis,[52] 70% for chronic HP,[53] 63% to 81% for DIP,[47,48] 81% for both RB-ILD and LIP,[47] 72% for both PLCH and LAM,[47] 65% for acute interstitial pneumonia, and 79% for bronchiolitis obliterans organizing pneumonia.[48] However, when NSIP was considered the main diagnosis, HRCT was notoriously inaccurate (see **Fig. 2**).[48] In a study involving 96 patients with a histologic diagnosis of UIP (n = 76) or NSIP (n = 23), Flaherty and colleagues[50] noted that 59%

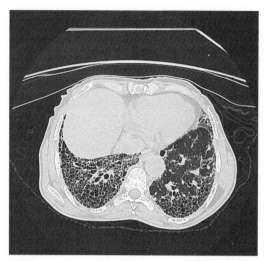

Fig. 4. UIP. HRCT demonstrates a honeycomb pattern exhibiting predominantly basal reticulation with architectural distortion and traction bronchiolectasis.

(26/44) of patients with typical HRCT findings of NSIP had a histologic diagnosis of UIP at surgical lung biopsy. This lack of reliability was confirmed by another study in which ground-glass opacities were the predominant HRCT findings, and which reported a broad range of diagnostic accuracies (range 44.2%–75.5%).[51] These data highlight the significant limitations of HRCT in definitively diagnosing NSIP; in the absence of CTD, a lung biopsy is warranted.

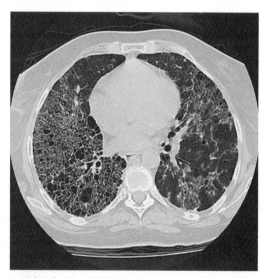

Fig. 5. UIP in rheumatoid arthritis. HRCT in a 44-year-old woman with rheumatoid arthritis shows areas of reticulation with honeycombing, ground-glass attenuation, traction bronchiectasis, and bronchiolectasis.

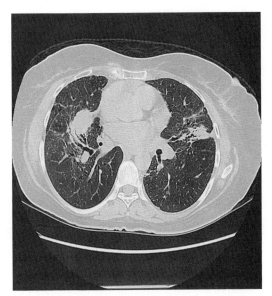

Fig. 6. Sarcoidosis. HRCT in a 52-year-old woman shows a conglomerate mass of fibrosis associated with traction bronchiectasis and reticulonodular changes along the bronchovascular bundles.

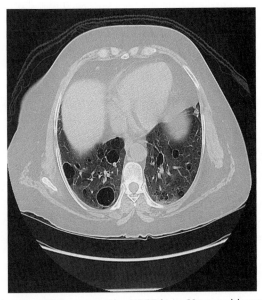

Fig. 7. Lymphocytic interstitial pneumonia. HRCT in a 60-year-old woman with systemic lupus erythematosus shows diffuse ground-glass opacities with multiple cysts of variable size.

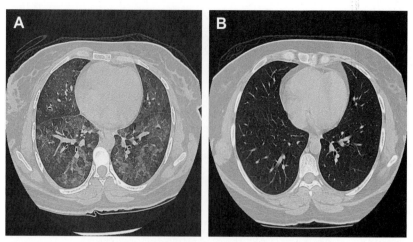

Fig. 8. Hypersensitivity pneumonitis in a 30-year-old woman with 3 months' exposure to pigeons at home. (*A*) HRCT demonstrates diffuse centrilobular nodules with ground-glass opacities associated with foci of trapped air. (*B*) Follow-up HRCT 12 weeks after removal of pigeons and corticosteroid therapy shows complete resolution of the abnormalities.

Bronchoscopy and Surgical Lung Biopsy

Fiberoptic bronchoscopy with bronchoalveolar lavage (BAL) and transbronchial biopsy can provide a definitive diagnosis in a wide array of parenchymal lung disorders, including infection, sarcoidosis, pulmonary alveolar proteinosis, pneumoconiosis, PLCH, diffuse alveolar hemorrhage, eosinophilic pneumonia, and malignancy. Although BAL lymphocytosis (>40%) is suggestive of HP, similar findings can be seen with sarcoidosis, berylliosis, miliary tuberculosis, and in asymptomatic exposed individuals, underscoring the importance of interpreting these results within the context of clinical and laboratory results, radiographic patterns, and physiologic features. The role of BAL and transbronchial lung biopsy in the initial evaluation of idiopathic interstitial pneumonias is unclear; according to the recently published

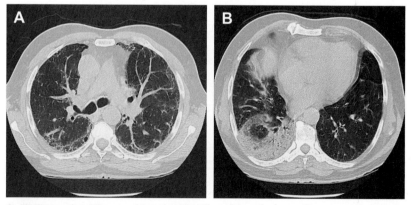

Fig. 9. HRCT scan in a 70-year-old man with idiopathic pulmonary fibrosis and histologically verified adenocarcinoma shows a honeycomb pattern with reticulation (*A*) and an area of consolidation involving the right lower lobe (*B*).

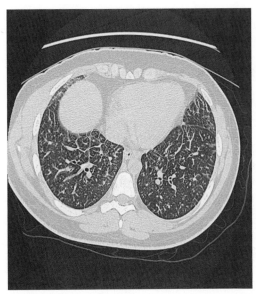

Fig. 10. Lymphangitic carcinomatosis caused by metastatic gastric adenocarcinoma in a 27-year-old man. HRCT demonstrates smooth and nodular interlobular septal thickening with diffuse pulmonary nodules.

international guidelines for IPF, these procedures may be of limited diagnostic value in confirming a confident diagnosis.[4]

A surgical lung biopsy is indicated when a confident diagnosis cannot be made based on the clinical, physiologic, and radiographic evaluations. Since the introduction of video-assisted thoracoscopy, morbidity and mortality have decreased compared with previous periods when the open lung biopsy approach predominated.[54,55] Several important points need to be taken into account when considering a surgical lung biopsy. Clinicians should consider the patient's age, comorbidities, and the likelihood that the biopsy results will alter the clinical course and the patient's potential to respond to drug therapy. Acute exacerbations of interstitial pneumonia in patients with preexisting ILD have been described following surgical lung biopsy.[56,57] It is not entirely clear why some patients develop it and others do not; however, until we have better understanding of the potential risks, careful selection of patients as well as strict preoperative, intraoperative, and postoperative monitoring is needed. Idiopathic NSIP is diagnosed by exclusion after secondary causes such as CTD, HP, drugs, and infection have been thoroughly evaluated. Of interest, both NSIP and UIP patterns can be seen in biopsies from the same patient; however, the clinical course in such patients is similar to that in patients with a UIP pattern in all lobes, supporting the notion that multiple surgical lung biopsies should be obtained from multiple lobes when NSIP or IPF is suspected.[4,58,59] Surgical lung biopsies have provided prognostic information in patients with idiopathic interstitial pneumonia, but little information is gained from patients with established CTD–associated ILD. As such, a surgical lung biopsy should be avoided unless patients present with an atypical HRCT appearance or a malignancy is suspected.[60] Finally, although surgical lung biopsies are considered the gold standard for the evaluation of patients with ILDs, pathologists occasionally encounter cases in which a histologic pattern cannot be ascribed to a specific disease, even if surgical biopsies were obtained away from severely affected areas; the term "nonclassifiable fibrosis" is applied to these cases. In such circumstances whereby a clear pathologic diagnosis is not available, the importance of a multidisciplinary approach is paramount, employing a pulmonologist, a rheumatologist, a radiologist, and a pathologist with expertise in ILD to reach an accurate diagnosis with sufficient confidence.[4,61–63]

COMORBIDITIES ASSOCIATED WITH ILD
Gastroesophageal Reflux Disease

Gastroesophageal reflux (GER) occurs in normal healthy individuals, but when reflux leads to symptoms or complications, the term GERD is applied. The association between GER and pulmonary fibrosis has long been reported, and microaspiration is considered the likely mechanism.[64] Although reflux events can occur at any time of the day, significant acid reflux has been reported to occur more frequently during the night in individuals who consume a late evening meal than in those who consume an early evening meal.[65] A recent study using 24-hour pH monitoring in IPF patients noted that the prevalence of acid GER was 87%, with 76% and 63% demonstrating abnormal distal and proximal esophageal acid exposures, respectively, implying that aspiration may play a role in the pathogenesis of IPF.[66] Of importance, the same study reported that only 47% of patients exhibited classic GERD symptoms (heartburn and regurgitation). Savarino and colleagues[67] noted a correlation between the degree of pulmonary fibrosis (HRCT score) and the number of proximal and distal reflux episodes in systemic sclerosis patients, underscoring the importance of GER in the development and/or progression of pulmonary fibrosis. Tcherakian and colleagues[68] compared 32 patients with asymmetric IPF (ie, lung fibrosis involving one side more than the other) with 64 matched controls with symmetric IPF. GER events were more frequent in asymmetric than in symmetric IPF (62.5% vs 31.3%, respectively). In 62.5% of patients with asymmetric IPF, fibrosis was predominantly on the right side, implying that fibrosis may potentially be related to recurrent microaspiration, and regardless of the site of fibrosis, in 94% of cases the sites of involvement were consistent with the preferred sleep posture. In 15 patients with asymmetric IPF, acute exacerbations were identified. Unilateral ground-glass opacities were identified in the most affected (fibrotic) areas of the lungs, suggesting that GER has a role in exacerbations.[68] However, it must be noted that these findings may be peculiar to a unique type of lung fibrosis patient and may not necessarily apply to patients with other types of pulmonary fibrosis. Furthermore, although prescribing acid suppression therapy may be logical, there is insufficient evidence to indicate that it prevents the progression of pulmonary fibrosis, perhaps because the current standard dose is not sufficient to prevent reflux events, as noted by Raghu and colleagues.[66] In this study, 63% of IPF patients treated with standard doses of proton-pump inhibitors (20–40 mg/d omeprazole) at the time of the esophageal pH probe studies demonstrated persistently elevated esophageal acid exposures. Alternatively, it may be related to the presence of a combination of acid and nonacid reflux, as shown in patients with systemic sclerosis, in whom a higher frequency of GER episodes (both acid and nonacid) reaching the proximal esophagus was noted in patients with systemic sclerosis–associated ILD compared with patients with systemic sclerosis without ILD.[67]

EXACERBATIONS OF ILD

An exacerbation refers to the progressive worsening of dyspnea, usually over 1 month, associated with deterioration in PFTs, worsening gas-exchange parameters, and new ground-glass opacities (or consolidation) on chest radiography or HRCT in the absence of infection, congestive heart failure, pulmonary embolism, or pneumothorax.[69–71] It has most commonly been reported in IPF patients.[69–73] However, it can occur with other forms of ILD including NSIP, CTD-associated ILD, and chronic HP.[57,74,75] Apart from surgical lung biopsies, which have been reported to induce exacerbation, specific triggers have not been identified.[56,57] During acute exacerbation, patients should receive supportive care. The efficacy of high-dose corticosteroids (including pulse therapy), cyclosporine, and anticoagulants has not been validated in clinical trials.[4]

Pulmonary Arterial Hypertension

Pulmonary arterial hypertension (PAH) in the context of ILD is associated with significant morbidity and mortality,[28,30,76–80] prompting increased research interest in understanding the pathogenesis of PAH in various forms of ILDs. The pathogenesis is complex, multifactorial, and varies among types of disorders. Some mechanisms that have been proposed in the pathogenesis of PAH include vascular remodeling due to chronic hypoxia, fibrotic destruction of the pulmonary vasculature, inflammation, thrombotic angiopathy, oxidant-antioxidant imbalance, cytokines, and growth factors, among others.[81–83] Significant variation exists in the reported prevalence of PAH association with ILD, due in part to differences in study designs and/or methods used to detect PAH (echocardiography versus the gold standard of right heart catheterization), and the use of different mean pulmonary artery pressure (mPAP) cutoff points as diagnostic criteria for PAH. Furthermore, diagnosing PAH in the setting of ILD can be very challenging, as manifestations are subtle and commonly share similar symptoms until signs of right heart failure develop.[81] Although echocardiography is commonly used for screening patients with PAH, this method is inaccurate in the setting of ILDs, with significant overestimations or, more dangerously, underestimations occurring in up to 47% of cases, a fact that may account for the late diagnosis in this group of patients.[84,85] Other investigators have found no correlation between pulmonary artery diameter based on HRCT and mPAP in IPF patients.[86,87] Alhamad and colleagues[88] measured mPAP based on right heart catheterization within 72 hours of HRCT scan in 100 consecutive patients with advanced ILD and compared it with that in 34 patients without ILD. In this study the sensitivity, specificity, positive predictive value, and negative predictive value of HRCT-based pulmonary artery diameter in detecting PAH among those with ILD was lower overall than among those without ILD (sensitivity, 86% vs 47%; specificity, 41% vs 93%; positive predictive value, 46% vs 90%; negative predictive value, 84% vs 58%). Similarly, measuring the degree of parenchymal involvement (HRCT score) did not differentiate patients with or without PAH and was not predictive of PAH,[86–88] implying the lack of an association between the degree of pulmonary fibrosis and PAH. Others have suggested that a DLCO% of less than 40% in IPF patients,[30] a ratio of percent forced vital capacity to DLCO% of greater than 1.8 in systemic sclerosis,[89] and measuring plasma B-type natriuretic peptide in ILD[90] can identify patients with PAH. However, none of the noninvasive tests is sufficiently sensitive or specific in predicting PAH in the context of ILD; thus, right heart catheterization remains the reference standard for the diagnosis of PAH. It should be noted that left heart disease is one of the most common causes of pulmonary hypertension, and diagnosing these patients is usually straightforward. However, a subgroup of patients with diastolic heart failure may present with progressive dyspnea, peripheral edema, and pulmonary congestion; in these patients, ejection fraction obtained by echocardiography is well preserved.[91] This condition frequently occurs in older patients with comorbidities such as obesity, hypertension, diabetes mellitus, atrial fibrillation, and/or coronary artery disease.[92] In general, patient history, physical examination, and echocardiography are sufficient for making the diagnosis, but right and/or left heart catheterization may be needed to distinguish between PAH and pulmonary hypertension associated with left heart disease. The required treatment regimen for patients with pulmonary hypertension caused by left heart disease generally involves diuretics, oxygen supplementation, anticoagulants, and medication to control heart rate and blood pressure, but a specific therapy targeting the pulmonary vasculature is not indicated in this setting.[81,92] In addition, PAH-specific therapy has not been shown to improve exercise capacity or survival in IPF or systemic sclerosis patients with ILD complicated by PAH.[78,93,94] As such, given the substantial evidence of increased mortality in cases where PAH complicates ILD and the lack of specific therapy, whenever possible patients should be referred to expert centers for enrollment in new clinical trials and/or consideration for lung transplantation.

Sleep-Disordered Breathing

Several studies have reported poor quality of sleep secondary to nocturnal hypoxemia in patients with diffuse parenchymal lung disease.[95–97] The reported frequency ranges from 61% to 88% in IPF patients[98–100] and from 17% to 44% in sarcoidosis.[101,102] Health-related decreases in the quality of life are associated with poor sleep quality in IPF patients,[103] but no correlation was found between the severity of sleep-disordered breathing or poor sleep quality and pulmonary physiologic parameters.[100,103] Clinicians suspecting sleep-disordered breathing should refer patients for nocturnal polysomnography. Although there is no evidence-based recommendation,[98] improving sleep quality and sleep-disordered breathing may improve quality of life and affect outcome in patients with ILD.

LUNG CANCER–COMPLICATED ILD

An increased risk of lung cancer is well established in IPF, CTD, PLCH, and occupational lung diseases (see Fig. 9).[104–107] The most common histologic types are squamous cell carcinoma and adenocarcinoma. Lymphoproliferative malignancies are more frequently seen in CTD-ILD, particularly Sjögren syndrome.[108] One report noted that lung cancer occurred 3 times more frequently in patients with sarcoidosis[109]; however, a recent, large epidemiologic study found no increased risk of lung cancer among sarcoidosis patients.[107] Although studies have noted that pulmonary resection for lung cancer in patients with underlying pulmonary fibrosis is associated with higher morbidity and mortality, clinicians should consider lung resection in carefully selected patients.[110,111]

A MULTIDISCIPLINARY APPROACH

Diagnosing ILDs can be very challenging, and requires significant interest and expertise in pulmonary medicine, rheumatology, radiology, and pathology. A multidisciplinary approach is important because it will produce more precise diagnoses, guide physicians to request appropriate investigations, and modify treatment regimens. This idea has been confirmed by a study showing that accuracy of diagnosis is significantly improved when pulmonologists, radiologists, and pathologists interact, in comparison with that achieved by physicians working in isolation.[62] In a similar study, when rheumatologists participated in a multidisciplinary ILD clinic that included a pulmonologist, radiologist, and pathologist, the diagnosis was changed in 54% of patients attending the clinic; moreover, therapies were changed in 80% of patients with CTD-ILD and in 27% of patients with IPF.[63] Substantial evidence shows that implementation of a multidisciplinary approach provides a high standard of care for patients, improving the accuracy of clinical diagnosis and leading to a significant positive impact on patient outcome.

SUMMARY

Clinicians evaluating patients with ILD require a significant depth of knowledge about many forms of ILDs. In the last decade there have been significant improvements in the diagnosis of many forms of ILDs using patient history, physical examination, laboratory testing, HRCT scanning, bronchoscopy, and surgical lung biopsy. HRCT scanning, in particular, has proved to be a valuable tool that accurately provides specific patterns, obviating the need for surgical lung biopsy or providing guidance for additional testing. Furthermore, collaborations among pulmonologists, radiologists, and pathologists have significantly improved our understanding of the natural history of specific disease patterns and have led to the development of numerous high-quality clinical trials targeting a specific disease or associated comorbidities.

REFERENCES

1. American Thoracic Society/European Respiratory Society International Multidisciplinary Consensus Classification of the Idiopathic Interstitial Pneumonias. This joint statement of the American Thoracic Society (ATS), and the European Respiratory Society (ERS) was adopted by the ATS board of directors, June 2001 and by the ERS Executive Committee, June 2001. Am J Respir Crit Care Med 2002;165(2):277–304.
2. Craig PJ, Wells AU, Doffman S, et al. Desquamative interstitial pneumonia, respiratory bronchiolitis and their relationship to smoking. Histopathology 2004;45(3):275–82.
3. Ryu JH, Myers JL, Capizzi SA, et al. Desquamative interstitial pneumonia and respiratory bronchiolitis-associated interstitial lung disease. Chest 2005; 127(1):178–84.
4. Raghu G, Collard HR, Egan JJ, et al. An official ATS/ERS/JRS/ALAT statement: idiopathic pulmonary fibrosis: evidence-based guidelines for diagnosis and management. Am J Respir Crit Care Med 2011;183(6):788–824.
5. Statement on sarcoidosis. Joint Statement of the American Thoracic Society (ATS), the European Respiratory Society (ERS) and the World Association of Sarcoidosis and Other Granulomatous Disorders (WASOG) adopted by the ATS Board of Directors and by the ERS Executive Committee, February 1999. Am J Respir Crit Care Med 1999;160(2):736–55.
6. Alhamad EH, Alanezi MO, Idrees MM, et al. Clinical characteristics and computed tomography findings in Arab patients diagnosed with pulmonary sarcoidosis. Ann Saudi Med 2009;29(6):454–9.
7. Keane MP, Lynch JP 3rd. Pleuropulmonary manifestations of systemic lupus erythematosus. Thorax 2000;55(2):159–66.
8. Lee DM, Weinblatt ME. Rheumatoid arthritis. Lancet 2001;358(9285):903–11.
9. Steen VD, Medsger TA Jr. Severe organ involvement in systemic sclerosis with diffuse scleroderma. Arthritis Rheum 2000;43(11):2437–44.
10. Gribbin J, Hubbard RB, Le Jeune I, et al. Incidence and mortality of idiopathic pulmonary fibrosis and sarcoidosis in the UK. Thorax 2006;61(11): 980–5.
11. Raghu G, Weycker D, Edelsberg J, et al. Incidence and prevalence of idiopathic pulmonary fibrosis. Am J Respir Crit Care Med 2006;174(7):810–6.

12. Ryu JH, Moss J, Beck GJ, et al. The NHLBI lymphangioleiomyomatosis registry: characteristics of 230 patients at enrollment. Am J Respir Crit Care Med 2006; 173(1):105–11.
13. Alhamad EH. Familial interstitial lung disease in four members of one family: a case series. Cases J 2009;2:9356.
14. Garcia CK, Raghu G. Inherited interstitial lung disease. Clin Chest Med 2004; 25(3):421–33, v.
15. Flieder DB, Travis WD. Pathologic characteristics of drug-induced lung disease. Clin Chest Med 2004;25(1):37–45.
16. Walker T, McCaffery J, Steinfort C. Potential link between HMG-CoA reductase inhibitor (statin) use and interstitial lung disease. Med J Aust. Jan 15 2007; 186(2):91–4.
17. Wolff AJ, O'Donnell AE. Pulmonary effects of illicit drug use. Clin Chest Med 2004;25(1):203–16.
18. Glazer CS, Newman LS. Occupational interstitial lung disease. Clin Chest Med 2004;25(3):467–78, vi.
19. Baumgartner KB, Samet JM, Coultas DB, et al. Occupational and environmental risk factors for idiopathic pulmonary fibrosis: a multicenter case–control study. Collaborating Centers. Am J Epidemiol 2000;152(4):307–15.
20. American Thoracic Society. Idiopathic pulmonary fibrosis: diagnosis and treatment. International consensus statement. American Thoracic Society (ATS), and the European Respiratory Society (ERS). Am J Respir Crit Care Med 2000;161(2 Pt 1):646–64.
21. Avouac J, Airo P, Meune C, et al. Prevalence of pulmonary hypertension in systemic sclerosis in European Caucasians and metaanalysis of 5 studies. J Rheumatol 2010;37(11):2290–8.
22. Johnson SR, Gladman DD, Urowitz MB, et al. Pulmonary hypertension in systemic lupus. Lupus 2004;13(7):506–9.
23. Todd NW, Lavania S, Park MH, et al. Variable prevalence of pulmonary hypertension in patients with advanced interstitial pneumonia. J Heart Lung Transplant 2010;29(2):188–94.
24. Udayakumar N, Venkatesan S, Rajendiran C. Pulmonary hypertension in rheumatoid arthritis—relation with the duration of the disease. Int J Cardiol 2008; 127(3):410–2.
25. Wigley FM, Lima JA, Mayes M, et al. The prevalence of undiagnosed pulmonary arterial hypertension in subjects with connective tissue disease at the secondary health care level of community-based rheumatologists (the UNCOVER study). Arthritis Rheum 2005;52(7):2125–32.
26. Handa T, Nagai S, Miki S, et al. Incidence of pulmonary hypertension and its clinical relevance in patients with sarcoidosis. Chest 2006;129(5):1246–52.
27. Alhamad EH, Idrees MM, Alanezi MO, et al. Sarcoidosis-associated pulmonary hypertension: clinical features and outcomes in Arab patients. Ann Thorac Med 2010;5(2):86–91.
28. Shorr AF, Helman DL, Davies DB, et al. Pulmonary hypertension in advanced sarcoidosis: epidemiology and clinical characteristics. Eur Respir J 2005; 25(5):783–8.
29. Shorr AF, Wainright JL, Cors CS, et al. Pulmonary hypertension in patients with pulmonary fibrosis awaiting lung transplant. Eur Respir J 2007;30(4):715–21.
30. Lettieri CJ, Nathan SD, Barnett SD, et al. Prevalence and outcomes of pulmonary arterial hypertension in advanced idiopathic pulmonary fibrosis. Chest 2006;129(3):746–52.

31. McLaughlin VV, Archer SL, Badesch DB, et al. ACCF/AHA 2009 expert consensus document on pulmonary hypertension a report of the American College of Cardiology Foundation Task Force on Expert Consensus Documents and the American Heart Association developed in collaboration with the American College of Chest Physicians; American Thoracic Society, Inc.; and the Pulmonary Hypertension Association. J Am Coll Cardiol 2009;53(17):1573–619.
32. Fischer A, West SG, Swigris JJ, et al. Connective tissue disease-associated interstitial lung disease: a call for clarification. Chest 2010;138(2):251–6.
33. Hebert J, Beaudoin J, Laviolette M, et al. Absence of correlation between the degree of alveolitis and antibody levels to *Micropolysporum faeni*. Clin Exp Immunol 1985;60(3):572–8.
34. Pinon JM, Geers R, Lepan H, et al. Immunodetection by enzyme-linked immuno-filtration assay (ELIFA) of IgG, IgM, IgA and IgE antibodies in bird breeder's disease. Eur J Respir Dis 1987;71(3):164–9.
35. Ohtani Y, Saiki S, Sumi Y, et al. Clinical features of recurrent and insidious chronic bird fancier's lung. Ann Allergy Asthma Immunol 2003;90(6):604–10.
36. Lacasse Y, Selman M, Costabel U, et al. Clinical diagnosis of hypersensitivity pneumonitis. Am J Respir Crit Care Med 2003;168(8):952–8.
37. Alhamad EH, Lynch JP 3rd, Martinez FJ. Pulmonary function tests in interstitial lung disease: what role do they have? Clin Chest Med 2001;22(4):715–50, ix.
38. Kawut SM, O'Shea MK, Bartels MN, et al. Exercise testing determines survival in patients with diffuse parenchymal lung disease evaluated for lung transplantation. Respir Med 2005;99(11):1431–9.
39. Flaherty KR, Andrei AC, Murray S, et al. Idiopathic pulmonary fibrosis: prognostic value of changes in physiology and six-minute-walk test. Am J Respir Crit Care Med 2006;174(7):803–9.
40. Baughman RP, Sparkman BK, Lower EE. Six-minute walk test and health status assessment in sarcoidosis. Chest 2007;132(1):207–13.
41. Alhamad EH. The six-minute walk test in patients with pulmonary sarcoidosis. Ann Thorac Med 2009;4(2):60–4.
42. Alhamad EH, Shaik SA, Idrees MM, et al. Outcome measures of the 6 minute walk test: relationships with physiologic and computed tomography findings in patients with sarcoidosis. BMC Pulm Med 2010;10:42.
43. Schoindre Y, Meune C, Dinh-Xuan AT, et al. Lack of specificity of the 6-minute walk test as an outcome measure for patients with systemic sclerosis. J Rheumatol 2009;36(7):1481–5.
44. Epler GR, McLoud TC, Gaensler EA, et al. Normal chest roentgenograms in chronic diffuse infiltrative lung disease. N Engl J Med 1978;298(17):934–9.
45. Gaensler EA, Carrington CB. Open biopsy for chronic diffuse infiltrative lung disease: clinical, roentgenographic, and physiological correlations in 502 patients. Ann Thorac Surg 1980;30(5):411–26.
46. Ryu JH, Olson EJ, Midthun DE, et al. Diagnostic approach to the patient with diffuse lung disease. Mayo Clin Proc 2002;77(11):1221–7; quiz 1227.
47. Koyama M, Johkoh T, Honda O, et al. Chronic cystic lung disease: diagnostic accuracy of high-resolution CT in 92 patients. AJR Am J Roentgenol 2003;180(3):827–35.
48. Johkoh T, Muller NL, Cartier Y, et al. Idiopathic interstitial pneumonias: diagnostic accuracy of thin-section CT in 129 patients. Radiology 1999;211(2):555–60.
49. Hunninghake GW, Zimmerman MB, Schwartz DA, et al. Utility of a lung biopsy for the diagnosis of idiopathic pulmonary fibrosis. Am J Respir Crit Care Med. Jul 15 2001;164(2):193–6.

50. Flaherty KR, Thwaite EL, Kazerooni EA, et al. Radiological versus histological diagnosis in UIP and NSIP: survival implications. Thorax 2003;58(2):143–8.

51. Sundaram B, Gross BH, Martinez FJ, et al. Accuracy of high-resolution CT in the diagnosis of diffuse lung disease: effect of predominance and distribution of findings. AJR Am J Roentgenol 2008;191(4):1032–9.

52. Primack SL, Hartman TE, Hansell DM, et al. End-stage lung disease: CT findings in 61 patients. Radiology 1993;189(3):681–6.

53. Silva CI, Muller NL, Lynch DA, et al. Chronic hypersensitivity pneumonitis: differentiation from idiopathic pulmonary fibrosis and nonspecific interstitial pneumonia by using thin-section CT. Radiology 2008;246(1):288–97.

54. Bensard DD, McIntyre RC Jr, Waring BJ, et al. Comparison of video thoracoscopic lung biopsy to open lung biopsy in the diagnosis of interstitial lung disease. Chest 1993;103(3):765–70.

55. Tiitto L, Heiskanen U, Bloigu R, et al. Thoracoscopic lung biopsy is a safe procedure in diagnosing usual interstitial pneumonia. Chest 2005;128(4):2375–80.

56. Kondoh Y, Taniguchi H, Kitaichi M, et al. Acute exacerbation of interstitial pneumonia following surgical lung biopsy. Respir Med 2006;100(10):1753–9.

57. Park IN, Kim DS, Shim TS, et al. Acute exacerbation of interstitial pneumonia other than idiopathic pulmonary fibrosis. Chest 2007;132(1):214–20.

58. Flaherty KR, Travis WD, Colby TV, et al. Histopathologic variability in usual and nonspecific interstitial pneumonias. Am J Respir Crit Care Med 2001;164(9):1722–7.

59. Monaghan H, Wells AU, Colby TV, et al. Prognostic implications of histologic patterns in multiple surgical lung biopsies from patients with idiopathic interstitial pneumonias. Chest 2004;125(2):522–6.

60. Antoniou KM, Margaritopoulos G, Economidou F, et al. Pivotal clinical dilemmas in collagen vascular diseases associated with interstitial lung involvement. Eur Respir J 2009;33(4):882–96.

61. Flaherty KR, Andrei AC, King TE Jr, et al. Idiopathic interstitial pneumonia: do community and academic physicians agree on diagnosis? Am J Respir Crit Care Med 2007;175(10):1054–60.

62. Flaherty KR, King TE Jr, Raghu G, et al. Idiopathic interstitial pneumonia: what is the effect of a multidisciplinary approach to diagnosis? Am J Respir Crit Care Med 2004;170(8):904–10.

63. Castelino FV, Goldberg H, Dellaripa PF. The impact of rheumatological evaluation in the management of patients with interstitial lung disease. Rheumatology (Oxford) 2011;50(3):489–93.

64. Mays EE, Dubois JJ, Hamilton GB. Pulmonary fibrosis associated with tracheobronchial aspiration. A study of the frequency of hiatal hernia and gastroesophageal reflux in interstitial pulmonary fibrosis of obscure etiology. Chest 1976;69(4):512–5.

65. Piesman M, Hwang I, Maydonovitch C, et al. Nocturnal reflux episodes following the administration of a standardized meal. Does timing matter? Am J Gastroenterol 2007;102(10):2128–34.

66. Raghu G, Freudenberger TD, Yang S, et al. High prevalence of abnormal acid gastro-oesophageal reflux in idiopathic pulmonary fibrosis. Eur Respir J 2006;27(1):136–42.

67. Savarino E, Bazzica M, Zentilin P, et al. Gastroesophageal reflux and pulmonary fibrosis in scleroderma: a study using pH-impedance monitoring. Am J Respir Crit Care Med 2009;179(5):408–13.

68. Tcherakian C, Cottin V, Brillet PY, et al. Progression of idiopathic pulmonary fibrosis: lessons from asymmetrical disease. Thorax 2011;66(3):226–31.

69. Kondoh Y, Taniguchi H, Kawabata Y, et al. Acute exacerbation in idiopathic pulmonary fibrosis. Analysis of clinical and pathologic findings in three cases. Chest 1993;103(6):1808–12.

70. Akira M, Hamada H, Sakatani M, et al. CT findings during phase of accelerated deterioration in patients with idiopathic pulmonary fibrosis. AJR Am J Roentgenol 1997;168(1):79–83.

71. Kim DS, Park JH, Park BK, et al. Acute exacerbation of idiopathic pulmonary fibrosis: frequency and clinical features. Eur Respir J 2006;27(1):143–50.

72. Martinez FJ, Safrin S, Weycker D, et al. The clinical course of patients with idiopathic pulmonary fibrosis. Ann Intern Med 2005;142(12 Pt 1):963–7.

73. Azuma A, Nukiwa T, Tsuboi E, et al. Double-blind, placebo-controlled trial of pirfenidone in patients with idiopathic pulmonary fibrosis. Am J Respir Crit Care Med 2005;171(9):1040–7.

74. Miyazaki Y, Tateishi T, Akashi T, et al. Clinical predictors and histologic appearance of acute exacerbations in chronic hypersensitivity pneumonitis. Chest 2008;134(6):1265–70.

75. Olson AL, Huie TJ, Groshong SD, et al. Acute exacerbations of fibrotic hypersensitivity pneumonitis: a case series. Chest 2008;134(4):844–50.

76. Lederer DJ, Caplan-Shaw CE, O'Shea MK, et al. Racial and ethnic disparities in survival in lung transplant candidates with idiopathic pulmonary fibrosis. Am J Transplant 2006;6(2):398–403.

77. Launay D, Humbert M, Berezne A, et al. Clinical characteristics and survival in systemic sclerosis-related PH associated With ILD. Chest 2011. [Epub ahead of print].

78. Le Pavec J, Girgis RE, Lechtzin N, et al. Systemic sclerosis related pulmonary hypertension associated with interstitial lung disease: impact of pulmonary arterial hypertension therapies. Arthritis Rheum 2011;63(8):2456–64.

79. Mathai SC, Hummers LK, Champion HC, et al. Survival in pulmonary hypertension associated with the scleroderma spectrum of diseases: impact of interstitial lung disease. Arthritis Rheum 2009;60(2):569–77.

80. Condliffe R, Kiely DG, Peacock AJ, et al. Connective tissue disease-associated pulmonary arterial hypertension in the modern treatment era. Am J Respir Crit Care Med 2009;179(2):151–7.

81. Behr J, Ryu JH. Pulmonary hypertension in interstitial lung disease. Eur Respir J 2008;31(6):1357–67.

82. Patel NM, Lederer DJ, Borczuk AC, et al. Pulmonary hypertension in idiopathic pulmonary fibrosis. Chest 2007;132(3):998–1006.

83. Polomis D, Runo JR, Meyer KC. Pulmonary hypertension in interstitial lung disease. Curr Opin Pulm Med 2008;14(5):462–9.

84. Fisher MR, Forfia PR, Chamera E, et al. Accuracy of Doppler echocardiography in the hemodynamic assessment of pulmonary hypertension. Am J Respir Crit Care Med 2009;179(7):615–21.

85. Arcasoy SM, Christie JD, Ferrari VA, et al. Echocardiographic assessment of pulmonary hypertension in patients with advanced lung disease. Am J Respir Crit Care Med 2003;167(5):735–40.

86. Zisman DA, Karlamangla AS, Ross DJ, et al. High-resolution chest CT findings do not predict the presence of pulmonary hypertension in advanced idiopathic pulmonary fibrosis. Chest 2007;132(3):773–9.

87. Devaraj A, Wells AU, Meister MG, et al. The effect of diffuse pulmonary fibrosis on the reliability of CT signs of pulmonary hypertension. Radiology 2008;249(3):1042–9.

88. Alhamad EH, Al-Boukai AA, Al-Kassimi FA, et al. Prediction of pulmonary hypertension in patients with or without interstitial lung disease: reliability of CT findings. Radiology 2011;260(3):875–83.

89. Chang B, Wigley FM, White B, et al. Scleroderma patients with combined pulmonary hypertension and interstitial lung disease. J Rheumatol 2003;30(11): 2398–405.

90. Leuchte HH, Neurohr C, Baumgartner R, et al. Brain natriuretic peptide and exercise capacity in lung fibrosis and pulmonary hypertension. Am J Respir Crit Care Med 2004;170(4):360–5.

91. Zile MR, Brutsaert DL. New concepts in diastolic dysfunction and diastolic heart failure: part I: diagnosis, prognosis, and measurements of diastolic function. Circulation 2002;105(11):1387–93.

92. Hoeper MM, Barbera JA, Channick RN, et al. Diagnosis, assessment, and treatment of non-pulmonary arterial hypertension pulmonary hypertension. J Am Coll Cardiol 2009;54(Suppl 1):S85–96.

93. Zisman DA, Schwarz M, Anstrom KJ, et al. A controlled trial of sildenafil in advanced idiopathic pulmonary fibrosis. N Engl J Med 2010;363(7):620–8.

94. King TE Jr, Brown KK, Raghu G, et al. BUILD-3: a randomized, controlled trial of bosentan in idiopathic pulmonary fibrosis. Am J Respir Crit Care Med 2011; 184(1):92–9.

95. Bye PT, Issa F, Berthon-Jones M, et al. Studies of oxygenation during sleep in patients with interstitial lung disease. Am Rev Respir Dis 1984;129(1):27–32.

96. Perez-Padilla R, West P, Lertzman M, et al. Breathing during sleep in patients with interstitial lung disease. Am Rev Respir Dis 1985;132(2):224–9.

97. McNicholas WT, Coffey M, Fitzgerald MX. Ventilation and gas exchange during sleep in patients with interstitial lung disease. Thorax 1986;41(10):777–82.

98. Mermigkis C, Chapman J, Golish J, et al. Sleep-related breathing disorders in patients with idiopathic pulmonary fibrosis. Lung 2007;185(3):173–8.

99. Mermigkis C, Stagaki E, Tryfon S, et al. How common is sleep-disordered breathing in patients with idiopathic pulmonary fibrosis? Sleep Breath 2010; 14(4):387–90.

100. Lancaster LH, Mason WR, Parnell JA, et al. Obstructive sleep apnea is common in idiopathic pulmonary fibrosis. Chest 2009;136(3):772–8.

101. Turner GA, Lower EE, Corser BC, et al. Sleep apnea in sarcoidosis. Sarcoidosis Vasc Diffuse Lung Dis 1997;14(1):61–4.

102. Verbraecken J, Hoitsma E, van der Grinten CP, et al. Sleep disturbances associated with periodic leg movements in chronic sarcoidosis. Sarcoidosis Vasc Diffuse Lung Dis 2004;21(2):137–46.

103. Krishnan V, McCormack MC, Mathai SC, et al. Sleep quality and health-related quality of life in idiopathic pulmonary fibrosis. Chest 2008;134(4):693–8.

104. Bouros D, Hatzakis K, Labrakis H, et al. Association of malignancy with diseases causing interstitial pulmonary changes. Chest 2002;121(4):1278–89.

105. Park J, Kim DS, Shim TS, et al. Lung cancer in patients with idiopathic pulmonary fibrosis. Eur Respir J 2001;17(6):1216–9.

106. Aubry MC, Myers JL, Douglas WW, et al. Primary pulmonary carcinoma in patients with idiopathic pulmonary fibrosis. Mayo Clin Proc 2002;77(8): 763–70.

107. Le Jeune I, Gribbin J, West J, et al. The incidence of cancer in patients with idiopathic pulmonary fibrosis and sarcoidosis in the UK. Respir Med 2007;101(12): 2534–40.

108. Fox RI. Sjogren's syndrome. Lancet 2005;366(9482):321–31.

109. Brincker H, Wilbek E. The incidence of malignant tumours in patients with respiratory sarcoidosis. Br J Cancer 1974;29(3):247–51.
110. Kumar P, Goldstraw P, Yamada K, et al. Pulmonary fibrosis and lung cancer: risk and benefit analysis of pulmonary resection. J Thorac Cardiovasc Surg 2003; 125(6):1321–7.
111. Watanabe A, Higami T, Ohori S, et al. Is lung cancer resection indicated in patients with idiopathic pulmonary fibrosis? J Thorac Cardiovasc Surg 2008; 136(5):1357–63, 1363, e1351–2.

Interventional Pulmonology

David Hsia, MD[a],*, Ali I. Musani, MD, FCCP[b]

KEYWORDS

- Interventional pulmonology • Bronchoscopy • Airway
- Pleural disease • Procedure

Interventional pulmonology is a rapidly growing procedural-based field that bridges the gap between pulmonary medicine and thoracic surgery. Focusing on minimally invasive methods of diagnosis and treatment, interventional pulmonology spans a wide range of areas within pulmonary medicine, including both malignant and benign diseases. The expansion of this field in recent years has largely been driven by advances in technology and development of novel devices. As a result, in the last several years, interventional pulmonology has extended beyond prior boundaries of therapeutic interventions for central airway and pleural disease to include new diagnostic tools for diagnosing lung lesions and novel therapeutic interventions such as bronchial thermoplasty (BT) for asthma and bronchoscopic lung volume reduction for chronic obstructive pulmonary disease (COPD). **Box 1** summarizes the wide range of diagnostic and therapeutic modalities at the disposal of the trained interventional pulmonologist and the variety of diseases that can be treated. Although not all these interventional pulmonary techniques are discussed, the authors aim to introduce prominent interventions within the context of the diseases encountered by the interventionalist.

DIAGNOSIS OF PULMONARY LESIONS
Peripheral Lung Lesions

Diagnosis of pulmonary lesions has always been a primary concern of the pulmonologist. Lung cancer remains the most common cause of malignancy-related death, with more than 150,000 deaths annually in the United States.[1] One in 500 chest radiographs demonstrates a pulmonary nodule,[2] with a higher incidence reported on

David Hsia has nothing to disclose. Ali I. Musani is a Consultant for Olympus USA, Spiration, Super Dimension, and Cardinal health; he has received honorarium as speaker from Olympus USA, Super Dimension, Bronchus, Asthmatics, and Cardinal health. Received unrestricted educational grants from Olympus USA. Received industry support for a industry sponsored clinical trials from Cardinal Health, Spiration, Asthmatics and Bronchus Inc.

[a] Division of Respiratory and Critical Care Physiology and Medicine, Harbor–University of California, Los Angeles Medical Center, 1000 West Carson Street, Box #405, Torrance, CA 90509, USA
[b] Interventional Pulmonology Program, National Jewish Health, University of Colorado, J 225, Molly Blank, 1400 Jackson Street, Denver, CO 80206, USA
* Corresponding author.
E-mail address: dhsia@labiomed.org

doi:10.1016/j.mcna.2011.08.002
0025-7125/11/$ – see front matter © 2011 Elsevier Inc. All rights reserved.

Box 1
Disease states and related interventional pulmonary procedures

Diagnosis of pulmonary lesions
- Peripheral lung lesion
  - Electromagnetic navigation
  - Radial endobronchial ultrasonography
- Mediastinal adenopathy
  - Linear endobronchial ultrasonography
- Early detection of lung cancer
  - Autofluorescence bronchoscopy
  - Narrow band imaging
  - Confocal bronchoscopy

Central airway obstruction
- Mechanical debulking and dilation
  - Rigid bronchoscopy
  - Balloon bronchoplasty
  - Microdebridement
  - Stent placement
- Ablation therapies
  - Endobronchial laser
  - Argon plasma coagulation
  - Electrocautery
  - Cryotherapy
  - Brachytherapy
  - Photodynamic therapy

Artificial airway
- Percutaneous tracheostomy
- Minitracheostomy
- Transtracheal oxygen catheter

Pleural disease
- Medical pleuroscopy and pleurodesis
- Indwelling pleural catheter
- Thoracic ultrasonography

Other diseases
- Asthma
  - Bronchial thermoplasty
- Emphysema
  - Endobronchial valve

computerized tomographic (CT) imaging.[3] In the United States alone, more than 150,000 patients with lung nodules are assessed annually, and this number will likely increase, given results from the National Lung Cancer Screening Trial demonstrating a 20% reduction in mortality with CT scan screening in a high-risk population.[4] Nevertheless, routine bronchoscopy has a sensitivity of only 34% for lesions smaller than 20 mm and 63% for lesions larger than 20 mm.[5] Diagnostic yield with only fluoroscopic guidance is also notably poor for peripheral lesions, with yields of only 14% for lesions smaller than 20 mm in the outer third compared with 31% for lesions within the proximal two-thirds of the lung parenchyma.[6] New technologies have been shown to dramatically increase bronchoscopic diagnostic yield for small peripheral lung lesions.

Electromagnetic navigation bronchoscopy
Electromagnetic navigation (EMN) bronchoscopy is a relatively new technology that allows real-time procedural guidance for sampling of peripheral pulmonary lesions. The system uses a high-resolution CT scan of the chest to create a virtual bronchoscopic image of the patient's tracheobronchial tree. The patient is placed within an electromagnetic field, and the virtual airway map is aligned with the patient's anatomic airway. The steerable sensor probe is then navigated to the target lesion under virtual real-time guidance. **Fig. 1** demonstrates the virtual images created for navigational guidance and the computerized tracking of the distance, direction, and orientation between the steerable sensor probe and the lesion. On reaching the lesion, a guide sheath catheter is left in place, which is used as an extended working channel for obtaining biopsy samples.

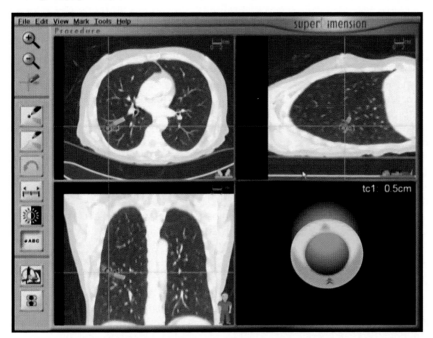

Fig. 1. EMN bronchoscopy. A steerable sensor probe is navigated to the target lesion using a virtual map of the tracheobronchial tree generated from the patient's high-resolution CT scan. Different image displays assist in the navigation process (coronal, axial, and sagittal CT images shown). The system indicates direction, distance, and orientation of the steerable probe to the lesion (*bottom right*). In this case, the steerable probe (represented by a solid bar on CT images) has been navigated within 0.5 cm of the lesion.

EMN bronchoscopy can be performed under moderate or deep procedural sedation in the bronchoscopy suite. An early study demonstrated EMN to only add an additional 15 minutes to a conventional bronchoscopic procedure.[7] EMN bronchoscopy increases diagnostic yield of peripheral lung nodules to a range of 59% to 77%.[7–12]

EMN bronchoscopy has also been used for navigational guidance for transbronchial needle aspiration (TBNA) of mediastinal lymph nodes, but its role in lymph node biopsy and mediastinal staging of cancer has largely been overshadowed by linear endobronchial ultrasonography (EBUS)-guided TBNA, which is less expensive and more readily available. EMN has also been used to guide placement of fiducial markers for localized radiation therapy for malignancies and surgical resection. Future uses of navigation techniques such as EMN may merge diagnostic bronchoscopy with therapeutic modalities, such as brachytherapy, to allow minimally invasive diagnosis and therapy for malignant lesions in patients for whom surgical options are limited.

Radial EBUS

Radial EBUS produces a 360° image of airways and surrounding structures such as lung parenchyma, blood vessels, lymph nodes, or abnormal lesions (**Fig. 2**). Radial EBUS images are processed using a processor different from that of the bronchoscopic video image. A 20-MHz mechanical EBUS probe is inserted into a guide sheath catheter and advanced through the flexible bronchoscope working channel. Once the lesion has been located, the guide sheath is left in place and the radial EBUS probe is removed, allowing the guide sheath to be used as an extended working channel for biopsy instruments to obtain tissue samples.[13] As with EMN, fluoroscopy can also be used to help visually confirm stability of the guide sheath placement during the biopsy process.

Diagnostic bronchoscopic yields of peripheral lung nodules with radial EBUS navigation range from 46% to 88%,[13–17] with a recent meta-analysis reporting a pooled sensitivity of 73%.[17] Although radial EBUS does not have the benefit of a steerable catheter such as EMN, it has the advantage of real-time radiographic confirmation of localization of the target lesion, whereas EMN is dependent on a virtual target location. Errors in EMN registration between the virtual image and the patient's anatomy may result in erroneous guide sheath catheter placement and thus biopsy sampling errors. In addition, EMN requires a significant amount of time in the preprocedural planning phase and has the additional cost of the disposable steerable probe. Radial EBUS, on the other hand, uses a reusable probe. Despite their differences, these 2 navigation technologies can be used together as complimentary systems with a higher combined diagnostic yield of 88%.[9]

On-site analysis of radiographic EBUS images has also been used to predict benign from malignant lesions with an accuracy of nearly 90%.[13] However, few bronchoscopists have this level of expertise with image interpretation.

Mediastinal Adenopathy

TBNA is an effective technique for diagnosing mediastinal adenopathy or extraluminal lung masses as well as staging lung cancer. This technique was first described for use with rigid bronchoscopy and adapted for flexible bronchoscopy by Wang and colleagues[18] in 1978. There is a wide range of diagnostic yield reported in the literature ranging from 15% to 85%,[19,20] and, despite the demonstrated safety and efficacy, this technique has largely been underutilized.[21,22] Several modifiable factors have been shown to improve diagnostic yield, including operator experience,[23,24] number of aspirates obtained,[25] use of rapid on-site cytology,[25,26] and larger needle gauge.[27–29]

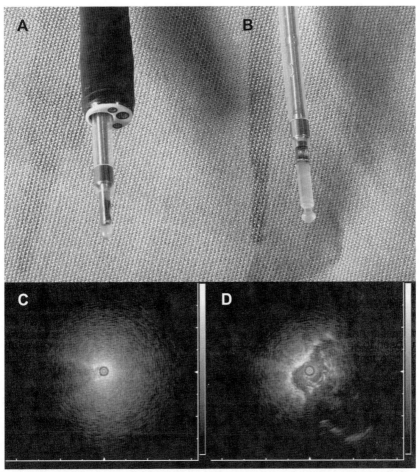

Fig. 2. Radial EBUS. (*A*) Therapeutic bronchoscope with a 2.8-mm diameter working channel. The radial EBUS probe and guide sheath (2.6-mm outer diameter) are shown extending beyond the distal tip of the flexible bronchoscope. (*B*) Example of a different model radial EBUS probe within a guide sheath. (*C*) Typical snowstorm pattern seen in normal lung. (*D*) Radial EBUS image of adenocarcinoma.

However, one of the most significant recent advances affecting diagnostic yield is the incorporation of linear EBUS into the procedure.

Linear EBUS

Endoscopic ultrasonography (EUS) has been used in gastroenterology, but the miniaturization of ultrasound transducers permit the technique's use in interventional pulmonology as a radial EBUS probe or by integrating the transducer into a bronchoscope for radiographic evaluation and biopsy of mediastinal lesions. Current EBUS bronchoscopes use a linear (convex) transducer placed in contact with the airway wall. A saline-filled balloon is used to improve contact between the bronchoscope and airway wall, thereby improving image acquisition. These bronchoscopes allow real-time ultrasonography of the mediastinum along with real-time needle aspiration and tissue sampling (**Fig. 3**). Given the unique characteristics of the EBUS

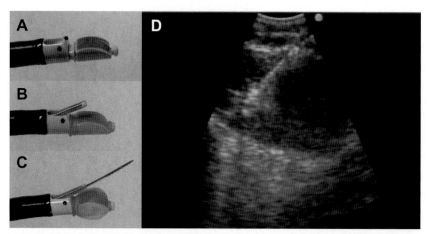

Fig. 3. Linear EBUS. (*A*) EBUS bronchoscope. The linear ultrasound transducer is located in the distal portion of the bronchoscope. Visual optics are oriented at 35° (not shown). (*B*) EBUS bronchoscope with balloon inserted and catheter deployed. (*C*) EBUS bronchoscope with saline-filled balloon and needle deployed. (*D*) Ultrasonographic image of needle aspiration of a lymph node.

bronchoscope, specific training and practice are required to maximize diagnostic yield with this technique.

Diagnostic yield of EBUS-guided TBNA has a sensitivity of more than 95%, specificity of 100%, and accuracy of 90%.[30] One study reported a sensitivity of 95.3% for non–small cell lung cancer and a negative predictive value of 97.6% after 3 successful aspirations of a lymph node.[31] When prospectively compared with conventional TBNA, EBUS-guided TBNA yields were similar for the subcarinal region and higher for all other nodal stations.[32]

Transesophageal EUS using a specialized endoscope with radial ultrasound transducer has been used by gastroenterologists for biopsy and staging of subcarinal and paraesophageal lesions. A meta-analysis of 18 studies using EUS-guided fine-needle aspiration (FNA) for non–small cell lung cancer staging demonstrated a pooled sensitivity of 83% and specificity of 97%.[33] EUS-guided FNA, however, is unable to access the hilar, infrahilar, and intralobar nodes, and, therefore, EBUS and EUS-guided sampling should be considered as complimentary modalities. Studies have now shown that both transbronchial and transesophageal lymph node biopsy can be performed using the same EBUS bronchoscope; this allows an operator to evaluate most mediastinal lymph node stations using the same endoscope in one procedure.[34,35]

Early Detection of Lung Cancer

Early airway cancers and precancerous lesions may not appear obvious under standard white light imaging but can be accentuated by specialized imaging modalities. Although these conditions primarily involve squamous cell carcinomas and carcinoma in situ, other abnormal epithelial findings such as squamous dysplasia may eventually develop into cancers. The rate of transformation of premalignant lesions into cancer is not well defined but has been observed to occur only in 6.1% of cases.[36] The bronchoscopy imaging modalities discussed in this article are approved by the US Food and Drug Administration (FDA) to help identify abnormal lesions for the early detection of cancer.

Autofluorescence imaging

Light fluorescence characteristics of abnormal bronchial epithelium have been shown to differ from those of normal tissue, with slightly weaker fluorescence for red wavelengths of light and much weaker fluorescence for green and blue wavelengths. This difference is thought to be related to an increase in epithelial thickness associated with increased blood flow and/or reduced concentration of fluorophores in abnormal tissue.[37] Autofluorescence bronchoscopy (AFB) uses a blue light filter to remove other wavelengths of light returning to the bronchoscope. Additional differences in fluorescence characteristics between normal and abnormal tissue can be highlighted using exogenous fluorescent compounds, such as hematoporphyrin derivatives such as 5-aminolevulinic acid. Although AFB has been shown to be superior to white light bronchoscopy alone in detecting early epithelial cancers,[37–40] these comparisons were primarily performed with fiberoptic imaging technology, and it is unclear if the benefit is still as notable when compared with higher-resolution video bronchoscopy systems. AFB also requires a separate bronchoscopy system, increasing procedure time and expense; this makes AFB more suitable for a dedicated interventional pulmonology suite.

Narrow band imaging

Narrow band imaging (NBI) capitalizes on the increased absorption of blue (415 nm) and green (540 nm) wavelengths of light by hemoglobin. As demonstrated in **Fig. 4**, atypical mucosal epithelium is associated with increased angiogenesis. These areas are differentially highlighted when white light bronchoscopy is viewed with specific filters.[41] Small studies using NBI have demonstrated increased detection rates of dysplasia or malignancy in up to 23% of cases not found using white light bronchoscopy.[42] Unlike AFB, NBI is integrated into newer bronchoscope processors, and the transition between white light bronchoscopy and NBI is nominal. NBI technology, however, is proprietary and only available through one manufacturer.

Confocal bronchoscopy

Fibered confocal fluorescence microscopy uses a blue laser (440–500 nm) to induce fluorescence. This technology is able to produce dynamic high-resolution microimaging of the respiratory epithelial cells, goblet cells, cilia, smooth muscle, subepithelial

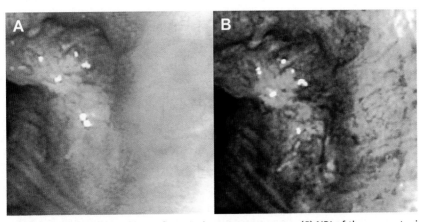

Fig. 4. NBI. (*A*) White light image of atypical squamous mucosa. (*B*) NBI of the same atypical mucosa demonstrating the ability of NBI to highlight angiogenesis associated with mucosal malignancies and premalignancies.

microvasculature, and alveolar ducts and sacs (termed alveoscopy) up to depths of 200 μm.[43] This high degree of resolution provides a real-time view of living tissue at almost histologic resolution through a 1-mm fiberoptic miniprobe. The miniprobe incorporates the light source and detector and is introduced through the working channel of the bronchoscope; in the future, the confocal endomicroscope may be incorporated directly into a flexible bronchoscope. Future uses of confocal bronchoscopy may include characterization of airway remodeling in patients with asthma and COPD and detection of dysplastic and malignant changes in airway epithelium.[44] In the meantime, confocal bronchoscopy is tempered by the limited areas that can be explored at any given time given the high resolution.

Future investigations using advanced imaging modalities may involve use of AFB or NBI to scan large sections of mucosa for areas of abnormality before more detailed investigation by confocal bronchoscopy. Additional imaging technologies, such as optical coherence tomography for use with clinical bronchoscopy, are also being explored.[45] At present, most detected lesions represent squamous metaplasia or dysplasia and the significance of intervention for these lesions has not been clearly demonstrated, although patients may be subjected to a greater number of unnecessary biopsies. The role of these adjunct imaging modalities is still being defined, and evidence demonstrating the clinical impact of these advanced imaging technologies is clearly needed.

CENTRAL AIRWAY OBSTRUCTION

Central airway obstructions of the trachea, mainstem bronchi, or other large airways can result from several different diseases, although bronchogenic carcinoma is the most common cause. The incidence of central airway obstruction is not known, but lung cancer trends suggest that the incidence is increasing,[46] and approximately 20% to 30% of patients with lung cancer will develop large airway-related complications associated with their disease.[47] Aside from malignancy, nonmalignant causes of central airway obstructions include stenosis, strictures, webs, and granulation tissue resulting from endotracheal intubation, tracheostomy, and inflammatory processes such as Wegener granulomatosis, sarcoidosis, relapsing polychondritis, or infections (eg, tuberculosis, histoplasmosis).[48] Aside from classifying based on underlying cause, central airway obstructions are also categorized based on the origin of obstruction (ie, endoluminal, extraluminal, mixed) because this affects what therapeutic modalities might be most appropriate for a specific situation.

Mechanical Debulking and Dilation

Rigid bronchoscopy

Rigid bronchoscopy was initially used by Gustav Killian in 1898 for a foreign body extraction,[49] but its popularity as a means to access the airways had waned after the introduction of the flexible bronchoscope in 1967. However, rigid bronchoscopy has several distinct advantages when dealing with central airway obstructions, including the ability to ventilate the patient through the rigid bronchoscope, the ability to use large-caliber suction catheters to aspirate blood and debris, and the ability to use the shaft of the rigid bronchoscope itself to mechanically debulk obstructing tissue and recanulate the airway. The specific safety advantages of rigid bronchoscopy in maintaining the patency of the patient's airway during a procedure makes it essential in many cases given the potential dire complications associated with therapeutic interventions for central airway obstructions.

Aside from mechanical debulking and serial dilation using the rigid bronchoscope to physically remove or compress obstructing tissue, rigid bronchoscopy can also be used in conjunction with other ablative modalities, including ablative therapies controlled via flexible bronchoscopy. Rigid bronchoscopy is also used for placement and removal of airway stents, foreign body extraction, and therapeutic interventions for massive hemoptysis. Rigid bronchoscopy is performed in an operating room setting with general anesthesia. Given the complexity, interventional pulmonologists require specific training on the proper use of rigid bronchoscope.

Balloon bronchoplasty

Mechanical debridement and dilation with rigid bronchoscopy can be complicated by the development of mucosal injury and granulation tissue formation.[50] Saline-filled balloons are used with either rigid or flexible bronchoscopy to dilate and restore airway patency with lower risk of mucosal trauma and have been effectively used to treat benign stenosis[51–53] and malignant obstructions.[54] Complications, although rare, include tracheobronchial laceration,[55] pneumothorax, pneumomediastinum, and mediastinitis.[56] Although balloon bronchoplasty is effective at increasing airway diameter, recurrent stenosis and or granulation tissue often requires the use of other airway interventions, such as stent placement, to maintain long-term lumen patency.[57]

Microdebridement

Microdebriders have been used previously in otolaryngological procedures and recently in conjunction with rigid bronchoscopy for mechanical debulking. These debriders are composed of a serrated blade rotating at 1000 to 3000 rpm attached to a hollow suction tube and have been used in both malignant and nonmalignant disease.[58] Procedures had been limited to the trachea and proximal mainstem bronchi because of the length of the microdebrider (37 cm), but a longer 45-cm device has recently been used to resect a distal left mainstem malignancy.[59] One of the benefits of microdebriders is that they are not associated with potential airway fires that can be triggered by thermal ablation modalities used in conjunction with supplemental oxygen.[58] However, microdebriders have been associated with inadvertent resection of normal tissue[60] and development of pneumomediastinum when used with jet ventilation.[61]

Stent placement

There are several indications for therapeutic placement of airway stents, including extrinsic compression or mixed extrinsic/intrinsic airway lesions, recurrent endoluminal airway obstructions, inoperable nonmalignant disease, and tracheoesophageal fistulas.[62,63] Stents are frequently used in conjunction with other therapies, such as mechanical debulking and/or ablative therapies, to help maintain airway patency.[64] Stents are made of silicone, expandable metal mesh (steel or nitinol), or a hybrid combination of covered metal mesh. Self-expanding metal stents and covered metal stents can be placed by either rigid or flexible bronchoscope.[65] Silicone stents, however, require rigid bronchoscopy for placement.

Like all airway therapeutics, stents have potentially serious associated risks. Epithelialization or tumor growth through the mesh wall of an uncovered stent can result in reobstruction and makes stent removal difficult (**Fig. 5**). This risk is alleviated by use of a covered metal stent, although granulation tissue can still form at the proximal and distal ends.[66] Metal stents are also difficult to remove, with one series of 25 patients (30 stents) requiring piecemeal extraction in 73% of cases. Complications of removal included retained stent pieces, mucosal tearing and bleeding, reobstruction requiring temporary silicone stent placement, need for postoperative mechanical

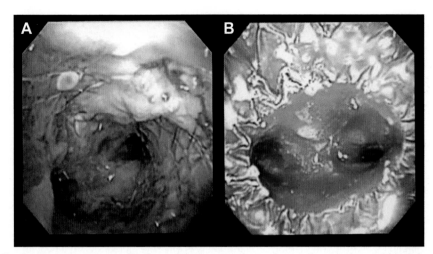

Fig. 5. Airway stent complications. (*A*) Uncovered metal stent in a patient with tracheal obstruction from adenocarcinoma. Stent patency has been compromised by growth of tumor through the stent wall, mucous occlusion, and stent fracture with exposed metal wires. (*B*) After rigid bronchoscopy with removal of uncovered metal stent, laser ablation, and replacement with a covered metal stent.

ventilation, and tension pneumothorax.[67] In 2005, the FDA issued a black box warning against the use of metal stents in patients with nonmalignant disease unless alternative therapies were unavailable.[68] Silicone stents, on the other hand, are easier to remove but more likely to migrate, with a migration rate of 9.5% in the largest described series of 677 patients (926 stents).[69] Other complications include mucous plugging and development of granulation tissue.[70] However, despite these potential complications, airway stents remain an important therapeutic tool for the trained interventional pulmonologist in the management of central airway obstructions.

Ablation Therapies

Laser, electrocautery, and argon plasma coagulation (APC) rely on thermal energy for tissue destruction. These modalities can be used with rigid or flexible bronchoscopy to debulk malignant and nonmalignant central airway masses, remove stenotic lesions, and coagulate areas of bleeding. Nonthermal ablative therapies are also available, although many have delayed effects, which limit their utility in the management of acute airway compromise. Each therapy has unique advantages, however, such as the ability of cryotherapy probes to freeze and attach to foreign bodies, assisting in removal. A comparison of ablative therapies is outlined in **Table 1**.

Endobronchial laser

Endobronchial lasers generate a monochromatic beam of light to produce thermal energy resulting in tissue vaporization, necrosis, and coagulation. There are several types of lasers available, and the Nd:YAG laser is the most commonly used by interventional pulmonologists. This laser is ideal because it provides deep tissue penetration (3–5 mm) as well as good coagulation and hemostasis. The Nd:YAG laser has been shown to successfully recanalize large airway obstructions more than 90% of the time, although success was lower for peripheral lesions (50%–70%) and for lesions with a component of extrinsic airway compression.[71] The neodymium:yttrium-aluminum-perovskite laser

Table 1
Comparison of ablation therapies

Therapy	Mechanism of Action	Advantages	Disadvantages
Nd:YAG laser	Noncontact, thermal energy from laser light	Deep tissue penetration and hemostasis, good for major tissue debulking	Potential damage to adjacent tissue
Nd:YAP laser	Noncontact, thermal energy from laser light	Better hemostasis than that of Nd:YAG laser	Less tissue penetration than that of Nd:YAG laser
Carbon dioxide laser	Noncontact, thermal energy from laser light	More precise ablation than that of other lasers, shallow penetration	Minimal hemostasis, bulky equipment limits use in airways
Argon plasma coagulation	Noncontact, thermal energy from ionized argon gas	Good hemostasis, preferential flow to uncoagulated tissue, bends around corners	Shallow penetration, not ideal for major tissue debulking
Electrocautery	Contact, thermal electrical energy	Inexpensive, multiple accessory types for different situations, good hemostasis	Requires frequent cleaning of contact device, less precision than laser
Cryotherapy	Repeated cycles of freezing and thawing	Good for foreign body removal, no risk of airway fire	Not for acute airway use because of delayed tissue destruction, requires follow-up bronchoscopic tissue removal
Brachytherapy	Direct implantation of radiation source into target lesion	Concentrated, long-lasting, localized tissue effect	Higher risk of hemorrhage and other complications
Photodynamic therapy	Preferential uptake of photosensitizer by malignant cells with nonthermal laser–activated phototoxic reaction	Potentially curative for early mucosal squamous cell cancers	Requires follow-up bronchoscopic tissue removal, 4–6 wk of skin photosensitivity
Microdebrider	Mechanical removal of tissue by rotating blade and suction	No risk of airway fire	Device length limits to proximal airway use

Abbreviation: Nd:YAP, neodymium:yttrium-aluminum-perovskite.

has decreased cutting but improved coagulation. The carbon dioxide (CO_2) laser is primarily used by otolaryngologists and has a shallow tissue penetration (0.1–0.5 mm) with very precise cutting but minimal hemostasis; the poor hemostasis qualities and size of the equipment limit CO_2 laser use in interventional pulmonology.[72,73]

Argon Plasma Coagulation

APC uses an argon gas source and electrical generator to create a stream of ionized gas that generates shallow tissue effects (<5 mm) but good hemostasis. Coagulated tissue has higher resistance to current flow compared with uncoagulated tissue, so APC has additional advantages in generating hemostasis. APC preferentially flows toward uncoagulated tissue, including around corners, making it helpful in airways that are anatomically difficult to reach. The relatively decreased ablative qualities, however, make it less ideal for debulking large amounts of tissue.[74]

Electrocautery

Although laser and APC are noncontact therapeutic modalities, electrocautery is a contact modality that generates thermal energy by the flow of electrons from an electrical generator. In addition to tissue ablation from contact with the electrocautery probe, specialized accessories permit a range of interventions, including cutting of strictures with a cautery knife, biopsy combined with hemostasis with cautery forceps, and resection of polypoid lesions with a cautery snare. Although not as precise as a laser, electrocautery has been shown to be effective in palliation of symptoms related to central airway obstruction with a significantly decreased cost.[75] Electrocautery generators often serve a dual use as an APC generator and are commonly found in endoscopy suites for use in both pulmonary and gastroenterology procedures.

Caution must be used with all thermal ablation therapies to avoid damage of normal adjacent tissue, perforation of the airways, or hemorrhage.[76] In addition, thermal ablation therapies can also damage metal or silicone stents, and extreme caution should be used when these devices are present. Thermal ablation modalities are also contraindicated in patients requiring large amounts of supplemental oxygen given the risk of airway fires, although the risk is low.[77,78] Cases of air emboli have been described with APC and Nd:YAG laser.[79]

PLEURAL DISEASE

Interventional pulmonologists have a wide range of diagnostic and therapeutic pleural procedures at their disposal. Some procedures, such as medical thoracoscopy, have been available for many years and have recently regained interest because of the emphasis on minimally invasive interventions. Other procedures involve adaptations of older devices for novel uses.

Medical Thoracoscopy

Medical thoracoscopy, also referred to as pleuroscopy, was initially described by Jacobeus[80] in 1910. Medical thoracoscopy can be performed by the interventional pulmonologist under local anesthesia and moderate procedural sedation in an ambulatory procedure suite, unlike video-assisted thoracic surgery (VATS), which requires general anesthesia with double-lumen intubation in an operating room.[81,82] Only a single site is required to enter the thoracic cavity rather than multiple incisions required by VATS. Both rigid and semirigid thoracoscopes are available and allow the operator to evaluate the pleural space, obtain targeted pleural biopsies under direct visualization, remove pleural fluid, lyse adhesions, and perform chemical pleurodesis. Diagnostic accuracy of medical thoracoscopy is higher than closed-needle biopsy and has been reported to be as high as 97% for malignant effusions, mesothelioma, and tuberculous-related pleural disease.[83] Successful pleurodesis with talc poudrage is achieved in more than 95% of cases at 90 days.[84] Lung biopsy[85] and management of spontaneous pneumothorax[86] have also been described. Potential complications include bleeding, persistent pneumothorax, or damage to intercostals nerves or blood vessels.[81]

Indwelling Pleural Catheter

Indwelling pleural catheters allow for outpatient management and periodic drainage of malignant and other recurrent pleural effusions. Catheters can be placed in an outpatient setting using local anesthesia and minimal procedural sedation. Up to 100% of patients have control of their effusion-related symptoms, and pleurodesis occurs in approximately 60% of patients over a 4- to 6-week period without additional chemical pleurodesis.[87–89] Complication rates are low (<1%) and include pain, cellulitis, and empyema.[87,89]

OTHER DISEASES
Bronchial Thermoplasty

In 2010, BT was approved by the FDA as the first nonpharmacologic treatment of patients with moderate and severe asthma. As shown in **Fig. 6**, a flexible bronchoscope is used to position an expandable basket to make contact with the walls of the bronchial tree and perform radiofrequency ablation (RFA). Prior animal studies demonstrated that RFA delivered in this manner resulted in a decrease in smooth muscle mass of the airway wall and decreased airway responsiveness to methacholine.[90] A total of 3 bronchoscopy procedures are performed to systematically deliver RFA to the bilateral upper and lower lobe bronchi with more than 3 mm in diameter. Clinical trials have recently demonstrated a 32% decrease in severe exacerbations,

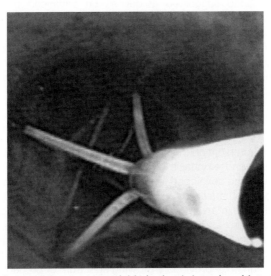

Fig. 6. Bronchial thermoplasty. An expandable basket is introduced into the large airways and used to contact airway walls and perform radiofrequency ablation of smooth muscle in patients with moderate and severe asthma.

84% decrease in emergency room visits, 66% decrease in days lost from work/school/activities, and a 36% decrease in patient-reported asthma symptoms with BT compared with sham bronchoscopy.[91] Benefit from BT is maintained for at least 2 years postprocedure with additional follow-up evaluation ongoing.[92]

Endobronchial Valve Placement

In 2003, the National Emphysema Treatment Trial demonstrated that lung volume reduction surgery (LVRS) decreased mortality, improved exercise tolerance, and improved quality of life in certain populations of patients with severe emphysema.[93] It was then theorized that endoscopically placed endobronchial valves (EBV) would allow 1-way flow of air and secretions, thereby promoting distal airway atelectasis and emulating the effects of LVRS. Results of a prospective randomized trial of unilateral EBV in patients with severe COPD recently demonstrated a mild improvement in lung function and exercise tolerance; however, there was a significantly greater incidence of COPD exacerbations, pneumonia, and hemoptysis in the treatment group compared with the medically treated control group.[94] At present, EBV placement for patients with COPD is not yet available for routine use. There are also ongoing evaluations of different valve designs,[95] biologic adhesives,[96,97] and airway bypass formation.[98,99]

Of note, EBV placement has also been used to treat bronchopleural fistulas[100,101] and are currently approved for postsurgical cases on a humanitarian use basis.

INTERVENTIONAL PULMONOLOGY TRAINING

Appropriate use of these advanced interventions requires additional training above and beyond the typical experience provided by most pulmonary and critical care fellowship training programs. At present, there is no structured method of demonstrating competency in these advanced procedures, although the American College of Chest Physicians, the American Thoracic Society, and the European Respiratory Society have published suggested guidelines on advanced procedural competency.[76,102] Although formal training in interventional pulmonology is not a requirement to learn specific procedures within the field, additional structured training in advanced interventional pulmonology procedures is becoming recognized as an important, and almost necessary, requirement to ensure competency of the interventional pulmonologist.[103] Operator competency, in turn, is essential to ensure optimized procedural efficacy, efficiency, and safety.

SUMMARY

In the last decade, interventional pulmonology has grown rapidly fueled by technologic advancements and emphasis on noninvasive procedural interventions. Novel modalities are now being developed for diseases not previously treated by procedural intervention, such as asthma and COPD. In the future, new modalities will undoubtedly become available to the interventional pulmonologist, with current exploratory studies investigating areas such as bronchoscopic use of optical coherence tomography, vibration resonance imaging, and RFA of tumors. In addition, established technologies are being adapted for new indications, such as ablative therapies for pleural diseases. Interventional pulmonology provides a growing spectrum of procedural interventions that supplement standard pulmonologists, radiologists, thoracic surgeons, and otolaryngologists.

REFERENCES

1. Howlader N, Noone AM, Krapcho M, et al, editors. SEER Cancer Statistics Review, 1975–2008. Bethesda (MD): National Cancer Institute; 2011. Available at: http://www.seer.cancer.gov/csr/1975_2008/. based on November 2010 SEER data submission, posted to the SEER web site, 2011. Accessed August 5, 2011.
2. Tan B, Flaherty K, Kazerooni E, et al. The solitary pulmonary nodule. Chest 2003; 123:89S–96S.
3. Menezes R, Robert H, Paul N, et al. Lung cancer screening using low-dose computed tomography in at-risk individuals: the Toronto experience. Lung Cancer 2010;67(2):177–83.
4. The National Lung Screening Trial Research Team. Reduced lung-cancer mortality with low-dose computed tomographic screening. N Engl J Med 2011;365(5):395–409.
5. Rivera MP, Mehta AC. Initial diagnosis of lung cancer: ACCP evidence-based clinical practice guidelines (2nd edition). Chest 2007;132:131S–48S.
6. Baaklini WA, Reinoso MA, Gorin AB, et al. Diagnostic yield of fiberoptic bronchoscopy in evaluating solitary pulmonary nodules. Chest 2000;117(4):1049–54.
7. Schwarz Y, Greif J, Becker HD, et al. Real-time electromagnetic navigation bronchoscopy to peripheral lung lesions using overlaid CT images: the first human study. Chest 2006;129(4):988–94.
8. Gildea TR, Mazzone PJ, Karnak D, et al. Electromagnetic navigation diagnostic bronchoscopy: a prospective study. Am J Respir Crit Care Med 2006;174(9):982–9.
9. Eberhardt R, Anantham D, Ernst A, et al. Multimodality bronchoscopic diagnosis of peripheral lung lesions: a randomized controlled trial. Am J Respir Crit Care Med 2007;176(1):36–41.
10. Makris D, Scherpereel A, Leroy S, et al. Electromagnetic navigation diagnostic bronchoscopy for small peripheral lung lesions. Eur Respir J 2007;29(6):1187–92.
11. Eberhardt R, Anantham D, Herth F, et al. Electromagnetic navigation diagnostic bronchoscopy in peripheral lung lesions. Chest 2007;131(6):1800–5.
12. Lamprecht B, Porsch P, Pirich C, et al. Electromagnetic navigation bronchoscopy in combination with PET-CT and rapid on-site cytopathologic examination for diagnosis of peripheral lung lesions. Lung 2009;187(1):55–9.
13. Kurimoto N, Miayzawa T, Okimasa S, et al. Endobronchial ultrasonography using a guide sheath increases the ability to diagnose peripheral pulmonary lesions endoscopically. Chest 2004;126:959–65.
14. Yoshikawa M, Sukoh N, Yamazaki K, et al. Diagnostic value of endobronchial ultrasonography with a guide sheath for peripheral pulmonary lesions without x-ray fluoroscopy. Chest 2007;131:1788–93.
15. Kikuchi E, Yamazaki K, Sukho N, et al. Endobronchial ultrasonography with guide-sheath for peripheral pulmonary lesions. Eur Respir J 2004;24:533–7.
16. Eberhardt R, Ernst A, Herth FJ. Ultrasound-guided transbronchial biopsy of solitary pulmonary nodules less than 20 mm. Eur Respir J 2009;34:1284–7.
17. Steinfort DP, Khor YH, Manser RL, et al. Radial probe endobronchial ultrasound for the diagnosis of peripheral lung cancer: systematic review and meta-analysis. Eur Respir J 2011;37:902–10.
18. Wang KP, Terry PB, Marsh BR. Bronchoscopic needle aspiration biopsy of paratracheal tumors. Am Rev Respir Dis 1978;118:17–21.

19. Shure D, Fedullo PF. The role of transcarinal needle aspiration in the staging of bronchogenic carcinoma. Chest 1984;86(5):693–6.
20. Schenk DA, Bower JH, Bryan CL, et al. Transbronchial needle aspiration staging of bronchogenic carcinoma. Am Rev Respir Dis 1986;134(1):146–8.
21. Prakash UB, Offord KP, Stubbs SE. Bronchoscopy in North America: the ACCP survey. Chest 1991;100:1668–75.
22. Haponik EF, Shure D. Underutilization of transbronchial needle aspiration: experiences of current pulmonary fellows. Chest 1997;112:251–3.
23. Rodriguez de Castro F, Diaz Lopez F, Serda GJ, et al. Relevance of training in transbronchial fine-needle aspiration technique. Chest 1997;111:103–5.
24. Hsu LH, Liu CC, Ko JS. Education and experience improve the performance of transbronchial needle aspiration: a learning curve at a cancer center. Chest 2004;125:532–40.
25. Chin R Jr, McCain TW, Lucia MA, et al. Transbronchial needle aspiration in diagnosing and staging lung cancer: how many aspirates are needed? Am J Respir Crit Care Med 2002;166:377–81.
26. Baram D, Garcia RB, Richman PS. Impact of rapid on-site cytologic evaluation during transbronchial needle aspiration. Chest 2005;128:869–75.
27. Schenk DA, Chambers SL, Derdak S, et al. Comparison of the Wang 19-gauge and 22-gauge needles in the mediastinal staging of cancer. Am Rev Respir Dis 1993;147:1251–8.
28. Bilaceroglu S, Cagiotariotaciota U, Gunel O, et al. Comparison of rigid and flexible transbronchial needle aspiration in the staging of bronchogenic carcinoma. Respiration 1998;65:441–9.
29. Harrow EM, Abi-Saleh W, Blum J, et al. The utility of transbronchial needle aspiration in the staging of bronchogenic carcinoma. Am J Respir Crit Care Med 2000;161:601–7.
30. Krimsky W, Sarkar S, Kurimoto N, et al. Endobronchial ultrasound: current applications and future directions: are we ready for prime time? J Bronchology 2007;14(1):63–9.
31. Lee HS, Lee GK, Lee HS, et al. Real-time endobronchial ultrasound-guided transbronchial needle aspiration in mediastinal staging of non-small cell lung cancer: how many aspirations per target lymph node station? Chest 2008;134(2):368–74.
32. Herth F, Becker HD, Ernst A. Conventional vs endobronchial ultrasound-guided transbronchial needle aspiration: a randomized trial. Chest 2004;125(1):322–5.
33. Micames CG, McCrory DC, Pavey DA, et al. Endoscopic ultrasound-guided fine-needle aspiration for non-small cell lung cancer staging: a systematic review and metaanalysis. Chest 2007;131:539–48.
34. Hwangbo B, Lee GK, Lee HS, et al. Transbronchial and transesophageal fine-needle aspiration using an ultrasound bronchoscope in mediastinal staging of potentially operable lung cancer. Chest 2010;138(4):795–802.
35. Herth FJ, Krasnik M, Kahn N, et al. Combined endoscopic-endobronchial ultrasound-guided fine-needle aspiration of mediastinal lymph nodes through a single bronchoscope in 150 patients with suspected lung cancer. Chest 2010;138(4):790–4.
36. Bota S, Jean-Bernard A, Paris C, et al. Follow-up of bronchial precancerous lesions and carcinoma in situ using fluorescence endoscopy. Am J Respir Crit Care Med 2001;164:1688–93.
37. Kusunoki Y, Imamura F, Uda H, et al. Early detection of lung cancer with laser-induced fluorescence endoscopy and spectrofluorometry. Chest 2000;118(6):1776–82.

38. Lam S, Kennedy T, Unger M, et al. Localization of bronchial intraepithelial neoplastic lesions by fluorescence bronchoscopy. Chest 1998;113:696–702.
39. Hirsch FR, Prindiville SA, Miller YE, et al. Fluorescence versus white-light bronchoscopy for detection of preneoplastic lesions: a randomized study. J Natl Cancer Inst 2001;93:1385–91.
40. Lee P, Brokx HA, Postmus PE, et al. Dual digital video-autofluorescence imaging for detection of pre-neoplastic lesions. Lung Cancer 2007;58(1):44–9.
41. Shibuya K, Hoshino H, Chiyo M, et al. High magnification bronchovideoscopy combined with narrow band imaging could detect capillary loops of angiogenic squamous dysplasia in heavy smokers at high risk for lung cancer. Thorax 2003; 58(11):989–95.
42. Vincent BD, Fraig M, Silvestri GA. A pilot study of narrow-band imaging compared to white light bronchoscopy for evaluation of normal airways and premalignant and malignant airways disease. Chest 2007;131(6):1794–9.
43. Thiberville L, Salaun M, Lachkar S, et al. Human in vivo fluorescence microimaging of the alveolar ducts and sacs during bronchoscopy. Eur Respir J 2009; 33(5):974–85.
44. Musani A, Sims M, Sareli C, et al. A pilot study of the feasibility of confocal endomicroscopy for examination of the human airway. J Bronchology Interv Pulmonol 2010;17(2):126–30.
45. Tsuboi M, Hayashi A, Ikeda N, et al. Optical coherence tomography in the diagnosis of bronchial lesions. Lung Cancer 2005;49(3):387–94.
46. Ayers ML, Beamis JF Jr. Rigid bronchoscopy in the twenty-first century. Clin Chest Med 2001;22:355–64.
47. Ginsberg RJ, Vokes EE, Ruben A. Non-small cell lung cancer. In: DeVita VT, Hellman S, Rosenberg SA, editors. Cancer principles and practice of oncology. Philadelphia: Lippincott-Raven; 1997. p. 858–911.
48. Ernst A, Feller-Kopman D, Becker HD, et al. Central airway obstruction. Am J Respir Crit Care Med 2004;169(12):1278–97.
49. Killian G. Uber direkte bronchoskopie. Munch Med Wochenschr 1898;27:844–7 [in German].
50. Rea F, Callegaro D, Loy M, et al. Benign tracheal and laryngotracheal stenosis: surgical treatment and results. Eur J Cardiothorac Surg 2002;22(3):352–6.
51. Keller C, Frost A. Fiberoptic bronchoplasty. Description of a simple adjunct technique for the management of bronchial stenosis following lung transplantation. Chest 1992;102:995–8.
52. Sheski FD, Mathur PN. Long-term results of fiberoptic bronchoscopic balloon dilation in the management of benign tracheobronchial stenosis. Chest 1998; 114:796–800.
53. Mayse ML, Greenheck J, Friedman M, et al. Successful bronchoscopic balloon dilation of nonmalignant tracheobronchial obstruction without fluoroscopy. Chest 2004;126(2):634–7.
54. Carlin BW, Harrell JH, Moser KM. The treatment of endobronchial stenosis using balloon catheter dilatation. Chest 1988;93:1148–51.
55. Kim JH, Shin JH, Song HY, et al. Tracheobronchial laceration after balloon dilation for benign strictures: incidence and clinical significance. Chest 2007;131(4):1114–7.
56. Kaloud H, Smolle-Juettner FM, Prause G, et al. Iatrogenic ruptures of the tracheobronchial tree. Chest 1997;112(3):774–8.
57. Noppen M, Schlesser M, Meysman M, et al. Bronchoscopic balloon dilatation in the combined management of postintubation stenosis of the trachea in adults. Chest 1997;112(4):1136–40.

58. Lunn W, Garland R, Ashiku S, et al. Microdebrider bronchoscopy. A new tool for the interventional bronchoscopist. Ann Thorac Surg 2005;80(4):1485–8.

59. Kennedy MP, Morice RC, Jimenez CA, et al. Treatment of bronchial airway obstruction using a rotating tip microdebrider: a case report. J Cardiothorac Surg 2007;2:16.

60. Kuhnel T, Hosemann W, Rothammer R. Evaluation of powered instrumentation in out-patient revisional sinus surgery. Rhinology 2001;39:215–9.

61. Sims HS, Lertsburapa K. Pneumomediastinum and retroperitoneal air after removal of papillomas with the microdebrider and jet ventilation. J Natl Med Assoc 2007;99:1068–70.

62. Makris D, Marquette CH. Tracheobronchial stenting and central airway replacement. Curr Opin Pulm Med 2007;13:278–83.

63. Lund ME, Garland R, Ernst A. Airway stenting: applications and practice management considerations. Chest 2007;13:278–83.

64. Mayazawa T, Yamakido M, Ikeda S, et al. Implantation of Ultraflex nitinol stents in malignant tracheobronchial stenoses. Chest 2000;118(4):959–65.

65. Dasgupta A, Dolmatch BL, Abi-Saleh WJ, et al. Self-expandable metallic airway stent insertion employing flexible bronchoscopy: preliminary results. Chest 1998;114(1):106–9.

66. Madden BP, Loke TK, Sheth AC. Do expandable metallic airway stents have a role in the management of patients with benign tracheobronchial disease? Ann Thorac Surg 2006;82:274–8.

67. Lunn W, Feller-Kopman D, Wahidi M, et al. Endoscopic removal of metallic airway stents. Chest 2005;127(6):2106–12.

68. Lund ME, Force S. Airway stenting for patients with benign airway disease and the Food and Drug Administration advisory: a call for restraint. Chest 2007;132: 1107–8.

69. Dumon JP, Cavaliere S, Diaz-Jimenez JP, et al. Seven-year experience with the Dumon prosthesis. J Bronchology 1996;31:6–10.

70. Wood DE, Liu YH, Vallieres E, et al. Airway stenting for malignant and benign tracheobronchial stenosis. Ann Thorac Surg 2003;76:167–72.

71. Cavaliere S, Venuta F, Foccoli P, et al. Endoscopic treatment of malignant airway obstructions in 2008 patients. Chest 1996;110:1536–42 [erratum appears in Chest 1997;111:1476].

72. Turner JF Jr, Wang KP. Endobronchial laser therapy. Clin Chest Med 1999;20: 107–22.

73. Ramser ER, Beamis JF Jr. Laser bronchoscopy. Clin Chest Med 1995;16: 415–26.

74. Morice RC, Ece T, Ece F, et al. Endobronchial argon plasma coagulation for treatment of hemoptysis and neoplastic airway obstruction. Chest 2001;119: 781–7.

75. Boxem T, Muller M, Venmans B, et al. Nd-YAG laser vs bronchoscopic electro-cautery for palliation of symptomatic airway obstruction: a cost-effectiveness study. Chest 1999;116(4):1108–12.

76. Ernst A, Silvestri GA, Johnstone D. Interventional pulmonary procedures: guide-lines from the American College of Chest Physicians. Chest 2003;123(5): 1693–7.

77. Brutinel WM, Cortese DA, Edell ES, et al. Complications of Nd:YAG laser therapy. Chest 1988;94:902–3.

78. Niskanen M, Purhonen S, Koljonen V, et al. Fatal inhalation injury caused by airway fire during tracheostomy. Acta Anaesthesiol Scand 2007;51(4):509–13.

79. Tellides G, Ugurlu BS, Kim RW, et al. Pathogenesis of systemic air embolism during bronchoscopic Nd:YAG laser operations. Ann Thorac Surg 1998;65(4):930–4.
80. Jacobeus HC. Ueber die möglichkeit die zytoskope bei untersuchung seröser höhlungen anzuwenden. Munch Med Wochenschr 1910;40:2090–2 [in German].
81. Colt HG. Thoracoscopy: window to the pleural space. Chest 1999;116:1409–15.
82. Mathur PN, Astoul P, Boutin C. Medical thoracoscopy: technical details. Clin Chest Med 1995;16:479–86.
83. Sakuraba M, Masuda K, Hebisawa A, et al. Diagnostic value of thoracoscopic pleural biopsy for pleurisy under local anaesthesia. ANZ J Surg 2006;76(8):722–4.
84. Hartman DL, Gaither JM, Kesler KA, et al. Comparison of insufflated talc under thoracoscopic guidance with standard tetracycline and bleomycin pleurodesis for control of malignant pleural effusions. J Thorac Cardiovasc Surg 1993; 105(4):743–7.
85. Mathur P, Loddenkemper R. Medical thoracoscopy: role in pleural and lung diseases. Clin Chest Med 1995;16:479–86.
86. Boutin C, Astoul P, Rey F, et al. Thoracoscopy in the diagnosis and treatment of spontaneous pneumothorax. Clin Chest Med 1995;16:497–503.
87. Musani AI, Haas AR, Seijo L, et al. Outpatient management of malignant pleural effusions with small-bore, tunneled pleural catheters. Respiration 2004;71(6): 559–66.
88. Tremblay A, Mason C, Michaud G. Use of tunneled catheters for malignant pleural effusions in patients fit for pleurodesis. Eur Respir J 2007;30(4):759–62.
89. Tremblay A, Michaud G. Single-center experience with 250 tunneled pleural catheter insertions for malignant pleural effusion. Chest 2006;129(2):362–8.
90. Danek CJ, Lombard CM, Dungworth DL, et al. Reduction in airway hyperresponsiveness to methacholine by the application of RF energy in dogs. J Appl Physiol 2004;97(5):1946–53.
91. Castro M, Rubin AS, Laviolette M, et al. Effectiveness and safety of bronchial thermoplasty in the treatment of severe asthma: a multicenter, randomized, double-blind, sham-controlled clinical trial. Am J Respir Crit Care Med 2010; 181(2):116–24.
92. Castro M, Rubin A, Laviolette M, et al. Persistence of effectiveness of bronchial thermoplasty in patients with severe asthma. Ann Allergy Asthma Immunol 2011; 107(1):65–70.
93. National Emphysema Treatment Trial Research Group. A randomized trial comparing lung-volume-reduction surgery with medical therapy for severe emphysema. N Engl J Med 2003;348:2049–73.
94. Sciurba FC, Ernst A, Herth FJ, et al. A randomized study of endobronchial valves for advanced emphysema. N Engl J Med 2010;363(13):1233–44.
95. Wood DE, McKenna J, Yusen RD, et al. A multicenter trial of an intrabronchial valve for treatment of severe emphysema. J Thorac Cardiovasc Surg 2007; 133(1):65–73.
96. Washko G, Kenney L, Pinto-Plata V, et al. Initial experience with a tissue engineering approach to bronchoscopic lung volume reduction in humans with emphysema [abstract]. Chest 2005;180:A230.
97. Reilly J, Washko G, Pinto-Plata V, et al. Biological lung volume reduction: a new bronchoscopic therapy for advanced emphysema. Chest 2007;131:1108–13.
98. Lausberg HF, Chino K, Patterson GA, et al. Bronchial fenestration improves expiratory flow in emphysematous human lungs. Ann Thorac Surg 2003;75: 393–7.

99. Macklem PT, Cardosa P, Snell G, et al. Airway bypass: a new treatment for emphysema [abstract]. Proc Am Thorac Soc 2006;167:A726.

100. Ferguson JS, Sprenger K, Van Natta T. Closure of a bronchopleural fistula using bronchoscopic placement of an endobronchial valve designed for the treatment of emphysema. Chest 2006;129(2):479–81.

101. Feller-Kopman D, Bechara R, Garland R, et al. Use of a removable endobronchial valve for the treatment of bronchopleural fistula. Chest 2006;130(1):274–5.

102. Bolliger CT, Mathur PN, Beamis JF, et al. ERS/ATS statement on interventional pulmonology. European Respiratory Society/American Thoracic Society. Eur Respir J 2002;19(2):356–73.

103. Lamb C, Feller-Kopman D, Ernst A, et al. An approach to interventional pulmonary fellowship training. Chest 2010;137(1):195–9.

Asthma

Rodolfo M. Pascual, MD*, Stephen P. Peters, MD, PhD

KEYWORDS

- Asthma • Airway • Inflammation • Diagnosis
- Treatment • Adult

Asthma is an important public health problem with a lifetime prevalence of approximately 10% in the United States. The morbidity of asthma is disproportionately borne by populations with a lower income, minorities, and children who live in the inner city[1] and individually by patients with more severe disease. Asthma is characterized by inflammation of the airways that leads to widespread and variable airflow obstruction. Asthmatic inflammation is heterogeneous, and many cells and mediators are involved. Key asthma effector inflammatory cells include mast cells, plasma cells, and eosinophils. Mast cell degranulation is responsible, in part, for immediate bronchospasm after exposure to antigen, a process that is regulated by IgE. Abnormal regulation and responses of eosinophils are hallmarks of allergic asthma, and eosinophils are particularly sensitive to glucocorticoid treatment. These effector cells are regulated by T lymphocytes, of which T-helper (TH) cells are particularly important. The airway inflammation of asthma is mediated by activated TH2 lymphocytes; however, TH1 lymphocytes, regulatory T cells, and TH17 lymphocytes also play a role.[2–4] There are complex interactions among different subpopulations of T cells, and this is a focus of active research, including attempts to identify targets for clinical intervention. Another important area of interest is the modulation of the immune system by airway resident cells, including epithelial cells; human airway smooth muscle cells; and, particularly, antigen-presenting cells, including dendritic cells. Abnormal responses of resident cells to infections and antigens may cause asthma in early life and may chronically perpetuate asthma. The many mediators involved in asthmatic inflammation explain why antiinflammatory drugs with broad activity such as corticosteroids tend to be

Supported in part by grants 5 U10 HL098103 to SPP and 1K12HL 089992 to RMP.
Disclosures: Dr Peters has participated in advisory boards sponsored by AstraZeneca, Aerocrine, Airsonett AB, Delmedica, Merck, and TEVA and in speakers' bureaus sponsored by Integrity CME and Merck. Dr Pascual has participated in clinical trials supported by Actelion, Forest, Boehringer Ingelheim, Genentech, GlaxoSmithKline, AstraZeneca, MedImmune, and Cephalon and has also participated in advisory boards sponsored by Actelion.
Section on Pulmonary, Critical Care, Allergy & Immunologic Diseases, Department of Internal Medicine, Center for Genomics and Personalized Medicine Research, Wake Forest University School of Medicine, Medical Center Boulevard, Winston-Salem, NC 27157, USA
* Corresponding author.
E-mail address: rpascual@wakehealth.edu

Med Clin N Am 95 (2011) 1115–1124
doi:10.1016/j.mcna.2011.09.001
0025-7125/11/$ – see front matter © 2011 Elsevier Inc. All rights reserved.

more effective, whereas agents that target a more narrow pathway or specific mediator have tended to be less effective. The natural history of asthma remains poorly understood. It is believed that chronic airway inflammation leads to structural changes in the airway or airway remodeling, but it is not known if this change occurs in all patients or if it is reversible.[5,6] In addition, most studies of airway inflammation in humans have been cross-sectional, so it is not known if inflammatory mechanisms change in time.

Asthma is a very common disease encountered in internal medicine practice. In most cases, the diagnosis and management of asthma is straightforward; however, the management of severe asthma may require subspecialty consultation. In this article, the authors focus on the diagnosis and management of asthma in adults.

DIAGNOSIS

The clinical presentation of asthma is quite heterogeneous in terms of symptoms, triggers, degree of impairment, and response to treatment. Asthma symptoms can be specific, such as wheezing after exposure to certain triggers, or nonspecific, such as chronic cough without an identified trigger. The cough associated with asthma is typically nonproductive and is episodic; concomitant rhinitis or sinusitis is very common and may contribute to the cough. Similarly, wheezing or chest tightness is episodic except in very severe asthma. A trigger is a discrete environmental exposure, activity, or event, which reliably causes coughing, wheezing, chest tightness, or shortness of breath in patients with asthma. Examples of common triggers include cold air, exercise, emotional situations, cat dander, pollen, and fumes. It is important to explore triggers in patients with asthma because avoidance of triggers can reduce symptoms. Some patients with asthma primarily experience exertional shortness of breath without much cough or wheeze, although this is highly unusual. Hence, asthma should be considered in the differential diagnosis for unexplained dyspnea, which is a symptom of many cardiac or pulmonary diseases. Similarly, some patients with asthma experience cough and do not wheeze or report exertional dyspnea, so asthma should be considered in the differential diagnosis for unexplained cough. The diagnosis of asthma is more likely in patients who have most of the symptoms mentioned earlier, but important differential diagnoses include rhinitis, interstitial lung disease, bronchitis related to smoking, or bronchiectasis. Asthma occurs with some uncommon lung diseases, including chronic eosinophilic pneumonia, allergic bronchopulmonary aspergillosis, or Churg-Strauss syndrome. Asthma may be diagnosed at any age, but, in most patients, asthma develops in childhood. However, children with asthma are often underdiagnosed. Clues that asthma may have been present in childhood, but not diagnosed, include a history of recurrent episodes of bronchitis; history of recurrent wheezing; family history of asthma, especially in the mother; and the presence of fixed airflow obstruction on initial diagnosis.

Asthma is an important comorbidity in patients with atopy or allergic disease. Asthma often occurs with allergic rhinitis or allergic sinusitis, so asthma should be considered in patients with those conditions who do not have satisfactory responses to treatment of conditions. Many clinicians perform testing to exclude asthma in patients with atopy even if rhinitis seems to be the predominant problem. The symptoms of asthma and chronic obstructive pulmonary disease (COPD) substantially overlap, so it is important to explore for a history of exposures that increase the risk of COPD, particularly cigarette smoking. Conversely, comorbid illnesses such as seasonal or perennial allergic rhinitis, gastroesophageal reflux disease (GERD), sinusitis, vocal cord dysfunction, and cigarette smoking should be considered that might worsen symptoms that might be attributed to asthma. Deconditioning and obesity are important cofactors because both affect quality of life in patients with asthma, although it is not clear if either factor worsens asthma per se. Comorbid illnesses are relevant because treatment of these conditions often improves the patient's quality of life, even though treatment may not specifically improve asthma.

In some patients, the symptoms of asthma might only be present during an asthma exacerbation. An asthma exacerbation is characterized by increased airway inflammation, reduced lung function, and increased bronchial hyperresponsiveness that is episodic and accompanied by worsened symptoms that typically last for several days to a few weeks. Often there is a preceding upper respiratory tract infection causing an exacerbation, so it is important to question patients about the typical courses of these exacerbations. The authors also ask patients if they have prolonged chest colds or bronchitis after upper respiratory tract infections.

Physical examination findings can vary significantly among patients and within a given patient depending on whether the patient is at his/her baseline state or is experiencing an exacerbation. Patients with stable, mild intermittent or mild persistent asthma are likely to have a normal lung examination. End expiratory musical wheezes are typically heard in patients with asthma experiencing exacerbations and may be a consistent finding in those with severe disease, although, rarely, patients with a severe exacerbation with very poor air exchange may present with a silent chest. Crackles or signs of consolidation or signs of congestive heart failure or hypoxemia are uncommon in asthma and should prompt consideration of other diagnoses. However, the diagnosis of asthma will not be accurate if it is not confirmed by objective testing.[7]

Spirometry is the gold standard test for diagnosing asthma, and it should be performed in all patients in whom asthma is suspected. In many patients with asthma, spirometry demonstrates airflow obstruction defined by a reduced ratio of forced expiratory volume in the first second to forced vital capacity ($FEV_1:FVC$), with a disproportionate reduction in FEV_1 compared with FVC. There should be substantial improvement (reversal) of at least 12% and 200 mL in the FEV_1 after treatment with short-acting bronchodilators; typically 4 to 8 puffs of albuterol are used. Although observing an acute bronchodilator response is perhaps the most commonly used test to diagnose asthma, variability of spirometry over time, either in response to treatment or after a triggering event, is also consistent with the diagnosis of asthma. Spirometry may be normal or nondiagnostic in an untreated patient in the absence of current symptoms or an exacerbation. In a patient who has been taking asthma medications, including inhaled steroids, FEV_1 reversibility may not be present. In such cases, a bronchial provocation test may be diagnostic. Most commonly inhaled methacholine challenge spirometry testing is used for this purpose, and it has an excellent negative predictive value. Usually a provocative concentration of 16 mg/mL or less of methacholine, of 8 mg/mL or less to 16 mg/mL, which causes a decrease of at least 20% in FEV_1, is considered diagnostic of asthma.[8] Sometimes an exercise challenge test for asthma is required in the rare patient who has intermittent symptoms and predominantly exercise-induced bronchospasm. Sometimes patients who experience significant air trapping or hyperinflation have reduced FVC, and this may also be reversible with short-acting bronchodilators. If coexisting diseases that cause pulmonary restriction are a consideration, then formal lung volume testing should be performed to prove that true pulmonary restriction is present. Unlike many other lung diseases, the diffusing capacity should not be reduced in a patient with asthma.

RISK STRATIFICATION

Once the diagnosis of asthma has been established, the patient should be assessed for current disease control (impairment) and risk of disease progression or serious complications or death from asthma. Current control and risk can both change over time, so both should be considered at every follow-up visit.[9,10] Validated questionnaires have been used to assess for current control, and these instruments typically assess the frequency and severity of symptoms, recent use of rescue medications, frequency of nocturnal symptoms, and impairment or limitation in activity towing to asthma symptoms. Examples of validated questionnaires include the Asthma Control Questionnaire (ACQ)[11] and the Asthma Control Test (QualityMetric, Lincoln, RI, USA).

Indicators of increased risk of death,[12] or frequent exacerbations from asthma, include prior severe exacerbations, frequent visits to the emergency department, prior respiratory failure due to asthma, chronic use of oral steroid, and severely reduced baseline FEV_1. Patients who are at particular risk include those with poor access to health care and lower levels of income and those who are poorly adherent to treatment recommendations. Both the control and risk should be considered in an integrated manner when deciding on an initial treatment plan and also at every reassessment visit. Spirometry should be repeated at least on an annual basis because accelerated loss of lung function indicates poor asthma control and might indicate poor adherence to treatment recommendations or the need for more treatment.

ASTHMA SEVERITY

Some guidelines have stressed the assessment of asthma severity based on the initial measured FEV_1 or the intensity of current asthma treatment, but this strategy had several important limitations.[10,13,14] Firstly, the natural history of asthma can be highly variable among patients. For example, some patients seem to have more labile disease than others as defined by greater fluctuations of lung function during exacerbations. Some patients who have had asthma for many years may have lower FEV_1 values but can be relatively asymptomatic, can use little health care, and can have infrequent exacerbations. Conversely, a younger patient may have relatively preserved lung function but poorly controlled asthma, requiring frequent urgent visits, hospitalizations, and rescue oral steroid use. Thus, the severity of asthma just based on lung function measurement may not forecast what will happen in the near term. Secondly, there is a paucity of data about whether effective antiinflammatory or maintenance medications prevent loss of lung function over long periods so that the effect of maintenance medications on severity in terms of reversing already low lung function or preventing loss of lung function over the long term is not known.[5] Lastly, some patients seem to use more medications than others despite having similar symptoms or degree of impairment. Medication use can be driven by psychosocial factors, comorbid conditions, and different physician practices. Hence, more recent guidelines have focused on assessing current asthma control during follow-up appointments.

ASTHMA CONTROL

Asthma can be considered well controlled or not well controlled because this allows for a simple dichotomous measurement that is useful to the clinician faced with treatment decisions. Asthma control is also typically a highly subjective and imprecise measurement because it often includes symptom recall and recall of recent rescue medication use. Not-well-controlled asthma should be initially treated with more aggressive antiinflammatory medication regimens, which usually means with higher doses of glucocorticoid steroids. It is important to explore possible reasons for poorly controlled symptoms, including nonadherence, improper use of inhaler devices, exposures, triggers, and comorbid factors. Comorbid factors that might cause symptoms that could be attributed to asthma include coexisting rhinitis, sinusitis, GERD, and obesity.

TREATMENT

Key steps in asthma care are listed in **Box 1**. Asthma treatment goals include reducing the frequency and severity of symptoms, preventing exacerbations, improving quality of life, and minimizing medication side effects. Occasionally, a patient has very mild symptoms that occur only intermittently and usually after a limited set of clearly defined triggers. These patients have intermittent asthma, and they may be treated with short-acting bronchodilator inhalers on an as-needed basis. All other patients, usually defined as having symptoms more than twice a week or nocturnal awakenings for asthma more than twice a month, are considered to have persistent asthma and should be treated with both maintenance and reliever medications. Drugs that are approved by the Food and Drug Administration (FDA) for maintenance treatment of asthma have only been tested in patients who have either reversible airflow obstruction on spirometry or positive responses to bronchial provocation tests. For persistent asthma, it is clear that inhaled corticosteroids (ICS) are the first-line drugs. ICS should be used at the lowest dose that achieves well-controlled asthma. Some patients achieve well-controlled asthma with low-dose ICS alone, but those who do not should have the ICS dose escalated until high doses are being used or until the

---

Box 1
Steps in asthma care

1. Initial asthma diagnosis
   a. Determine type, frequency, and severity of symptoms
   b. Determine risk
      i. Determine baseline lung function
      ii. History of severe exacerbations
   c. List triggers
   d. Discuss treatment goals
   e. Select initial treatment
   f. Schedule follow-up visit
2. Asthma follow-up visits
   a. Assess for asthma control
      i. Determine type, frequency, and severity of symptoms
      ii. Rescue medication use
      iii. Inquire about exacerbations and interventions by other health care providers
   b. Assess maintenance and rescue medication adherence and technique
   c. Determine risk
   d. Adjust medications; consider clinical trials

well-controlled state occurs. If control is not achieved with high-dose ICS, then subspecialty consultation should be considered. If an adherent patient is taking high-dose inhaled steroids and has not achieved good control, then there are 2 basic options. The first option is to use a course of systemic steroids, and, in many cases, this achieves control within several days. Systemic steroids have a faster onset of action than other controllers and are preferred in severe exacerbations. The second option is to add a second nonsteroid controller agent that could include a long-acting inhaled β-agonist, a leukotriene antagonist, or theophylline. The anti-IgE antibody omalizumab is usually reserved for atopic patients with asthma who fail treatment regimes containing multiple controllers. These drugs have been shown to have steroid-sparing effects and can reduce symptoms more than ICS alone.[15–19] Postmarketing experience has revealed some important side effects of nonsteroid controllers, which may limit their use.[20] One area of controversy in asthma care involves the use of long-acting β-agonists in asthma as controller or maintenance medications. Concerns about the safety of these β-adrenergic agonists have been raised because they have been infrequently associated with respiratory failure and death. These drugs are effective bronchodilators and, when used in combination with ICS, improve lung function and reduce the frequency of exacerbations and symptoms in many, but not all, patients. Another therapeutic option that might be useful in very carefully selected patients is bronchial thermoplasty. This treatment was approved by the FDA and is thought to work by reducing the amount of airway wall smooth muscle by the application of thermal energy. In a sham-controlled clinical trial, it was shown that thermoplasty may improve asthma-related quality of life and subsequent asthma exacerbations, although the procedure may cause acute exacerbations and adverse events immediately after treatment.[21,22]

For selected individuals, it is appropriate to teach the patient to deal with symptoms using nonpharmacologic approaches such as activity modification, avoidance of triggers, and modification of the environment. These approaches can empower the patient and may relieve symptoms safely while minimizing medication exposure. Recent reports illustrate that there is a substantial placebo effect in asthma treatment[23] and that the presentation of a treatment in a way that enhances expectation of benefit can modify subjective outcomes such as perceived asthma control.[24] Also important to consider is the cost of the treatment regimen, its complexity, and the ability of the individual patient to adhere to the treatment plan. The treatment plan, including an action plan, which addresses deterioration in asthma control, should be tailored to maximize patient acceptance and adherence. Treatment of asymptomatic GERD has not been shown to improve asthma control.[25] Therefore, comorbid conditions, including GERD and obesity, should be treated as separate important conditions. In addition, it may be especially important to identify and aggressively treat environmental tobacco smoke (ETS) exposure, including secondhand exposures, because ETS may influence treatment response[26] or worsen asthma severity.[27] Annual influenza vaccination with inactivated virus is recommended and has been shown to be safe and efficacious,[28] even with severe asthma, especially because asthma is a risk factor for death from pandemic influenza.[29,30]

It is important to discuss treatment goals and the role of the various drugs used to treat asthma with the patient at each visit. Asthma is a disease that is most effectively managed when the patient learns to recognize, report, and manage symptoms. If the patient understands that controller medications are used to treat inflammation, sustained bronchodilation should be provided, and, to prevent symptoms, these patients may be more likely to take controllers regularly and to understand that they do not provide immediate relief. Similarly, the patient needs to be taught that reliever medications do not treat inflammation but rather only provide bronchodilation. This concept may not be readily grasped because these short-acting drugs typically provide more immediate relief from symptoms, which is a feedback that reinforces their use and, often, overuse. It is important for the patient and the clinician to realize that frequent need for reliever medication indicates poor control of inflammation. One way to prevent unrecognized overuse of reliever medication is to not prescribe refills. Because the typical inhaler contains 200 metered doses or enough medication for 4 puffs weekly over a year, a well-controlled patient should only need 1 or 2 inhalers annually.

SUBSPECIALTY CONSULTATION

Subspecialty consultation should be considered when a patient has severe obstruction on spirometry, when there is a poor response to inhaled controller therapy, if an associated lung disease is suspected, or if the risk for significant morbidity or mortality is high. If another lung disease is suspected, then a pulmonary disease specialist should be consulted. Allergy specialists are also trained to care for patients with severe asthma and are especially effective when patients have significant allergic disease.

EMERGING THERAPEUTICS

As discussed previously, the pathobiology of asthma is complex, and it is likely that it involves different genes, mediators, and environmental exposures among various patients. Recent reports have explored more detailed phenotyping of characteristics of patients with asthma and have demonstrated that there are different subsets of asthma.[31–34] It is logical to assume that response to various treatments or the natural history of the disease varies by such subset. Also, it has become apparent that biological response rates to treatments studied in clinical trials are highly variable and that responder analyses should be performed more often during these studies. Some elegant work has shown that airway biomarkers might be useful in directing therapy. For example, Woodruff and colleagues[35] demonstrated that molecular evidence of TH2 airway inflammation was associated with responsiveness to ICS, whereas there was no response to ICS when the TH2 pattern was absent. In another example, Haldar and colleagues[36] showed that eosinophilic airway inflammation was associated with good responses to the anti–interleukin (IL)-5 monoclonal antibody mepolizumab. However, with the exception of IgE, there are no other clinically useful serum biomarkers. This is important because clinical trials that have narrowly targeted biological mediators, such as tumor necrosis factor α,[37] IL-4/IL-13,[38] or IL-5,[39] without selecting patients with a particular molecular phenotype have yielded disappointing results. The development of biomarkers that can direct the use of targeted drug or biological treatments would be desirable to maximize effectiveness while minimizing side effects.

Other therapeutic targets have shown promise. The inhaled anticholinergic drug tiotropium was shown to be noninferior to salmeterol when added to ICS in patients with not-well-controlled asthma.[40] Epidemiologic evidence associating vitamin D deficiency and asthma[41,42] has led to the launch of a clinical trial sponsored by the National Heart, Lung, and Blood Institute AsthmaNet clinical trials group to investigate vitamin D supplementation in asthma (NCT01248065). Studies of the chemoattractant receptor of TH2 cells,[43] a novel target that might specifically modulate TH2-mediated inflammation, are underway. Phosphodiesterase subtype 4 inhibitors may also prove useful in asthma,[44] and 1 drug from this class is approved for COPD treatment.

SUMMARY

Asthma is encountered frequently in internal medicine clinics, and it is a heterogeneous disease that is characterized by both exacerbations and variability in symptoms over time. The accurate diagnosis and risk assessment of asthma requires pulmonary function testing because historical findings and symptoms are subjective, and the physical examination is often nondiagnostic. Patients with asthma who are at high risk of recurrent or severe exacerbations should be considered for specialty care and should receive more intensive antiinflammatory therapy. Inhaled glucocorticoid steroids are the cornerstone of asthma treatment and should be used in all patients with persistent asthma. Other asthma controllers may be used as add-on treatment after careful consideration of potential side effects and should only be continued if they provide meaningful benefit. Novel treatments are being studied and may provide important benefits in the future.

REFERENCES

1. Lieu TA, Lozano P, Finkelstein JA, et al. Racial/ethnic variation in asthma status and management practices among children in managed Medicaid. Pediatrics 2002;109:857–65.
2. Moore WC, Pascual RM. Update in asthma 2009. Am J Respir Crit Care Med 2010;181:1181–7.
3. Robinson DS. The role of regulatory T lymphocytes in asthma pathogenesis. Curr Allergy Asthma Rep 2005;5:136–41.
4. Robinson DS. Regulatory T cells and asthma. Clin Exp Allergy 2009;39:1314–23.
5. Durrani SR, Viswanathan RK, Busse WW. What effect does asthma treatment have on airway remodeling? Current perspectives. J Allergy Clin Immunol 2011;128(3):439–48.
6. Pascual RM, Peters SP. Airway remodeling contributes to the progressive loss of lung function in asthma: an overview. J Allergy Clin Immunol 2005; 116:477–86.
7. Lugogo NL, Kraft M. Diagnosis of asthma in adults. In: Castro M, Kraft M, editors. Clinical asthma. Philadelphia (PA): Mosby; 2008. p. 67.
8. Crapo RO, Casaburi R, Coates AL, et al. Guidelines for methacholine and exercise challenge testing-1999. This official statement of the American Thoracic Society was adopted by the ATS Board of Directors, July 1999. Am J Respir Crit Care Med 2000;161:309–29.
9. Pascual RM, Peters SP. Management of persistent asthma in adults. In: Castro M, Kraft M, editors. Clinical asthma. Philadelphia (PA): Mosby; 2008. p. 189.
10. Busse WW, Boushey HA, Camargo CA, et al. National Asthma Education and Prevention Program, Expert Panel Report 3, guidelines for the diagnosis and management of asthma. Bethesda (MD): U.S. Department of Health and Human Services, National Institutes of Health, National Heart, Lung, and Blood Institute; 2007.
11. Juniper EF, O'Byrne PM, Guyatt GH, et al. Development and validation of a questionnaire to measure asthma control. Eur Respir J 1999;14:902–7.
12. Alvarez GG, Schulzer M, Jung D, et al. A systematic review of risk factors associated with near-fatal and fatal asthma. Can Respir J 2005;12:265–70.
13. O'Byrne P, Bateman ED, Bousquet J, et al. MCR Vision. In: Global strategy for asthma management and prevention. Edgewater (NJ): Global Initiative for Asthma; 2006.

14. Proceedings of the ATS workshop on refractory asthma: current understanding, recommendations, and unanswered questions. American Thoracic Society. Am J Respir Crit Care Med 2000;162:2341–51.

15. Busse W, Corren J, Lanier BQ, et al. Omalizumab, anti-IgE recombinant humanized monoclonal antibody, for the treatment of severe allergic asthma. J Allergy Clin Immunol 2001;108:184–90.

16. Evans DJ, Taylor DA, Zetterstrom O, et al. A comparison of low-dose inhaled budesonide plus theophylline and high-dose inhaled budesonide for moderate asthma. N Engl J Med 1997;337:1412–8.

17. Greening AP, Ind PW, Northfield M, et al. Added salmeterol versus higher-dose corticosteroid in asthma patients with symptoms on existing inhaled corticosteroid. Allen & Hanburys Limited UK Study Group. Lancet 1994;344:219–24.

18. Virchow JC, Mehta A, Ljungblad L, et al. Add-on montelukast in inadequately controlled asthma patients in a 6-month open-label study: the MONtelukast In Chronic Asthma (MONICA) study. Respir Med 2010;104:644–51.

19. Lazarus SC, Boushey HA, Fahy JV, et al. Long-acting beta2-agonist monotherapy vs continued therapy with inhaled corticosteroids in patients with persistent asthma: a randomized controlled trial. JAMA 2001;285:2583–93.

20. Nelson HS, Weiss ST, Bleecker ER, et al. The Salmeterol Multicenter Asthma Research Trial: a comparison of usual pharmacotherapy for asthma or usual pharmacotherapy plus salmeterol. Chest 2006;129:15–26.

21. Castro M, Rubin A, Laviolette M, et al. Persistence of effectiveness of bronchial thermoplasty in patients with severe asthma. Ann Allergy Asthma Immunol 2011;107:65–70.

22. Castro M, Rubin AS, Laviolette M, et al. Effectiveness and safety of bronchial thermoplasty in the treatment of severe asthma: a multicenter, randomized, double-blind, sham-controlled clinical trial. Am J Respir Crit Care Med 2010;181:116–24.

23. Wechsler ME, Kelley JM, Boyd IO, et al. Active albuterol or placebo, sham acupuncture, or no intervention in asthma. N Engl J Med 2011;365:119–26.

24. Wise RA, Bartlett SJ, Brown ED, et al. Randomized trial of the effect of drug presentation on asthma outcomes: the American Lung Association Asthma Clinical Research Centers. J Allergy Clin Immunol 2009;124:436–8.

25. Mastronarde JG, Anthonisen NR, Castro M, et al. Efficacy of esomeprazole for treatment of poorly controlled asthma. N Engl J Med 2009;360:1487–99.

26. Lazarus SC, Chinchilli VM, Rollings NJ, et al. Smoking affects response to inhaled corticosteroids or leukotriene receptor antagonists in asthma. Am J Respir Crit Care Med 2007;175:783–90.

27. Comhair SA, Gaston BM, Ricci KS, et al. Detrimental effects of environmental tobacco smoke in relation to asthma severity. PLoS One 2011;6:e18574.

28. The safety of inactivated influenza vaccine in adults and children with asthma. N Engl J Med 2001;345:1529–36.

29. Chowell G, Bertozzi SM, Colchero MA, et al. Severe respiratory disease concurrent with the circulation of H1N1 influenza. N Engl J Med 2009;361:674–9.

30. Jain S, Kamimoto L, Bramley AM, et al. Hospitalized patients with 2009 H1N1 influenza in the United States, April-June 2009. N Engl J Med 2009;361:1935–44.

31. Fitzpatrick AM, Teague WG, Meyers DA, et al. Heterogeneity of severe asthma in childhood: confirmation by cluster analysis of children in the National Institutes of Health/National Heart, Lung, and Blood Institute Severe Asthma Research Program. J Allergy Clin Immunol 2011;127:382–9.

32. Haldar P, Pavord ID, Shaw DE, et al. Cluster analysis and clinical asthma phenotypes. Am J Respir Crit Care Med 2008;178:218–24.

33. Moore WC, Bleecker ER, Curran-Everett D, et al. Characterization of the severe asthma phenotype by the National Heart, Lung, and Blood Institute's Severe Asthma Research Program. J Allergy Clin Immunol 2007;119:405–13.

34. Moore WC, Meyers DA, Wenzel SE, et al. Identification of asthma phenotypes using cluster analysis in the Severe Asthma Research Program. Am J Respir Crit Care Med 2009;181:315–23.

35. Woodruff PG, Modrek B, Choy DF, et al. T-helper type 2-driven inflammation defines major subphenotypes of asthma. Am J Respir Crit Care Med 2009;180:388–95.

36. Haldar P, Brightling CE, Hargadon B, et al. Mepolizumab and exacerbations of refractory eosinophilic asthma. N Engl J Med 2009;360:973–84.

37. Wenzel SE, Barnes PJ, Bleecker ER, et al. A randomized, double-blind, placebo-controlled study of tumor necrosis factor-alpha blockade in severe persistent asthma. Am J Respir Crit Care Med 2009;179:549–58.

38. Corren J, Busse W, Meltzer EO, et al. A randomized, controlled, phase 2 study of AMG 317, an IL-4Ralpha antagonist, in patients with asthma. Am J Respir Crit Care Med 2010;181:788–96.

39. Flood-Page P, Swenson C, Faiferman I, et al. A study to evaluate safety and efficacy of mepolizumab in patients with moderate persistent asthma. Am J Respir Crit Care Med 2007;176:1062–71.

40. Peters SP, Kunselman SJ, Icitovic N, et al. Tiotropium bromide step-up therapy for adults with uncontrolled asthma. N Engl J Med 2010;363:1715–26.

41. Brehm JM, Schuemann B, Fuhlbrigge AL, et al. Serum vitamin D levels and severe asthma exacerbations in the Childhood Asthma Management Program study. J Allergy Clin Immunol 2010;126:52–8.

42. Sutherland ER, Goleva E, Jackson LP, et al. Vitamin D levels, lung function, and steroid response in adult asthma. Am J Respir Crit Care Med 2010;181:699–704.

43. Barnes N, Pavord I, Chuchalin A, et al. A randomized, double-blind, placebo-controlled study of the CRTH2 antagonist OC000459 in moderate persistent asthma. Clin Exp Allergy 2011. [Epub ahead of print].

44. Fan CK. Phosphodiesterase inhibitors in airways disease. Eur J Pharmacol 2006;533:110–7.

Chronic Obstructive Pulmonary Disease: A Concise Review

Ron Balkissoon, MD, DIH, MSc, FRCP(C)*, Steve Lommatzsch, MD,
Brendan Carolan, MD, Barry Make, MD

KEYWORDS

- Chronic obstructive pulmonary disease • Guidelines
- Chronic bronchitis • Emphysema

DEFINITIONS

Writing on the definition of chronic obstructive pulmonary disease (COPD), Dr Nicholas Gross once compared it to defining love, "everybody knows what it is, but each individual describes it differently."[1–3] In 1997, the US National Heart Lung and Blood Institute and the World Health Organization held an international workshop that led to the first Global Initiative on Obstructive Lung Disease (GOLD) report. The most recent iteration of the GOLD guidelines defines COPD as

> ...a preventable and treatable disease with some significant extra-pulmonary effects that may contribute to the severity in individual patients. Its pulmonary component is characterized by chronic airflow limitation that is not fully reversible. The airflow limitation is usually both progressive and associated with an abnormal inflammatory response of the lungs to noxious particles and gases.[4]

Previously COPD was defined in terms of the presence of chronic bronchitis and emphysema, but now we understand it has a more complex pathogenesis, and objective measures of lung function are performed to make the diagnosis.

PATHOGENESIS OF COPD

A comprehensive review of the pathogenesis of COPD is beyond the scope of this article; however, it is important to appreciate that there are complex interactions between several host factors (gender, airway hyperresponsiveness, genetics, epigenetics) and environmental factors (eg, exposures and diet) that influence susceptibility

Conflict of Interest: R. Balkissoon: Advisory Boards: Astra Zeneca, Glaxo SmithKline. Speakers Bureau: Astra Zeneca, Glaxo SmithKline, Boehringer Ingelheim, Pfizer, Novartis.
National Jewish Health, Pulmonary Division, Department of Medicine, 1400 Jackson Street, Denver, CO 80206, USA
* Corresponding author.
E-mail address: balkissoonr@NJHealth.org

Med Clin N Am 95 (2011) 1125–1141
doi:10.1016/j.mcna.2011.08.009
0025-7125/11/$ – see front matter © 2011 Published by Elsevier Inc.

medical.theclinics.com

and the numerous pathogenic mechanisms (inflammatory cell recruitment, inflammatory mediator release, oxidative stress, tissue destruction, protease/antiprotease imbalance, defective cell repair, apoptosis, and fibrosis), involved in the development of COPD (**Fig. 1**).

Risk Factors

Cigarette smoke, containing more than 6000 molecules and 10^{14} free radicals per puff, can initiate an inflammatory response in many ways.[5] While tobacco smoke remains the most recognized cause for COPD globally, there are other exposures that can cause COPD related to occupation (various organic and inorganic dusts, chemical fumes, smoke)[2,6] and biomass fuels in lesser developed countries.[7] There are studies demonstrating that cannabis smoke may contribute to COPD.[8] Although it is quite

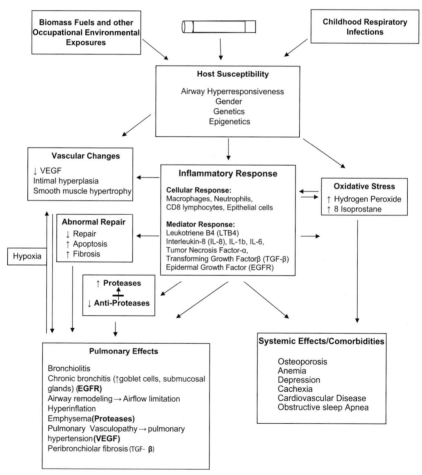

Fig. 1. The pathogenesis of COPD is complex, and involves multiple mechanisms and pathways with resulting lung inflammation, cell damage, tissue destruction, and disordered repair responses, leading to a heterogeneous disease with pulmonary and systemic consequences with varying individual susceptibility and clinical manifestations. ICS, inhaled corticosteroid.

clear that air pollution has a significant impact on exacerbations, it is still unclear as to what extent COPD is caused by air pollution.[9]

Given that only 20% to 30% of individuals who smoke appear to develop evidence of COPD, it seems clear that there are likely COPD susceptibility genes and probably genes that might influence severity and response to various medications (**Table 1**).[10,12,14,15] Indeed, the current COPDGene[16] study funded by the National Institutes of Health (NIH) will help to unravel this complex question.

Airway hyperresponsiveness increases the risk of developing COPD by as much as 12-fold, such that asthma patients who smoke or those simply with airway hyperresponsiveness even without the clinical diagnosis of asthma are more susceptible.[17] Female smokers may be more susceptible to effects of cigarette smoke, as they have more extensive emphysema and airway disease and worse quality of life than male COPD patients.[18,19] It has been proposed that perhaps the higher dose of exposure to tobacco smoke relative to lung size and hormonal influences may explain these observations.[20]

Pathobiology

Several studies have documented the presence of increased levels of proinflammatory cytokines in specimens from individuals with COPD including interleukin (IL)-8, tumor necrosis factor α (TNF-α), CXC motif ligand 1, and monocyte chemoattractant factor protein 1,[21] to name just a few. The most susceptible and hence earliest morphologic changes in COPD are observed in small-airway injury, producing a bronchiolitis.[22] The identification of α1-antitrypsin deficiency led to the initial concept of protease-antiprotease imbalance leading to tissue destruction; however, research now supports the idea that an imbalance between mediators that promote inflammation and mediators that protect tissues from inflammation lead to the development of emphysema.[21] Oxidants are also part of the inflammatory consequences of cigarette smoke and, while the lung produces and tightly regulates a large array of antioxidants to protect itself, the endogenous antioxidant system also becomes overwhelmed, leading to cellular damage and lung destruction.[23] Reduced levels of vascular endothelial growth factor and increased apoptosis, along with inefficient removal of apoptotic cells, may cause emphysema independent of inflammation.[23,24]

Systemic Effects and Comorbidities

The inflammatory response of COPD does not remain confined to the lungs and signs of inflammation including increases in TNF-α, IL-6, and oxygen-derived free radicals have been demonstrated in the systemic circulation, and may play a role in the systemic manifestations of COPD such as osteoporosis, depression, and chronic normochromic, normocytic anemia.[23,25,26] Cachexin proteins have been identified in the systemic circulation of COPD patients and likely contribute to muscle wasting seen in these patients.[27]

Table 1 Summary of candidate genes for COPD	
α1-Antitrypsin deficiency	SERPINA1
Susceptibility genes for developing COPD or lower lung function	(EPHX1, GST, MMP12, TGFB1, SERPINE2),[10] (HHIP and FAM13A, XRCC5),[11] (Surfactant protein B)[12]
Nicotine dependence and lung cancer	CHRNA3/5[13]

Obstructive sleep apnea has been identified as being very common in COPD, and the term "overlap syndrome" has been incorporated to indicate patients with both conditions. Such patients are at greater risk for cardiac dysrhythmias and pulmonary hypertension as opposed to those with either condition alone.[26,28]

The pathogenesis of COPD is complex, and involves multiple mechanisms and pathways. Understanding the complex and heterogeneous nature of COPD pathogenesis is critical to identifying new therapeutic targets for this disease.

DIAGNOSIS AND STAGING OF COPD
History

Cough and/or dyspnea are the presenting symptoms for most patients with COPD. Many patients presume shortness of breath early on is part of aging and general deconditioning, which is undoubtedly partially correct because many lead relatively sedentary lifestyles. Many patients do not seek attention until they have dyspnea with exertion that is disabling, and this is usually when the disease is already quite advanced and less reversible. A cough that is productive should not be suppressed, and chronic daily cough is predictive of frequent exacerbations.[29] Many report an increase in cough and sputum immediately after smoking cessation, but this gradually improves following long-term smoking cessation.[30] Enquiries regarding other symptoms such as fatigue, chest pain, weakness, hemoptysis, weight loss, and ankle swelling should be made to address issues of advanced disease, complications of the disease, comorbidities, and lung cancer.

Spirometry

The GOLD Guidelines use the post bronchodilator Forced Expiratory Volume in one second (FEV-1)/Forced Vital Capacity (FVC) ratio of less than 70% as the criteria to define significant airflow limitation for COPD and the FEV-1 value (% predicted) to stage severity stage I>80%, stage II 50-80%, stage III 30-50%, stage IV <30%. Somewhat perplexing is that within this framework it is possible for patients to have chronic bronchitis and/or emphysema and not meet the GOLD criteria for COPD (ie, FEV-1/FVC <70%). Further there is debate as to whether the absolute value of 70% or using the lower limit of normal (LLN) of the FEV-1/FVC ratio as the cutoff to define airflow limitation is the most reliable and accurate measure to optimally identify COPD patients.[31] It is important to appreciate that the goal of the GOLD Guidelines and staging system is to increase awareness and provide a framework for general health care providers to approach therapy. A precise definition was not the aim of the committee.

MANAGEMENT OF COPD
Assessing Outcomes

COPD can accelerate the rate of decline in FEV_1, and progression to disability and death. COPD management goals include preventing or slowing the progressive loss of lung function, relieving symptoms, improving exercise tolerance and the patient's health status, preventing and treating exacerbations and complications, minimizing side effects of treatment, and reducing mortality (**Fig. 2**). While lung function is important for diagnosis and classification of the severity of COPD, clinicians and patients are also very interested in so-called patient-centered outcomes such as symptoms, ability to function, quality of life, and health status.[32] In recent years there has been an emphasis on identifying the minimal clinically important difference for various outcome

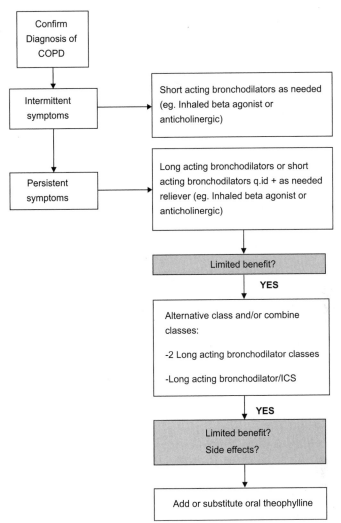

Fig. 2. American Thoracic Society/European Respiratory Society algorithm for management of COPD. Symptoms include cough, wheeze, dyspnea. If the FEV_1 is less than 50% and exacerbations of COPD require oral corticosteroids or antibiotics at least once in the past 12 months, then consider adding regular inhaled corticosteroid. Theophylline should be reserved for patients who still are quite symptomatic despite combination therapy. VEGF, vascular endothelial growth factor. (*Adapted from* Celli BR, MacNee W. Standards for the diagnosis and treatment of patients with COPD: a summary of the ATS/ERS position paper. Eur Respir J 2004;23(6):936; with permission.)

measures such as lung function, exercise endurance, dyspnea scores, and quality-of-life measures.[33]

Nonpharmacologic Management

Smoking cessation

In 2009 the United States implemented the Family Smoking Prevention and Tobacco Control Act, with the goals of greater regulation of tobacco marketing and the implementation of public health strategies to reduce tobacco-related morbidity and mortality. Nicotine chewing gum was introduced in 1982 after it was shown to increase smoking cessation rates by approximately 1.5- to 2-fold after 12 months.[34] Alternatives to nicotine replacement therapy (NRT) are bupropion, which inhibits the neuronal uptake of noradrenaline and dopamine, and varenicline, a partial agonist at nicotinic $\alpha 4$ $\beta 2$ receptors. A Cochrane analysis of multiple studies concluded that more participants quit successfully with varenicline than with bupropion, and in a comparison with NRT suggested a modest benefit of varenicline; however, confidence intervals did not rule out equivalence.[35] The main adverse effect of varenicline is nausea, which is mostly mild to moderate in severity and tends to subside over time. Possible links with serious adverse events, including depressed mood, agitation, and suicidal thoughts, have been reported but are so far unsubstantiated. Counseling has been shown to augment the effects of pharmacologic intervention alone.

Pulmonary rehabilitation

Pulmonary rehabilitation is an important nonpharmacologic therapeutic in COPD, yet it remains underutilized by providers. Typical components include patient assessment, exercise training, education, nutritional intervention, and psychosocial support. Several studies have demonstrated that pulmonary rehabilitation therapy has positive impacts on health-related quality of life, reduced symptoms, improved peripheral muscle strength, exercise endurance, reduced number of hospital days, and improved psychosocial status.[36] Recent results from a large, randomized 1-year trial of a comprehensive disease management program at 5 Veterans Affairs medical centers demonstrated a reduction in hospitalizations and emergency room visits.[37]

Oxygen therapy

Oxygen therapy is well established to increase survival, and is indicated for patients with an arterial oxygen tension (PaO_2) of less than 55 mm Hg. The therapeutic goal is to maintain saturations greater than 90% during rest, sleep, and exertion, as it is now well established that such measures increase survival and that 24 hours is more effective than 12 hours.[38,39] Following an acute exacerbation, patients should be reevaluated with blood gases and walk oximetry 30 to 90 days later.

Pharmacologic Management

A detailed review of the agents available for treating COPD is beyond the scope of this article, but there are now several guidelines providing direction for pharmacologic management of COPD (**Table 2**).[2,35,40,41] Given that airflow obstruction is the primary concern in COPD, it follows that short-acting and long-acting bronchodilators form the cornerstone of pharmacologic management. Inhaled short-acting $\beta 2$ agonists such as albuterol have a more rapid onset of effect and shorter duration of action than short-acting anticholinergic agents such as ipratropium bromide, and thus are more often prescribed as "rescue" medications to relieve acute bronchospasm.[24,42,43] Patients that have persistent symptoms and require daily use of short-acting agents are recommended to switch to long-acting (12 hours) bronchodilators such as salmeterol and formoterol and the anticholinergic or long-acting antimuscurinic agent (LAMA), tiotropium (24 hours).[2] Several studies have identified the long-acting $\beta 2$ agonists (LABAs) to be effective in reducing symptoms, and improving lung function and health-related quality of life in patients with COPD.[43] The use of $\beta 2$ agonists has been associated with an increase in asthma-related deaths[44,45] and while there remain questions as to the exact nature of the relationship between $\beta 2$ agonists and asthma-related deaths, the black-box warning by the US Food and Drug Administration (FDA)

Table 2
Summary of major COPD guideline recommendations

Agent	GOLD Stage (1)	ERS/ATS (2)	ACP (3)
Short-acting bronchodilators	I FEV$_1$ >80%	Mild FEV$_1$ >80%	FEV$_1$ <80%
Long-acting bronchodilators	II–IV FEV$_1$ <80%	Moderate FEV$_1$ <80%	FEV$_1$ <60% (or combination of bronchodilators if still symptomatic)
Inhaled corticosteroids (combined with bronchodilators)	III–IV Exacerbation requiring oral steroids and/or antibiotics in past 12 months	FEV$_1$ <50% Exacerbation requiring oral steroids and/or antibiotics in past 12 months	FEV$_1$ <60% Symptomatic patients with stable COPD
Theophylline	III–IV	Very severe FEV$_1$ <30%	Not included
Phosphodiesterase-4 inhibitors	Not included	Not included	Not included

FEV$_1$ is expressed as percent predicted.
Abbreviations: ACP, American College of Physicians Guidelines[40]; ERS/ATS, European Respiratory Society/American Thoracic Society Guidelines[41]; GOLD, Global Initiative for Chronic Obstructive Pulmonary Disease (COPD) Guidelines.[4]

has been extended to COPD patients. To date there have not been any studies that have shown an increase in deaths in COPD patients treated with β2 agonists in comparison with placebo or any other agent. Nonetheless, stimulation of β2-receptors can produce resting sinus tachycardia and can potentially trigger disturbances of cardiac rhythm in very susceptible individuals. Further, older patients treated with higher doses of β2 agonists may experience exaggerated somatic tremor that may limit their use.[46]

The Understanding the Potential Long-Term Impacts on Function with Tiotropium (UPLIFT) trial was a large, prospective, controlled study of 5993 patients with mean FEV$_1$ of 1.32 ± 0.44 L (48% of predicted) randomized to tiotropium or placebo over 4 years.[46] Subjects were allowed to use all respiratory medications except other inhaled anticholinergics. Tiotropium did not slow the rate of decline in pre- and post-bronchodilator FEV$_1$ (coprimary end points) over 4 years, but did significantly reduce exacerbations (hazard ratio 0.86, P<.001) compared with placebo.[46] UPLIFT was reassuring in that it did not show an association between the use of tiotropium and major cardiovascular-related events or indeed death, as had been suggested by a previous meta-analysis of anticholinergic use in COPD.[47] Some of the reported side effects of anticholinergic agents include worsening signs and symptoms of narrow-angle glaucoma, prostatic hyperplasia, or bladder-neck obstruction. Studies have shown additive effects of combining short-acting β2-agonists and anticholinergics,[48] and LABAs and LAMAs.[49]

Given the importance of inflammation in the pathogenesis of COPD, inhaled corticosteroids (ICS) are typically the next line of therapy recommended for patients. ICS should be added to bronchodilators and should not be used as monotherapy in COPD. Alsaeedi and colleagues[50] reviewed 9 randomized placebo-controlled trials of ICS given to patients with stable COPD for longer than 6 months, and found that use of inhaled corticosteroids led to about a 30% reduction in the total number of exacerbations. Systemic corticosteroids have proved useful in treating acute exacerbations, but are rarely indicated as part of maintenance therapy for patients with the most advanced disease.

For patients not optimally controlled in terms of symptoms with frequent use of rescue inhalers and with evidence of frequent exacerbations, combination therapy with ICS and either LABAs or long-acting anticholinergics are recommended in all major guidelines.[2,40,41] Previous studies with the combinations fluticasone propionate/salmeterol[51] and budesonide/formoterol[52–54] have shown improvement in lung function, reductions in symptoms, and improvement in patient-centered outcomes and quality of life in comparison with the monocomponents. In a study of 782 patients with COPD, fluticasone propionate/salmeterol 250/50 μg significantly reduced the annual rate of moderate to severe exacerbations by 30.5% compared with salmeterol alone (1.06 and 1.53 per subject per year, respectively; $P<.001$).[55]

The Toward a Revolution in COPD Health (TORCH) study,[56] a multicenter, double-blind, placebo-controlled, randomized clinical trial involving 6112 patients with COPD, demonstrated that treatment with combination fluticasone/salmeterol decreased the risk of all-cause mortality over the 3-year period by 17.5% compared with placebo ($P = .052$). Although TORCH did not reach statistical significance in terms of reduced mortality, it did show statistically significant improvement in health status (St. George's Respiratory Questionnaire [SGRQ] total score), postbronchodilator FEV_1, and reductions in the frequency of exacerbations compared with placebo or the monocomponents. Recently, another combination inhaler containing mometasone and formoterol has gained an indication by the FDA in the United States for use in patients with COPD, despite limited published data.

The INSPIRE (Investigating New Standards for Prophylaxis in Reducing Exacerbations) trial studied 1323 patients randomized for 2 years to fluticasone/salmeterol 500/50 μg twice a day versus tiotropium 18 μg once daily, and found no difference in exacerbation rate between salmeterol/fluticasone propionate and tiotropium. More patients failed to complete the study while receiving tiotropium, and there was a small statistically significant beneficial effect found on health status, with an unexpected finding of statistically significant lower death rate in salmeterol/fluticasone propionate–treated patients (3%) versus tiotropium (6%) ($P<.032$).[57]

The most common side effects seen with ICS include skin bruising, oropharyngeal candidiasis, and voice alterations. Less common but also associated with ICS use are cataracts and osteopenia, which are likely reflective of COPD patients' comorbidities and oral steroid use. More recently there have been concerns raised about an increase in rates of pneumonia in COPD patients on ICS.[56–59] In most of these studies there were typically fewer exacerbations overall in the steroid-treated groups. Sin and colleagues[60] conducted a meta-analysis of 7 large, randomized controlled trials with use of budesonide in patients with COPD, and demonstrated that budesonide treatment for 12 months did not increase the risk of pneumonia in patients with COPD during that time. It may be that inhaled corticosteroids reduce the proportion of noninfectious exacerbations and hence increase the likelihood of infectious exacerbations, which may have a longer more protracted course. It is clear that earlier identification and treatment of these events may preclude the development of pneumonia. There are likely multiple contributing factors to this observed phenomenon that require further research. The pneumonia risk is considered a class effect by the FDA and therefore, clinicians should consider the risk to be the same across all steroid containing formulations.

Investigators have also compared dual therapy with triple therapy comprising fluticasone/salmeterol/tiotropium, and have found that in those with very advanced disease the triple combination was superior to the use of the fluticasone/salmeterol or tiotropium/salmeterol in terms of improvements in bronchodilation, symptoms, and reduced rescue medication requirements.[61,62] A recent systematic review suggested that while there has been evidence of improvement in average health-related quality of life and lung function, it is uncertain whether triple therapy has an impact on mortality, hospitalization, exacerbations of COPD, or pneumonia.[63]

Theophylline
Due to its narrow therapeutic index and potential side effects, theophylline has been relegated to a third-tier option for COPD, but there has been renewed interest because recent studies have suggested that theophylline may restore steroid sensitivity.[64] The mechanism for this is not completely understood, but new evidence indicates that phosphoinositide-3-kinase (PI3K) inhibition may be part of that mechanism, and supports further investigation of more selective molecules targeted at PI3K.[65,66]

PHARMACOTHERAPY: BEYOND THE CURRENT GUIDELINES

There are several drugs both old and new that are being studied for a potential role in treating patients with COPD. At this point these drugs are not included in the various guidelines for COPD management, although some have gained indications by the FDA for treatment of patients with COPD in the United States. Indacaterol and other so-called ultralong-acting (24 hours) β2 agonists are in various stages of clinical study. Indacaterol (which demonstrates a rapid improvement in lung function similar to for-moterol) is the most advanced of these agents in terms of clinical research, and has been shown to have superior bronchodilation and clinical efficacy to twice-daily LABAs and at least equal bronchodilation with tiotropium.[67] It has recently gained FDA approval for use in COPD patients in the United States.

Phosphodiesterase-4 inhibitors decrease inflammation and promote airway smooth muscle relaxation and bronchodilation.[68] Roflumilast has been studied in COPD, and results in a modest improvement in the FEV_1 and reduced numbers of exacerba-tions.[69,70] Both the European Medicines Agency and the US FDA have approved roflu-milast for the treatment of severe COPD associated with chronic bronchitis and a history of frequent exacerbations. Side effects of diarrhea and weight loss may be a limiting factor to the use of this drug, and monitoring is required as the occurrence is not infrequent.

There are several other medications that currently do not have an FDA indication for COPD but are being studied for their potential efficacy in COPD. Macrolide anti-biotics have both antimicrobial and anti-inflammatory effects. The direct antibiotic effect of inhibiting bacterial protein synthesis has been well described, and the immunomodulatory effects, though not fully elucidated, appear to involve inhibition of inflammatory cell chemotaxis, cytokine synthesis, adhesion molecule expression, and reactive oxygen species production.[71-73] Recently a prospective double-blind, placebo-controlled trial was conducted in which 1142 patients with a clinical diag-nosis of COPD on supplemental oxygen and/or having exacerbations within the previous year were randomized to receive either azithromycin 250 mg or placebo daily for 1 year. Final results have not been published, but preliminary data presented in abstract form suggest a significant reduction in time to first exacerbation (hazard ratio 0.73, $P<.0001$), rate of acute exacerbations ($P = .008$), and quality-of-life scores using the SGRQ ($P<.006$).[74]

Statins have been shown to inhibit cytokine production, neutrophil infiltration, and fibrotic activity, and to have antioxidant and anti-inflammatory effects on skeletal muscle, reduce inflammatory responses to pulmonary infections, and inhibit epithelial-mesenchymal cell transition (lung cancer).[75] Dobler and colleagues[76] conducted a systematic review of studies that reported effects of statin treatment in COPD, and found potential benefits in terms of decreased all-cause mortality (odds ratio [OR]/hazard ratio, 0.48–0.67 in 3 studies; OR, 0.99 in one study), decreased COPD-related mortality (OR, 0.19–0.29), reduction in incidence of respiratory-related urgent care (OR, 0.74), fewer COPD exacerbations (OR, 0.43), fewer intubations for COPD exacerbations (OR, 0.1), and reduced decline in pulmonary function. Of interest, Mancini and colleagues[77] tested the effects of angiotensin-converting enzyme (ACE) inhibitors, angiotensin receptor blockers, and statins on cardiovascular events and pulmonary mortality/morbidity in a case-control study with two population-based retrospective cohorts ($n = 6214$): COPD—high risk (COPD + coronary revascularization) and COPD—low risk (COPD without myocardial infarction). The drugs reduced both cardiovascular and pulmonary outcomes, with the largest benefits occurring with the combination of statins and either ACE inhibitors or angiotensin receptor blockers not only in the high-risk but also in the low-risk group. The Statins in COPD Exacerbations [STATCOPE] trial currently under way (n >1000) is a prospective, randomized, placebo-controlled long-term trial (up to 37 months) sponsored by the National Heart, Lung, and Blood Institute, evaluating the effects of simvastatin (40 mg/d). This study will help to establish the potential contribution of statins in COPD patients.

Phosphodiesterase-5 (PDE-5) inhibitors such as sildenafil have been used in erectile dysfunction, but studies have shown that PDE-5 inhibition also leads to anti-inflammatory effects by decreasing leukocyte influx and nitrogen oxide (NO) generation.[78] Other studies have suggested varying benefits with regard to effects on pulmonary hemodynamics.[79]

Vitamin D is known to have both bone effects and potential extracalcemic effects such as an impact on tumor cell proliferation and angiogenesis, macrophage antimicrobial peptides, interaction between dendritic cells and T cells, CD4 T-cell activation, insulin secretion, renin synthesis, and skeletal muscle strength.[80–83] These effects may all play a role in COPD pathogenesis and systemic effects of COPD. Janssens and colleagues[80] analyzed serum levels of 25-hydroxyvitamin D in a sample of 414 smokers and ex-smokers, ranging from individuals with normal spirometry to those with GOLD IV COPD. The investigators found a GOLD-stage–dependent reduction of vitamin D levels. There currently is a large NIH-funded trial to assess the role for vitamin D supplementation in COPD.

TREATMENT OF ACUTE EXACERBATIONS

Acute exacerbations are associated with in-hospital mortality rates of about 10%, including intensive care unit and nonintensive care hospitalization.[84] Mortality rates for the 6 to 12 months after exacerbations with signs of respiratory failure have been reported to be between 30% and 40%.[85] Hence early and aggressive treatment of acute exacerbations is critical. Bronchodilators should be used aggressively during an acute exacerbation, and rapidly acting agents and nebulized formulations are recommended for those who are very ill and unable to generate the flows required for other modalities. Supplemental oxygen should be given to maintain the PaO_2 above 60 mm Hg and the SaO_2 above 90%. Up to 50% to 80% of exacerbations may be associated with pathogens known to colonize the respiratory tract, including various viruses and *Haemophilus influenzae*, *Streptococcus pneumoniae*, and *Moraxella catarrhalis*.[86] The more significant the symptoms of cough, sputum, and dyspnea and the more purulent the sputum, the more likely patients will benefit from empiric antibiotic therapy.[67] Systemic glucocorticoids have been shown to reduce recovery time, reduce hospital time, reduce treatment failures, decrease risk of relapse, and improve airflow limitation during acute exacerbations.[87] Initial doses may range from 30 to 60 mg/d, and there does not seem to be a difference between intravenous versus oral delivery in terms of outcomes.[87,88] Noninvasive positive-pressure ventilation has been shown to be able to negate the need for intubation and reduce mortality for severe exacerbations, and should be started early.[89]

LUNG VOLUME REDUCTION SURGERY VERSUS LUNG TRANSPLANTATION FOR COPD

In 1996 the National Emphysema Treatment Trial (NETT) enrolled 1218 patients in a multicenter, randomized controlled trial to receive rehabilitation therapy and lung volume reduction surgery (LVRS) or pulmonary rehabilitation alone, and followed them for a mean of 2.4 years.[90] It was identified that a subgroup defined by FEV_1 less than 20% predicted, and either diffusing capacity for carbon monoxide less than 20% predicted or homogeneous pattern of emphysema on computed tomography, was at high risk for death.[91] The LVRS non–high-risk group subjects were more likely to demonstrate improvements in functional status and physiologic parameters as well as quality of life than those in the medically treated group, and those with upper lobe–predominant emphysema and low baseline exercise tolerance showed the most favorable response to LVRS.[90] The 5-year survival advantage for LVRS over the medical arm showed a risk ratio for death of 0.47 ($P = .005$).[90] Therefore, in a carefully selected subgroup of individuals with low exercise tolerance post rehabilitation and upper lobe–predominant emphysema, LVRS offers substantial survival, functional, physiologic, and quality-of-life benefits. In these patients LVRS joins smoking cessation and long-term oxygen therapy as a means of improving survival. Lung transplantation can be considered in patients who do not meet criteria for LVRS but who are otherwise good candidates. NETT's upper lobe–predominant LVRS cohort also demonstrated better 5-year survival than transplantation for COPD.[92]

FUTURE DIRECTIONS

Numerous potential phenotypes have been proposed in COPD based on clinical and physiologic characteristics, radiological features, the presence of exacerbations, systemic inflammation, comorbidities, and now genetics.[93] Classification of patients into distinct prognostic and therapeutic subgroups will be helpful for both clinical and research purposes, but much research is needed before there is any meaningful consensus on how to group patients and what the significance of such grouping may be. With further understanding of the underlying pathobiology of COPD, new therapeutic targets to decrease inflammation such as TNF-α, CXCL8, IL-17, and neutrophil elastase, and to presumably impede disease progression such as PI3K and nuclear factor κB inhibitors, are now undergoing study.[93]

The currently available data on efficacy of bronchoscopic lung volume reduction are not conclusive, and subjective benefit in dyspnea scores is a more frequent finding than improvements in spirometry or exercise tolerance.[94] A range of different techniques such as endobronchial blockers, airway bypass, endobronchial valves, thermal vapor ablation, biologic sealants, and airway implants have been used on both homogeneous and heterogeneous emphysema. Safety-wise the data are more promising, with rare procedure-related mortality, few serious complications, and short length of stay in hospital.[94] This area continues to evolve, and ongoing prospective randomized trials will help to elucidate the true efficacy of such techniques.

SUMMARY

COPD will continue to be an increasing cause of morbidity and mortality worldwide. One of the greatest challenges is to educate providers to view COPD as a preventable and treatable disease rather than to maintain the futile and nihilistic attitudes that have been so prevalent in the past. Further, COPD should be viewed as a systemic disease with important pulmonary and extrapulmonary manifestations. Patients with COPD require a thorough and comprehensive evaluation to assess both pulmonary and systemic manifestations as well as severity of their disease, so that therapy can be adequately individualized. We now know that smoking cessation, oxygen for hypoxemic patients, lung reduction surgery for selected patients with emphysema, and noninvasive ventilation during severe exacerbations have an impact on mortality. Ultimately, the advent of newer and more effective therapies will lead to a decline in the global burden of illness attributed to this disease.

ACKNOWLEDGMENTS

Thanks to Ms Linda Brown for administrative assistance with preparation of the article.

REFERENCES

1. Miniño AM, Xu J, Kochanck KD. Preliminary data for 2008. Natl Vital Stat Rep 2010;59(7).
2. National Heart Lung and Blood Institute. Morbidity and mortality: 2009 chart book on cardiovascular, lung, and blood diseases. Bethesda (MD): National Heart, Lung, and Blood Institute; 2009.
3. Gross NJ. What is this thing called love?—or, defining asthma. Am Rev Respir Dis 1980;121(2):203–4.
4. Global Initiative for Chronic Obstructive Lung Disease (GOLD). Global Strategy for Diagnosis, Management and Prevention of COPD. GOLD; 2010. Available at: http://www.goldcopd.org/. Accessed August 27, 2011.
5. Wright DT, Cohn LA, Li H, et al. Interactions of oxygen radicals with airway epithelium. Environ Health Perspect 1994;102(Suppl 10):85–90.
6. Blanc PD, Iribarren C, Trupin L, et al. Occupational exposures and the risk of COPD: dusty trades revisited. Thorax 2009;64(1):6–12.
7. Po JY, FitzGerald JM, Carlsten C. Respiratory disease associated with solid biomass fuel exposure in rural women and children: systematic review and meta-analysis. Thorax 2011;66(3):232–9.
8. Lee MH, Hancox RJ. Effects of smoking cannabis on lung function. Expert Rev Respir Med 2011;5(4):537–47.
9. Ko FW, Hui DS. Outdoor air pollution: impact on chronic obstructive pulmonary disease patients. Curr Opin Pulm Med 2009;15(2):150–7.
10. Nakamura H. Genetics of COPD. Allergol Int 2011;60(3):253–8.
11. Pillai DR, Shahinas D, Buzina A, et al. Genome-wide dissection of globally emergent multi-drug resistant serotype 19A Streptococcus pneumoniae. BMC Genomics 2009;10:642.
12. Han MK. Update in chronic obstructive pulmonary disease in 2010. Am J Respir Crit Care Med 2011;183(10):1311–5.
13. Pillai SG, Ge D, Zhu G, et al. A genome-wide association study in chronic obstructive pulmonary disease (COPD): identification of two major susceptibility loci. PLoS Genet 2009;5(3):e1000421.

14. Sinderby C, Spahija J, Beck J. Changes in respiratory effort sensation over time are linked to the frequency content of diaphragm electrical activity. Am J Respir Crit Care Med 2001;163(4):905–10.
15. Seibold MA, Schwartz DA. The lung: the natural boundary between nature and nurture. Annu Rev Physiol 2011;73:457–78.
16. Regan EA, Hokanson JE, Murphy JR, et al. Genetic epidemiology of COPD (COPDGene) study design. COPD 2010;7(1):32–43.
17. Guerra S. Overlap of asthma and chronic obstructive pulmonary disease. Curr Opin Pulm Med 2005;11(1):7–13.
18. Camp PG, O'Donnell DE, Postma DS. Chronic obstructive pulmonary disease in men and women: myths and reality. Proc Am Thorac Soc 2009; 6(6):535–8.
19. Sin DD, Cohen SB, Day A, et al. Understanding the biological differences in susceptibility to chronic obstructive pulmonary disease between men and women. Proc Am Thorac Soc 2007;4(8):671–4.
20. Tam A, Morrish D, Wadsworth S, et al. The role of female hormones on lung function in chronic lung diseases. BMC Womens Health 2011;11:24.
21. Spurzem JR, Rennard SI. Pathogenesis of COPD. Semin Respir Crit Care Med 2005;26(2):142–53.
22. Hogg JC, Chu F, Utokaparch S, et al. The nature of small-airway obstruction in chronic obstructive pulmonary disease. N Engl J Med 2004;350(26): 2645–53.
23. Kirkham P, Rahman I. Oxidative stress in asthma and COPD: antioxidants as a therapeutic strategy. Pharmacol Ther 2006;111(2):476–94.
24. Gosselink JV, Hayashi S, Elliott WM, et al. Differential expression of tissue repair genes in the pathogenesis of chronic obstructive pulmonary disease. Am J Respir Crit Care Med 2010;181(12):1329–35.
25. Vogelmeier CF, Wouters EF. Treating the systemic effects of chronic obstructive pulmonary disease. Proc Am Thorac Soc 2011;8(4):376–9.
26. Lee SD, Ju G, Choi JA, et al. The association of oxidative stress with central obesity in obstructive sleep apnea. Sleep Breath 2011. [Epub ahead of print].
27. Buist AS, Nagy JM. Relationship between smoking and the single breath nitrogen washout. Scand J Respir Dis Suppl 1976;95:108–16.
28. Lee R, McNicholas WT. Obstructive sleep apnea in chronic obstructive pulmonary disease patients. Curr Opin Pulm Med 2011;17(2):79–83.
29. Seemungal TA, Donaldson GC, Paul EA, et al. Effect of exacerbation on quality of life in patients with chronic obstructive pulmonary disease. Am J Respir Crit Care Med 1998;157(5 Pt 1):1418–22.
30. Buist AS, Sexton GJ, Nagy JM, et al. The effect of smoking cessation and modification on lung function. Am Rev Respir Dis 1976;114(1):115–22.
31. Mohamed Hoesein FA, Zanen P, Lammers JW. Lower limit of normal or FEV1/FVC < 0.70 in diagnosing COPD: an evidence-based review. Respir Med 2011;105(6): 907–15.
32. Glaab T, Vogelmeier C, Buhl R. Outcome measures in chronic obstructive pulmonary disease (COPD): strengths and limitations. Respir Res 2010;11:79.
33. Sethi S, Evans N, Grant BJ, et al. New strains of bacteria and exacerbations of chronic obstructive pulmonary disease. N Engl J Med 2002;347(7):465–71.
34. Wu J, Sin DD. Improved patient outcome with smoking cessation: when is it too late? Int J Chron Obstruct Pulmon Dis 2011;6:259–67.
35. Cahill K, Stead LF, Lancaster T. Nicotine receptor partial agonists for smoking cessation. Cochrane Database Syst Rev 2011;2:CD006103.

36. Ries AL, Bauldoff GS, Carlin BW, et al. Pulmonary rehabilitation: joint ACCP/AACVPR evidence-based clinical practice guidelines. Chest 2007;131(Suppl 5):4S–42S.
37. Rice KL, Dewan N, Bloomfield HE, et al. Disease management program for chronic obstructive pulmonary disease: a randomized controlled trial. Am J Respir Crit Care Med 2010;182(7):890–6.
38. Long term domiciliary oxygen therapy in chronic hypoxic cor pulmonale complicating chronic bronchitis and emphysema. Report of the Medical Research Council Working Party. Lancet 1981;1(8222):681–6.
39. Anthonisen NR. Long-term oxygen therapy. Ann Intern Med 1983;99(4):519–27.
40. Qaseem A, Wilt TJ, Weinberger SE, et al. Diagnosis and management of stable chronic obstructive pulmonary disease: a clinical practice guideline update from the American College of Physicians, American College of Chest Physicians, American Thoracic Society, and European Respiratory Society. Ann Intern Med 2011;155(3):179–91.
41. Celli BR, MacNee W. Standards for the diagnosis and treatment of patients with COPD: a summary of the ATS/ERS position paper. Eur Respir J 2004;23(6):932–46.
42. Wise RA, Tashkin DP. Optimizing treatment of chronic obstructive pulmonary disease: an assessment of current therapies. Am J Med 2007;120(8 Suppl 1): S4–13.
43. Sin DD, McAlister FA, Man SF, et al. Contemporary management of chronic obstructive pulmonary disease: scientific review. JAMA 2003;290(17):2301–12.
44. Nelson HS, Weiss ST, Bleecker ER, et al. The Salmeterol Multicenter Asthma Research Trial: a comparison of usual pharmacotherapy for asthma or usual pharmacotherapy plus salmeterol. Chest 2006;129(1):15–26.
45. Salpeter SR, Ormiston TM, Salpeter EE. Meta-analysis: respiratory tolerance to regular beta2-agonist use in patients with asthma. Ann Intern Med 2004; 140(10):802–13.
46. Tashkin DP, Celli B, Senn S, et al. A 4-year trial of tiotropium in chronic obstructive pulmonary disease. N Engl J Med 2008;359(15):1543–54.
47. Singh S, Loke YK, Furberg CD. Inhaled anticholinergics and risk of major adverse cardiovascular events in patients with chronic obstructive pulmonary disease: a systematic review and meta-analysis. JAMA 2008;300(12):1439–50.
48. Dorinsky PM, Reisner C, Ferguson GT, et al. The combination of ipratropium and albuterol optimizes pulmonary function reversibility testing in patients with COPD. Chest 1999;115(4):966–71.
49. van Noord JA, Aumann JL, Janssens E, et al. Comparison of tiotropium once daily, formoterol twice daily and both combined once daily in patients with COPD. Eur Respir J 2005;26(2):214–22.
50. Alsaeedi A, Sin DD, McAlister FA. The effects of inhaled corticosteroids in chronic obstructive pulmonary disease: a systematic review of randomized placebo-controlled trials. Am J Med 2002;113(1):59–65.
51. Hanania NA, Darken P, Horstman D, et al. The efficacy and safety of fluticasone propionate (250 microg)/salmeterol (50 microg) combined in the Diskus inhaler for the treatment of COPD. Chest 2003;124(3):834–43.
52. Tashkin DP. Budesonide and formoterol in a single pressurized metered-dose inhaler for treatment of COPD. Expert Rev Respir Med 2010;4(6):703–14.
53. Rennard SI, Tashkin DP, McElhattan J, et al. Efficacy and tolerability of budesonide/formoterol in one hydrofluoroalkane pressurized metered-dose inhaler in patients with chronic obstructive pulmonary disease: results from a 1-year randomized controlled clinical trial. Drugs 2009;69(5):549–65.

54. Tashkin DP, Rennard SI, Martin P, et al. Efficacy and safety of budesonide and formoterol in one pressurized metered-dose inhaler in patients with moderate to very severe chronic obstructive pulmonary disease: results of a 6-month randomized clinical trial. Drugs 2008;68(14):1975–2000.

55. Ferguson GT, Anzueto A, Fei R, et al. Effect of fluticasone propionate/salmeterol (250/50 microg) or salmeterol (50 microg) on COPD exacerbations. Respir Med 2008;102(8):1099–108.

56. Calverley PM, Anderson JA, Celli B, et al. Salmeterol and fluticasone propionate and survival in chronic obstructive pulmonary disease. N Engl J Med 2007; 356(8):775–89.

57. Wedzicha JA, Calverley PM, Seemungal TA, et al. The prevention of chronic obstructive pulmonary disease exacerbations by salmeterol/fluticasone propionate or tiotropium bromide. Am J Respir Crit Care Med 2008;177(1):19–26.

58. Ernst P, Gonzalez AV, Brassard P, et al. Inhaled corticosteroid use in chronic obstructive pulmonary disease and the risk of hospitalization for pneumonia. Am J Respir Crit Care Med 2007;176(2):162–6.

59. Calverley PM, Stockley RA, Seemungal TA, et al. Reported pneumonia in patients with COPD: findings from the INSPIRE study. Chest 2011;139(3):505–12.

60. Sin DD, Tashkin D, Zhang X, et al. Budesonide and the risk of pneumonia: a meta-analysis of individual patient data. Lancet 2009;374(9691):712–9.

61. Aaron SD, Vandemheen KL, Fergusson D, et al. Tiotropium in combination with placebo, salmeterol, or fluticasone-salmeterol for treatment of chronic obstructive pulmonary disease: a randomized trial. Ann Intern Med 2007;146(8):545–55.

62. Singh D, Brooks J, Hagan G, et al. Superiority of "triple" therapy with salmeterol/ fluticasone propionate and tiotropium bromide versus individual components in moderate to severe COPD. Thorax 2008;63(7):592–8.

63. Gaebel K, McIvor RA, Xie F, et al. Triple therapy for the management of COPD: a review. COPD 2011;8(3):206–43.

64. Ford PA, Durham AL, Russell RE, et al. Treatment effects of low-dose theophylline combined with an inhaled corticosteroid in COPD. Chest 2010;137(6):1338–44.

65. To Y, Ito K, Kizawa Y, et al. Targeting phosphoinositide-3-kinase-delta with theophylline reverses corticosteroid insensitivity in chronic obstructive pulmonary disease. Am J Respir Crit Care Med 2010;182(7):897–904.

66. Rabe KF, Hiemstra PS. Theophylline for chronic obstructive pulmonary disease? Time to move on. Am J Respir Crit Care Med 2010;182(7):868–9.

67. Ram FS, Rodriguez-Roisin R, Granados-Navarrete A, et al. WITHDRAWN: Antibiotics for exacerbations of chronic obstructive pulmonary disease. Cochrane Database Syst Rev 2011;1:CD004403.

68. Lipworth BJ. Phosphodiesterase-4 inhibitors for asthma and chronic obstructive pulmonary disease. Lancet 2005;365(9454):167–75.

69. Puhan M. Phosphodiesterase 4 inhibitors for chronic obstructive pulmonary disease. Cochrane Database Syst Rev 2011;8:ED000028.

70. O'Byrne PM, Gauvreau G. Phosphodiesterase-4 inhibition in COPD. Lancet 2009; 374(9691):665–7.

71. Altenburg J, de Graaff CS, van der Werf TS, et al. Immunomodulatory effects of macrolide antibiotics—part 2: advantages and disadvantages of long-term, low-dose macrolide therapy. Respiration 2011;81(1):75–87.

72. Altenburg J, de Graaff CS, van der Werf TS, et al. Immunomodulatory effects of macrolide antibiotics—part 1: biological mechanisms. Respiration 2011;81(1):67–74.

73. Tamaoki J. The effects of macrolides on inflammatory cells. Chest 2004;125 (Suppl 2):41S–50S [quiz: 51S].

74. Albert R. Chronic azithromycin decreases the frequency of chronic obstructive pulmonary disease exacerbations. Am J Respir Crit Care Med 2011;183: A6416.

75. Young RP, Hopkins R, Eaton TE. Pharmacological actions of statins: potential utility in COPD. Eur Respir Rev 2009;18(114):222–32.

76. Dobler CC, Wong KK, Marks GB. Associations between statins and COPD: a systematic review. BMC Pulm Med 2009;9:32.

77. Mancini GB, Etminan M, Zhang B, et al. Reduction of morbidity and mortality by statins, angiotensin-converting enzyme inhibitors, and angiotensin receptor blockers in patients with chronic obstructive pulmonary disease. J Am Coll Cardiol 2006;47(12):2554–60.

78. Vestbo J, Tan L, Atkinson G, et al. A controlled trial of 6-weeks' treatment with a novel inhaled phosphodiesterase type-4 inhibitor in COPD. Eur Respir J 2009;33(5):1039–44.

79. Holverda S, Rietema H, Bogaard HJ, et al. Acute effects of sildenafil on exercise pulmonary hemodynamics and capacity in patients with COPD. Pulm Pharmacol Ther 2008;21(3):558–64.

80. Janssens W, Bouillon R, Claes B, et al. Vitamin D deficiency is highly prevalent in COPD and correlates with variants in the vitamin D-binding gene. Thorax 2010; 65(3):215–20.

81. Janssens W, Lehouck A, Carremans C, et al. Vitamin D beyond bones in chronic obstructive pulmonary disease: time to act. Am J Respir Crit Care Med 2009; 179(8):630–6.

82. Janssens W, Mathieu C, Boonen S, et al. Vitamin D deficiency and chronic obstructive pulmonary disease: a vicious circle. Vitam Horm 2011;86:379–99.

83. Black PN, Scragg R. Relationship between serum 25-hydroxyvitamin d and pulmonary function in the third national health and nutrition examination survey. Chest 2005;128(6):3792–8.

84. Connors AF Jr, Dawson NV, Thomas C, et al. Outcomes following acute exacerbation of severe chronic obstructive lung disease. The SUPPORT investigators (Study to Understand Prognoses and Preferences for Outcomes and Risks of Treatments). Am J Respir Crit Care Med 1996;154(4 Pt 1):959–67.

85. Sin DD, Tu JV. Inhaled corticosteroids and the risk of mortality and readmission in elderly patients with chronic obstructive pulmonary disease. Am J Respir Crit Care Med 2001;164(4):580–4.

86. Sethi S. Infectious etiology of acute exacerbations of chronic bronchitis. Chest 2000;117(5 Suppl 2):380S–5S.

87. Bakri F, Brauer AL, Sethi S, et al. Systemic and mucosal antibody response to *Moraxella catarrhalis* after exacerbations of chronic obstructive pulmonary disease. J Infect Dis 2002;185(5):632–40.

88. Abe Y, Murphy TF, Sethi S, et al. Lymphocyte proliferative response to P6 of *Haemophilus influenzae* is associated with relative protection from exacerbations of chronic obstructive pulmonary disease. Am J Respir Crit Care Med 2002; 165(7):967–71.

89. Murphy TF, Sethi S, Hill SL, et al. Inflammatory markers in bacterial exacerbations of COPD. Am J Respir Crit Care Med 2002;165(1):132.

90. Fishman A, Martinez F, Naunheim K, et al. A randomized trial comparing lung-volume-reduction surgery with medical therapy for severe emphysema. N Engl J Med 2003;348(21):2059–73.

91. Patients at high risk of death after lung-volume-reduction surgery. N Engl J Med 2001;345(15):1075–83.

92. Patel N, DeCamp M, Criner GJ. Lung transplantation and lung volume reduction surgery versus transplantation in chronic obstructive pulmonary disease. Proc Am Thorac Soc 2008;5(4):447–53.
93. Sethi S. The role of antibiotics in acute exacerbations of chronic obstructive pulmonary disease. Curr Infect Dis Rep 2003;5(1):9–15.
94. Ernst A, Anantham D. Bronchoscopic lung volume reduction. Pulm Med 2011; 2011:610802.

Community-Acquired Pneumonia: An Unfinished Battle

Girish B. Nair, MD[a], Michael S. Niederman, MD[b,c],*

KEYWORDS

- Community-acquired pneumonia • Mortality • Lungs
- Pneumococcus

Community-acquired pneumonia (CAP) is a common disease causing considerable morbidity and mortality in the United States. CAP is an alveolar infection that develops in the outpatient setting or within 48 hours of admission to a hospital. However, some patients developing pneumonia out of hospital have had recent contact with the health care environment, and these individuals are designated as having health care–associated pneumonia (HCAP), which may need to be managed differently from CAP. The clinical spectrum varies from a mild outpatient illness, with rapid resolution, to severe sepsis with multiorgan failure and death. The potential grave consequences are more likely with extremes of age and among patients with comorbid conditions.[1]

The annual incidence of CAP is between 5 and 11 per 1000 population, with the incidence being higher in elderly patients.[2] Mortality from CAP continues to be unchanged even though newer antimicrobial therapy has been introduced in the last several decades.[1] According to National Vital Statistics Report (2011), pneumonia, along with influenza, was the eighth leading cause of death in 2009.[3] In 2006, 1.2 million people in the United States were hospitalized with pneumonia and 55,477 people died of the disease.[4] Most cases of CAP occur in outpatients, in whom the mortality is less than 5%, but, when patients are admitted to the hospital, the mortality increases to more than 10%, and can exceed 30% when patients are admitted to the intensive care unit (ICU).[5] The data from the German CAPNETZ Network trial showed that the mortality among patients hospitalized with CAP ranged from 5% to 20%, but was up to 50% in patients admitted to the ICU.[6] Recently, investigators

---

Conflict of interest: Dr Nair has no potential conflicts of interest to declare. Dr Niederman has served as a consultant to Pfizer, Johnson and Johnson, and Merck.

a Pulmonary and Critical Care Medicine, Winthrop-University Hospital, Mineola, NY, USA
b Department of Medicine, Winthrop-University Hospital, 222 Station Plaza North, Suite 509, Mineola, NY 11501, USA
c Department of Medicine, SUNY at Stony Brook, Stony Brook, NY, USA
* Corresponding author. Department of Medicine, Winthrop-University Hospital, 222 Station Plaza North, Suite 509, Mineola, NY 11501.
E-mail address: mniederman@winthrop.org

Med Clin N Am 95 (2011) 1143–1161
doi:10.1016/j.mcna.2011.08.007
0025-7125/11/$ – see front matter © 2011 Elsevier Inc. All rights reserved.

have shown that patients with CAP in a Medicare population have a 1-year mortality of more than 40%, suggesting that pneumonia may be a surrogate marker of severe underlying comorbidity, or that it initiates a series of adverse consequences for some patients that leads to their eventual death.[7]

Despite the availability of different guidelines and treatment options, the economic burden associated with CAP remains high at more than $17 billion annually in United States alone.[8] Although most patients with CAP are outpatients, the greatest portion of the cost for this illness is borne by those admitted to hospital, making the decision about admission an important one for several reasons. A recent study noted that decreasing the length of stay by 1 day in a patient with CAP had a potential economic benefit of $2000.[9] With new health care reforms imminent and the emphasis on better health care delivery, cost-effective treatment of pneumonia will assume greater significance.

There are several challenges with the management of CAP, from the accurate diagnosis of lung infiltrates, decisions about the site of care, and the choice of appropriate antibiotics. The Infectious Disease Society of America (IDSA)/American Thoracic Society (ATS) guideline from 2007 provides a summary of the approach to the treatment of CAP directed mainly towards primary care physicians, hospitalists, and emergency medicine physicians.[1] Multiple validated severity assessment scores have been developed that stratify patients according to the risk of death and can be used as decision support tools to guide site-of-care decisions.[10,11] The emergence of drug-resistant organisms, particularly drug-resistant *Streptococcus pneumoniae* (DRSP), is another challenge in disease management. Biomarkers are increasingly being used to distinguish bacterial pneumonia from other causes and to help reduce the duration of antibiotic therapy.[12] This article reviews the recent advances in the diagnosis, management, and potential complications associated with CAP.

PATHOGENESIS

In CAP, the major route of infection is microaspiration from a previously colonized oropharynx, but inhalation of suspended aerosolized microorganisms is the mechanism of infection for viruses, *Legionella*, and tuberculosis. Interactions between the host immune response, the virulence of the infecting organism, and the size of the inoculums determine whether a patient develops pneumonia.[13] Defective cough, mucociliary clearance, and impaired local and humoral immunity predispose to severe pneumonia. Alcohol consumption and smoking are independent risk factors for the development of pneumonia. Medical comorbidities such as chronic obstructive pulmonary disease (COPD), congestive heart failure, chronic kidney disease, liver disease, and immune deficiency states have an increased predisposition for the development of CAP. Recent use of proton pump inhibitor therapy started within 30 days has been identified as a risk factor for CAP.[14] Elderly patients are at increased risk for development of pneumonia and, when it occurs, they are more likely to die than younger individuals.[2] Although many patients develop severe pneumonia because of immune impairment, others develop acute lung injury (acute respiratory distress syndrome [ARDS]) as a consequence of unilateral pneumonia because of an inability to localize the immune response to the initial site of infection, possibly because of the presence of a genetic variation in their immune responsiveness.[15,16]

CAUSES

The most common organism causing CAP, in all patient populations, is *S pneumoniae*, or pneumococcus. Other pathogens include *Hemophilus influenzae* (particularly in cigarette smokers), *Moraxella catarrhalis*, *Staphylococcus aureus* (after influenza and recently in the form of methicillin-resistant *S aureus* [MRSA]), viruses (including influenza, respiratory syncytial virus, parainfluenza, and epidemic viruses), and atypical pathogens such as *Mycoplasma pneumoniae*, *Chlamydophila pneumoniae*, and *Legionella pneumophila*. In most series, atypical pathogens are common, including in those admitted to the ICU, where they can account for up to 20% of the identified pathogens. In addition, many investigators have documented that atypical pathogens may coexist with bacterial pathogens, accounting for their presence in up to 60% of patients with CAP, when serologic testing is used.[17]

Gram-negative bacteria (*Pseudomonas aeruginosa*, *Klebsiella pneumoniae*, *Escherichia coli*, *Enterobacter* spp, *Serratia* spp, *Proteus* spp) are the causal agents in up to 10% of patients with CAP, but may be more common in patients who develop pneumonia out of the hospital and have HCAP risk factors. Gram-negative bacteria have been associated with severe CAP, and *K pneumoniae* was noted to be an independent risk factor for mortality in severe CAP.[18] In one study from Korea, in a multivariate analysis, the risk factors associated with gram-negative CAP were septic shock (with an odds ratio of 4.1), cardiac disease, smoking, hyponatremia, and dyspnea, emphasizing the association of these organisms with severe illness.[19] *Enterobacter* CAP behaves more like hospital-acquired pneumonia and is associated with prolonged mechanical ventilation, delay in initiation of antibiotics, and longer ICU stay.[20] Risk factors for community-acquired *P aeruginosa* pneumonia include bronchiectasis, immunocompromised state, use of multiple courses of antibiotics, prolonged glucocorticoids in patients with COPD, and recent hospitalization.[21] Anaerobic organisms should be considered when aspiration is suspected.

Influenza is a common viral cause of CAP, with a seasonal variation in frequency. Primary influenza pneumonia tends to cause severe pneumonia, which can be either caused by the virus itself or a result of secondary bacterial infection with pneumococcus, *S aureus*, or *H influenzae*. High-risk patients include those with chronic heart or lung disease, diabetes, immunosuppression, hemoglobinopathy, renal disease, and otherwise healthy individuals more than 65 years of age. Other viruses that cause CAP include Parainfluenza virus, respiratory syncytial virus (RSV), human metapneumovirus, severe acute respiratory syndrome virus, varicella, Hantavirus, and adenovirus. Many of these patients have viral infection as part of a mixed infection, often with bacterial pathogens.[22]

Emergence of DRSP and community-acquired MRSA is a matter of concern that has complicated the empiric therapy choices for patients with CAP. DRSP is seen most often in patients older than 65 years of age, and in those with a history of alcoholism, antibiotic therapy within 3 months, multiple medical comorbid conditions, exposure to children in day care, or those with immune-compromised states.[23] Community-associated MRSA (CA-MRSA) pneumonia occurs in patients with no prior health care exposure, usually after influenza, and may lead to a severe necrotizing pneumonia, although milder forms of illness have also been reported.[24] In patients with severe illness, the organism may produce a variety of exotoxins, including the Panton-Valentine leukocidin (PVL), which may contribute to lung necrosis.[25] Multidrug resistance has been reported with CA-MRSA strains but, in general, these organisms are more drug sensitive than their hospital-acquired counterparts.[26]

Other less common causes of CAP include *Mycobacterium tuberculosis*, *Coxiella burnetii* (Q fever), *Burkholderia pseudomallei* (melioidosis), *Chlamydophila psittaci* (psittacosis), endemic fungi (histoplasmosis, coccidioidomycosis, blastomycosis), *Pasteurella multocida*, *Bacillus anthracis*, *Actinomyces israeli*, *Francisella tularensis* (tularemia), and *Nocardia* spp. These organisms should be included in the differential diagnosis when evaluating a patient with CAP, depending on the presence of specific risk factors that are noted in the clinical history.

CLINICAL EVALUATION
Presentation

Patients with CAP usually present with an acute illness of 1 to 2 days duration. In those with intact immune response, systemic and respiratory symptoms such as cough, dyspnea, fever, and pleuritic chest pain predominate. Fever and chills have a sensitivity of 50% to 85%, and dyspnea a sensitivity of 70% for the diagnosis of CAP, whereas purulent sputum has a sensitivity of only 50%.[23] Hemoptysis suggests necrotizing infection, such as lung abscess, tuberculosis, or gram-negative pneumonia, but is also a common finding, even in patients with bronchitis. In patients with disease and age-associated impairments in the immune response, the clinical presentation may be subtle, and involve primarily nonrespiratory findings. In the elderly, chest pain and cough may be absent in the early course of the disease, and fever and confusion may be the only symptoms.[23] Other complaints such as lethargy, falling, poor oral intake, and decompensation of a chronic illness could also occur in patients with comorbid conditions and among the elderly.

History and Physical Examination

A good history and physical examination are essential for determining the possible causal agent and assessing the severity of illness, which in turn helps with management. Risk factors for HCAP, such as hospitalization or antibiotic therapy in the past 90 days, residence in a long-term care facility, chronic dialysis, outpatient wound care, or home infusion therapy, needs to be identified, because these patients are at risk for drug-resistant gram-negative organisms and *S aureus*. The history should identify risk factors for DRSP and gram-negative organisms, as discussed earlier. It is also important to elicit recent travel history and exposure to birds, bats, farm animals, and rabbits (**Table 1**).

On physical examination, patients may have tachypnea, tachycardia, crackles, bronchial breath sounds, and findings of pleural effusion. Clinicians should pay attention to other clues, such as relative bradycardia in relation to fever, which can be seen in infections caused by agents like *Legionella*, *Chlamydophila*, and *Mycoplasma*.[27] *Mycoplasma* can also cause cervical lymphadenopathy, arthralgia, and bullous myringitis. Poor outcomes are noted in patients with a respiratory rate greater than 30 breaths/min, diastolic blood pressure less than 60 mm Hg, systolic blood pressure less than 90 mm Hg, heart rate greater than 125 beats/min, and temperature less than 35°C or greater than 40°C.[23] These clinical findings can be used to determine the risk of death, by incorporating them into prognostic scoring, using the Pneumonia Severity Index (PSI), the CURB-65 criteria (a modification of the British Thoracic Society scoring system), or other tools (discussed later).

Other than raising clinical suspicion, no combination of symptoms and signs can accurately diagnose pneumonia in the clinical setting, and the definitive diagnosis requires a chest radiograph.[28] The clinical diagnosis has an overall sensitivity ranging from 70% to 90% and specificity between 40% and 70%. Therefore, whenever there is suspicion of CAP, a chest radiograph should be obtained for corroboration of the physical findings.[29] Certain chest radiographic findings can also suggest more severe illness, including the presence of multilobar infiltrates, rapid progression of infiltrates, pleural effusion, and findings of necrotizing pneumonia.

Diagnostic Approach

In the outpatient setting, extensive diagnostic testing is not routinely performed, because results are nonspecific, and antibiotic treatment should be initiated

Table 1
Pathogens by risk factors and underlying conditions

Underlying Conditions	Suspected Pathogens
Chronic obstructive lung disease	H influenza, P aeruginosa, Legionella species, S pneumonia, M pneumonia, C pneumoniae
Alcoholism	S pneumonia, oral anaerobes, K pneumonia, Acinetobacter species, M tuberculosis
HIV infection	S pneumoniae, H influenzae, Salmonella, Cytomegalovirus, Cryptococcus, P jiroveci, anaerobes, M tuberculosis
Aspiration	Anaerobes, enteric gram-negative bacilli, chemical pneumonitis
Exposure to bats	Histoplasma capsulatum
Exposure to birds	C psittaci, Cryptococcus neoformans, H capsulatum
Contact with farm animals	Coxiella burnetii (Q fever)
Exposure to rabbits	Francisella tularensis
Travel to southwest United States	Coccidioides immitis
Nursing home resident	S pneumoniae, gram-negative bacilli, anaerobes, H influenzae, MRSA, C pneumoniae, M tuberculosis
Recent influenza infection	S pneumoniae, S aureus (including MRSA), H influenzae
Structural disease of lung (bronchiectasis, cystic fibrosis)	P aeruginosa, P cepacia, S aureus
Bioterrorism	Bacillus anthracis, Yersinia pestis, Francisella tularensis
Cruise ship, sauna, hot tub, or hotel stay within 2 wk	Legionella species

Abbreviation: HIV, human immunodeficiency virus.

empirically.[1] Even for inpatients, the value of diagnostic testing is limited and, when outcomes were compared using pathogen-directed therapy, compared with empiric therapy, there was limited benefit of testing.[30] In one prospective study of 262 patients from the Netherlands, a pathogen was identified in 60% of cases. Adequate sputum samples were obtained from only 44 patients, Gram stain was diagnostic and confirmed by a positive sputum in 82%, urine pneumococcal antigen was positive in 54% of cases, blood cultures were positive in 16%, and bronchoscopic samples added benefit to diagnostic yield when sputum could not be expectorated.[31] In most studies, a specific causal diagnosis is obtained in less than 50% of patients with CAP, even with extensive diagnostic testing, and the major focus of laboratory testing should be to assess severity of illness and allow early identification of the presence of pneumonic complications.

White blood cell count may be normal on admission, and leukopenia is seen in patients with overwhelming pneumococcal pneumonia with sepsis and pneumonia caused by gram-negative organisms.[27] Thrombocytosis and thrombocytopenia are associated with worse 30-day mortality in patients admitted with CAP.[32] Hyponatremia (<130 mEq/L) is also associated with a poor outcome, if present on admission, in patients with CAP.[33] The IDSA/ATS guidelines recommended testing for patients with pneumonia (**Table 2**).

Table 2
Recommended tests per IDSA/ATS 2007 guidelines

Tests	Indications
Blood culture	ICU admission. Consider if multiple of: cavitary infiltrate, leucopenia, active alcohol abuse, chronic liver disease, asplenia, pneumococcal UAT positive, pleural effusion
Sputum culture	ICU admission, failure of outpatient antibiotics, cavitary infiltrate, severe COPD/structural disease, active alcohol abuse, legionella or pneumococcal UAT positive, pleural effusion
Legionella UAT	ICU admission, failure of outpatient antibiotics, active alcohol abuse, recent travel within 2 wk, pleural effusion
Pneumococcal UAT	ICU admission, failure of outpatient antibiotics, leukopenia, asplenia, active alcohol abuse, chronic liver disease, pleural effusion
Pleural fluid culture/ thoracentesis	Significant pleural effusion
Endotracheal aspirate/ bronchoscopic washings	ICU admission
Fungal culture and TB testing	Cavitary infiltrate
Special media for legionella	Positive UAT for legionella

Abbreviations: TB, tuberculosis; UAT, urinary antigen testing.

Radiographic Evaluation

Radiographic evidence of lung infiltration provides a sensitive, but not specific, confirmation of community-acquired pneumonia. Chest radiograph may show areas of consolidation, pleural effusion, lung abscess, necrotizing pneumonia, or multilobar illness. It may help in pattern recognition of the disease process: *H influenzae* has a peribronchial distribution of bronchopneumonia; *S pneumoniae* infection can have either lobar consolidation or bronchopneumonia; atypical pathogens may have an alveolar and interstitial pattern; aspiration most commonly involves the superior segment of the right lower lobe or the posterior segment of the right upper lobe; hematogenous dissemination follows the distribution of blood flow and may lead to bilateral nodular infiltrates.[27] Cavitation or necrotizing pneumonia suggests infection with anaerobes, gram-negative bacteria, or *S aureus*, including MRSA. Loculated effusion can be ruled out by decubitus film or computed tomography (CT). Chest ultrasound is increasingly being used to assess the size, and to identify a safe site for sampling of pleural fluid.

The usefulness of chest radiography is suboptimal in patients with very early infection, dehydration, severe granulocytopenia, structural changes such as with bullous emphysema, and in obese patients. It is reasonable to repeat a follow-up radiograph in 24 to 48 hours in patients who have had a negative initial finding, but have clinical signs of pneumonia.[1] There may be interobserver variability in chest radiographic interpretation of pneumonia. In a study that compared the readings of at least 2 radiologists, positive agreement (59%) was less frequent than negative agreement (94%).[34] CT has better sensitivity in diagnosing an infiltrate than chest radiography, but it is not routinely used, because there is a lack of evidence that use of CT scan improves outcomes.[35]

Sputum Examination

Sputum should be sent for Gram stain and culture before starting therapy, but primarily in patients suspected of infection with drug-resistant or unusual pathogens.

A good specimen contains no more than 10 squamous epithelial cells and more than 25 polymorphonuclear cells per low per field. The Gram stain pattern on sputum can help with tailoring of antibiotics, particularly if it shows a pathogen that would not be treated routinely (such as clumps of gram-positive cocci, suggesting *S aureus*). The sensitivity of identifying *S pneumonia* is only 50% to 60% and specificity is greater than 80%.[27] It is less likely to have *S aureus* or gram-negative pneumonia in the absence of these organisms on Gram stain of a good sputum sample, but this test is more valuable if positive than if negative. Routine culture of expectorated sputum is not useful in the absence of an informative Gram stain. The usefulness of real-time polymerase chain reaction testing of sputum samples has not been shown. Culture can be obtained from intubated patients by collecting an endotracheal aspirate.

Blood Culture

A positive blood or pleural culture is seen in less than 20% of patients with pneumonia but, if present, helps with establishing the diagnosis. Most positive cultures are of *S pneumoniae*. The IDSA/ATS guidelines recommend blood culture testing in patients admitted to ICU, and in those with multiple other risk factors, including active alcohol abuse, liver disease, cavitatory lung disease, asplenia, leukopenia, and pleural effusion. These recommendations are based, in part, on the data from 13,043 Medicare patients who showed that a true-positive blood culture was associated with no previous antibiotics, underlying liver disease, systolic blood pressure less than 90 mm Hg, fever less than 35°C or greater than 40°C, pulse greater than 125 beats/min, blood urea nitrogen greater than 10.71 mmol/L (30 mg/dL), serum sodium less than 130 mmol, and leukocyte count less than 5000 or greater than 20,000 cells/mL. The diagnostic yield of blood cultures increased in patients with 1 or more risk factor and in those who had not received antibiotics before blood was collected.[36]

Urinary Antigen Testing

Urinary antigen testing (UAT) is commercially available for detection of capsular polysaccharide of *S pneumoniae* and *L pneumophilia* serogroup 1. Pneumococcal urinary antigen tests have a sensitivity of 50% to 80% and specificity of more than 90%.[37] The degree of positivity is correlated with the PSI for *S pneumoniae*.[38] False-positive tests occur in patients who have had CAP from pneumococcus within the previous 3 months. UAT for *Legionella* has a sensitivity of 70% to 90% and a specificity of up to 99% for detection of infection with serogroup 1, by far the commonest species to infect humans.[27] However, it does not detect other types of *Legionella*, so a negative finding cannot rule out this infection. In one study, the use of UAT for *Legionella* had increased with time, leading to more diagnoses of serogroup 1 infection, but a decreased mortality from *Legionella*, suggesting that urinary antigen testing was finding milder illness than had been recognized previously.[39] Although one prospective study of 474 episodes of CAP from Spain found that *S pneumoniae* was diagnosed by urinary antigen test in 43.8% and helped physicians optimize antibiotic choice,[40] in general, it remains uncertain whether a positive result of any urinary antigen test changes CAP management, or whether it is primarily of epidemiologic interest.

Serology Testing

Serologic tests are of questionable importance in the initial setting, but are useful for the epidemiologic diagnosis of agents that are not readily cultured, although results are generally not available for weeks, and require the collection of both acute and convalescent serum samples. The diagnosis of most pathogens is based on acute and convalescent blood serologies showing a fourfold increase in immunoglobulin (Ig) G obtained 2 to 6 weeks apart, which applies to *C pneumoniae*, *C psittaci*, Q fever, and *M pneumoniae*. Ig M antibodies start to increase in the acute phase and are useful in the early course of the disease. Cold agglutinins are sometimes present in patients with *M pneumoniae*.

Polymerase Chain Reaction

Nucleic acid amplification tests provide rapid test results in CAP for atypical agents such as viruses, *Mycoplasma*, *Chlamydophila*, and *Legionella*. Polymerase chain reaction (PCR) assays were widely used for detecting influenza virus in the recent H1N1 epidemic. Direct immunofluorescence or enzyme immunoassay are available for detection of viral antigens like influenza, RSV, adenovirus and parainfluenza viruses. The usefulness of PCR assays in managing CAP has not been proven, and the concern with this method is that it is so sensitive that, if a respiratory sample is positive, it cannot distinguish colonization from infection unless the presence of a specific pathogen is itself diagnostic of infection (such as *M tuberculosis*). However, the test may be valuable if negative, because the absence of a suspected pathogen by PCR may permit a more focused antibiotic therapy approach.

Biomarkers

Several newer biomarkers have been developed (midregional proadrenomedullin, midregional proatrial natriuretic peptide, proarginin-vasopressin, proendothelin-1, procalcitonin [PCT], C-reactive protein [CRP]) to identify patients with bacterial infection and to define the prognosis of CAP. In one recent study, cardiac biomarkers, such as midregional proadrenomedullin, were better predictors of 28-day and 180-day mortality than inflammatory biomarkers such as PCT. In that study, biomarkers correlated with disease severity and mortality, but did not help with causal diagnosis.[41] In another prospective study evaluating the relationship between biomarkers and ICU admission, inflammatory biomarkers helped identify patients needing intensive care monitoring, including those requiring delayed ICU admission.[42]

The inflammatory biomarkers that have been studied most extensively are CRP and PCT, both of which are acute-phase reactants primarily produced by the liver in the presence of bacterial infection, but not viral illness. CRP may identify which patients with acute respiratory symptoms have infectious pneumonia; levels are higher in patients who require hospitalization and in those with pneumococcal and *Legionella* infection.[43] PCT is a hormokine, produced in response to microbial toxins and certain host responses associated with bacterial infection, but inhibited by viral-related cytokines. Serum levels tend to be high in patients with CAP, who benefit from antibiotic therapy, and in those with an increased risk of death from CAP. Serial measurements of serum levels have also been used to define when antibiotics can be safely stopped in the presence of CAP.[12,44,45] In one study of 302 patients with radiographic infiltrates and suspected CAP, initiation of antibiotics and duration of therapy were determined by randomizing patients to management by an algorithm dictated by serial PCT measurements versus management by clinical assessment. The PCT-guided group had significantly fewer antibiotic prescriptions on admission and less antibiotic usage, and the duration of therapy was reduced from 12 to 5 days with similar clinical success.[46]

SEVERITY ASSESSMENT

One of the most important decisions in the management of pneumonia is to assess the severity of the disease, which can be used to predict mortality risk and may be a surrogate measure to define the site of care (outpatient, hospital ward, or ICU). Proper site-of-care decisions can have an impact on mortality, with several studies showing that delayed admission to the ICU leads to a poor outcome.[47,48] The most widely used prognostic scoring systems are the PSI and the CURB-65 score. In clinical practice, the PSI is not widely used because it is complex and difficult to calculate a score.[49] In addition to these general scoring tools, some evaluations are designed to identify the need for ICU admission, including the IDSA/ATS criteria for severe CAP, and an Australian method called the SMART-COP, which is designed to predict the need for intensive respiratory or vasopressor support. Other prediction rules are available and their clinical application varies widely.

The PSI was developed to identify patients with a low risk of dying who could be safely discharged home and receive outpatient treatment. The PSI stratifies patients into 5 categories based on 30-day mortality, by using a scoring system based on 20 factors. It includes demographic characteristics, coexisting illnesses, physical examination findings, laboratory measurements, and radiographic finding.[50] Patients in classes IV (30-day mortality risk of 4%–10%) and V (27% risk of death at 30 days) are usually admitted to the hospital and often to the ICU. Those in low-risk classes I and II are often treated as outpatients, whereas it is a clinical judgment whether those in class III should be hospitalized. The PSI score includes age as an important determinant of point scoring and hence can overestimate the severity of illness in the elderly and in those with comorbidity. In one study of patients in PSI class V, only approximately 20% needed ICU admission, and these tended to be individuals who scored points based on acute illness features, and not on age and comorbid illness factors.[51] In contrast, the PSI may underestimate severity of illness in young patients without comorbid illness, especially if their vital sign abnormalities are slightly less than the cutoffs used in the scoring system.[52] This was a particular problem during recent influenza epidemics that have involved primarily younger populations, in which PSI scoring was not valuable for defining the need for ICU admission.

The CURB-65 score from the British Thoracic Society is an easy scoring system to use, with the score (0–5) being defined (1 point each) by the presence of confusion, blood urea nitrogen greater than 7.0 mol/L (19.6 mg/dL), respiratory rate of 30 breaths/min or greater, systolic blood pressure less than 90 mm Hg or diastolic blood pressure no greater than 60 mm Hg, and age 65 years or older. Patients with 2 of these criteria have a high enough risk of death that they should probably be admitted to the hospital, while those with 3 or more points should be considered for ICU admission. Modifications of this tool, without the laboratory measurement of blood urea nitrogen (CRB-65) have also been found to be similarly accurate.[53] The limitation of this approach is its focus on assessment of only clinical parameters, such as vital signs, but without measurement of oxygenation or serial measurement of severity of illness after the initial hospital admission, and that it does not evaluate the presence of comorbid illness and its decompensation from baseline.[54]

Serum biomarkers can be used to supplement data obtained by prognostic scoring.[55] Data from the German Competence Network for the Study of Community Acquired Pneumonia (CAPNETZ) Study Group, showed that all new biomarkers were good predictors of short-term and long-term all-cause mortality and correlated with CRB-65 score.[41] In other studies, low levels of PCT were able to define patients at low risk of death regardless of findings using severity scoring. Huang and colleagues[55] as well as Kruger and colleagues[56] found, that even in patients identified as high risk using CURB-65 or PSI, a low PCT value predicted a low chance of dying.[55,56]

IDSA/ATS 2007 criteria for severe CAP

Major criteria

1. Invasive mechanical ventilation

2. Septic shock with the need for vasopressors

Minor criteria

1. Respiratory rate 30 breaths/min

2. Alveolar oxygen partial pressure (Pao_2)/forced inspiratory oxygen (Fio_2) ratio 250

3. Multilobar infiltrates

4. Confusion/disorientation

5. Uremia (blood urea nitrogen level 1.1 mmol/L)

6. Leukopenia (white blood cells <4000 cells/mm^3)

7. Thrombocytopenia (platelet count <100,000 cells/mm^3)

8. Hypothermia (core temperature <36°C)

9. Hypotension requiring aggressive fluid resuscitation

Severe CAP

Scoring systems can also be used to help define which patients need ICU care, identifying those with severe illness. The IDSA/ATS guidelines and the PIRO (predisposition, insult, response, and organ dysfunction) scoring system were developed to help define mortality risk in patients with severe pneumonia. According to the 2007 IDSA/ATS guidelines, severe CAP is present if a patient needs invasive mechanical ventilation or requires vasopressors or has any 3 of 9 from the minor criteria listed later. Liapakou and colleagues[57] found that patients meeting the major criteria needed ICU admission, but those patients who had only minor criteria present had no increased mortality risk, regardless of how many criteria were met. More recently, Brown and colleagues[58] found that both the positive and negative predictive value of minor criteria exceeded 80% if 4 criteria were used to define the need for ICU admission rather than just 3 criteria.

The PIRO score is calculated within 24 hours of ICU admission, with 1 point given for each variable: comorbidities (COPD, immunocompromise), age greater than 70 years, multilobar opacities on chest radiograph, shock, severe hypoxemia, acute renal failure, bacteremia, and acute respiratory distress syndrome. The maximum score that can be achieved is 8. Patients are stratified into 4 levels of risk: (a) low, 0 to 2 points; (b) mild, 3 points; (c) high, 4 points; and (d) very high, 5 to 8 points. The PIRO score performed well as a 28-day mortality prediction tool in patients with CAP requiring ICU admission, with a better performance than APACHE II and IDSA/ATS criteria.[59] The SMART–COP tool was developed to identify the need for intensive respiratory or vasopressor support (IRVS), rather than a specific site-of-care decision. This tool uses a complex scoring system with the following values: low systolic blood pressure (<90 mm Hg) (2 points), multilobar pneumonia (1 point), low albumin level (<3.5 g/dL) (1 point), high respiratory rate ($\geq$25–30 breaths/min) (1 point), tachycardia (>125 beats/min) (1 point), confusion (1 point), poor oxygenation (2 points), and low arterial pH (<7.35) (2 points). When this method was used, the finding of a patient with a score of more than 3 points identified 92% of those needing IRVS, with a specificity of 62.3%, whereas the PSI and CURB-65 did not perform as well for this endpoint.[60] An algorithm for decision on site of care based on scoring system and treatment strategy is provided later (**Fig. 1**).

TREATMENT AND PROGNOSIS

Early diagnosis and timely administration of antibiotics are associated with improved outcomes in patients with CAP.[61,62] Although administration of therapy within 4 to 6 hours of arrival at the hospital can reduce mortality, it is important to only use antibiotics when the diagnosis is certain, because indiscriminate use of antibiotics in the absence of radiographic pneumonia has limited benefit and a real risk of

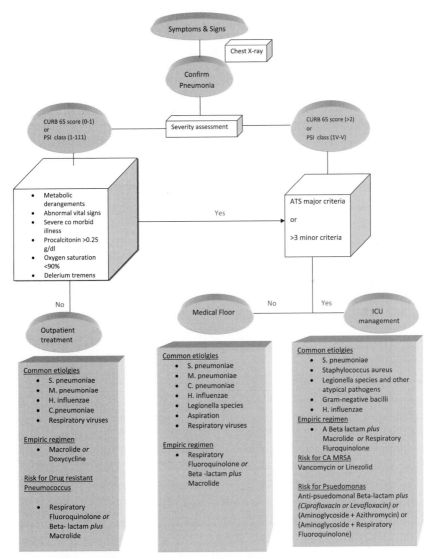

Fig. 1. A proposed algorithm for site of care and treatment of CAP and common organisms per the IDSA/ATS guidelines. CA, community acquired.

antibiotic-associated adverse events, including drug-induced infectious diarrhea. According to IDSA/ATS guidelines, the first dose of antibiotic should be given in the emergency department, preferably within 4 to 6 hours of arrival, but no time period is specified. Because no diagnostic testing can rapidly identify the causal pathogens in a patient with CAP, initial therapy is empiric, based on an epidemiologic assessment of patient risk factors for specific pathogens. This assessment requires a careful history of patient comorbidity, recent antibiotic therapy history (within the past 3 months), and identification of pathogen-specific risk factors (see **Table 1**; **Box 1**).

The IDSA/ATS guidelines recommend outpatient treatment with a macrolide or doxycycline for previously healthy adult patients with no risk factors for DRSP. In patients with risk factors for DRSP, a respiratory fluoroquinolone or a β-lactam antibiotic plus a macrolide or doxycycline is recommended. In choosing between these options, it is important to take a history about antibiotic usage in the past 3 months and to use an agent that is different from what has recently been used, because recent therapy may predispose to pneumococcal resistance to the agent used, rendering that therapy less effective.

For patients admitted to the hospital, but not to the ICU, an intravenous respiratory fluoroquinolone or a β-lactam plus a macrolide should be used. As mentioned earlier, the choice should be influenced by a history of which antibiotics have been used in the past 3 months, using agents from a different class, if possible. Doxycycline is an

---

Box 1
Treatment regimen per ATS/IDSA 2007 guidelines in different settings

Outpatient treatment

Previously healthy individual

- A macrolide or doxycycline.

Presence of comorbid disease or risk factors for DRSP

- A respiratory fluoroquinolone (gemfloxacin, levofloxacin, moxifloxacin) or a β-lactam (high-dose amoxicillin or amoxicillin-clavulanate) plus a macrolide (azithromycin, clarithromycin)

Inpatient non-ICU

- A respiratory fluoroquinolone (levofloxacin 750 mg or moxifloxacin) or
- β-lactam (cefotaxime, ceftriaxone, or ertapenem in selected patients) plus a macrolide (intravenous azithromycin)

Patients in ICU

No pseudomonal risk factors present

- A β-lactam (cefotaxime, ceftriaxone, or ampicillin-sulbactam) plus a macrolide (azithromycin) or respiratory fluoroquinolone (levofloxacin 750 mg or moxifloxacin).
- In patients allergic to penicillin – respiratory fluoroquinolone plus aztreonam.

If community-acquired MRSA is suspected

- Vancomycin (and possibly clindamycin) or linezolid alone added to above regimen.

If *Pseudomonas* is suspected

- A β-lactam with activity against *P aeruginosa* (piperacillin-tazobactam, cefepime, imipenem, or meropenem) plus either ciprofloxacin or levofloxacin, or
- A β-lactam with activity against *Pseudomonas* plus an aminoglycoside and azithromycin or a nonpseudomonal respiratory fluoroquinolone (moxifloxacin)

alternative to a macrolide. Ertapenem is an alternative to β-lactam agents such as cefotaxime, ceftriaxone, or ampicillin-sulbactam, and should be considered for patients with risk factors for infection with gram-negative pathogens other than *P aeruginosa*. All patients with CAP should have routine therapy directed at pneumococcus and atypical pathogens, plus other organisms, as dictated by specific risk factors. The routine coverage for atypical pathogens is based on outcome studies that show that the addition of a macrolide to a β-lactam, or the use of a quinolone alone, leads to better outcome than β-lactam monotherapy.[1] In addition, some studies have shown a high frequency of atypical pathogen coinfection in patients with bacterial CAP.

Current CAP guidelines do not recommend monotherapy with any agent, including a quinolone, for patients with severe CAP who are admitted to the ICU. In patients with bacteremia (pneumococcal and other), atypical pathogen coverage with a macrolide (monotherapy or combination) improves mortality compared with treatment regimens with a quinolone, particularly quinolone monotherapy.[63,64] Combination therapy with a β-lactam and a macrolide has a survival advantage compared with quinolones alone in patients in the ICU, and in the 1 prospective study that compared quinolone monotherapy with a β-lactam/quinolone combination therapy the monotherapy arm was not as effective.[65] In addition, in patients with pneumococcal bacteremia, especially in those with severe illness, the use of dual therapy (usually by adding a macrolide to a β-lactam) is associated with better outcome than with monotherapy, implying benefit from atypical pathogen coverage or from the antiinflammatory effect of the macrolide.[64] In a prospective study by Rodriguez and colleagues[66] on 279 patients with CAP and shock requiring vasopressors, combination therapy with either a β-lactam and a macrolide or a β-lactam and a quinolone had a 28-day survival advantage compared with monotherapy with a β-lactam or a quinolone alone.

Based on these data, in patients in the ICU, an intravenous β-lactam plus either a macrolide or respiratory fluoroquinolone is recommended for patients without pseudomonal risk factors. In patients with risk factors for pseudomonal infection, an antipseudomonal β-lactam should be combined with either levofloxacin or ciprofloxacin, or the antipseudomonal β-lactam can be combined with both an aminoglycoside and either azithromycin or a respiratory quinolone. In patients allergic to penicillin, a respiratory fluoroquinolone should be used with aztreonam as an alternative regimen. When CA-MRSA is suspected, vancomycin or linezolid should be added to the other recommended agents. However, it may be necessary to add an anti–toxin producing agent, because part of the illness caused by CA-MRSA is mediated by bacterial exotoxin production. To stop toxin production, it may be necessary to add clindamycin to vancomycin, or to use linezolid alone.

Duration of Therapy

Outpatients with mild-to-moderate CAP are treated for 7 days or fewer with oral antibiotics, and therapy is stopped if they are afebrile and clinical features of pneumonia are resolving (cough, dyspnea, and sputum production). For inpatients, antibiotics are switched from intravenous to oral once the patient is afebrile for at least 2 occasions 8 hours apart, is able to take food by mouth, and there are clinical signs of improvement (in parameters such as cough, dyspnea, sputum production, oxygenation, and vital sign abnormalities), and this usually happens by the second or third hospital day. The switch to oral antibiotics can also be done for bacteremic patients, although it may take longer for these patients to reach clinical stability compared with nonbacteremic patients.[67] Use of PCT as a guide to decide on the duration of antibiotic use is supported by clinical trial data.[46] The duration of therapy should be a minimum of 5 days, providing that the patient is afebrile for 48 to 72 hours, there is no sign of extrapulmonary infection, the correct therapy was used initially, and the organism identified is not *S aureus* or *P aeruginosa*.

Complications

With appropriate antibiotic treatment, most cases of CAP resolve without complications. However, the treating physician should be alert to potential complications that, if not detected early, can lead to adverse outcomes. If the patient is responding well to therapy, no immediate follow-up radiograph is needed, and imaging is only done 4 to 6 weeks after discharge to define a new radiographic baseline. In most patients, the chest radiograph usually clears within 4 weeks, especially in patients younger than 50 years without underlying pulmonary disease or bacteremia. However, resolution may be delayed for 12 weeks or longer in older individuals and those with underlying lung disease and bacteremia.

Treatment Failure

In about 15% of patients, there is a lack of response or clinical deterioration despite antibiotic therapy. The IDSA/ATS guidelines define early failure as progressive pneumonia or clinical deterioration, occurring in the first 72 hours of therapy, usually with respiratory failure or septic shock, and is a consequence of inappropriate antibiotic therapy or an incorrect initial diagnosis. Later failure or nonresponse is often caused by a nosocomial infection, a disease-related or therapy complication, or a noninfectious process (eg, pulmonary embolism, inflammatory lung disease).

If the patient has persistent fever, worsening dyspnea, unresolving pneumonia symptoms, and continued debility, a repeat radiograph should be done focusing on a broad differential diagnosis, including therapy for an unusual or drug-resistant pathogen (tuberculosis, endemic fungus, or a zoonosis), a pneumonic complication (empyema), an antibiotic complication (drug-induced colitis) or a nonpneumonic diagnosis (inflammatory lung disease, malignancy). Diagnostic testing can include a chest CT scan, bronchoscopy, and, in some cases, open lung biopsy. Organizing pneumonia is a complication of viral lung infection and other processes, and is characterized by fibroblast proliferation and diagnosed by a combination of radiographic findings, bronchoscopic lung biopsy, and the absence of ongoing infection. It is often managed with a therapeutic trial of steroids. The definitive investigation is an open lung biopsy.

Parapneumonic effusion and empyema are complications that can lead to apparent treatment failure. The chest radiograph shows an effusion, which should be sampled, and, if a low pleural fluid pH is present (<7.2 if previously healthy, but <7.3 if chronically ill) or if organisms are present, chest tube drainage and prolonged antibiotic therapy is required. A connection between the pleural space and the lung can develop and result in a bronchopleural fistula, which can be caused by erosion of the lung infection to the pleural surface. Bronchopleural fistula is initially treated conservatively with antibiotics and a chest tube, but sometimes requires surgical repair. Localized bronchiectasis can be a long-term sequela of CAP, as a result of injury and dilation of the bronchus, and can be seen on CT scan of the chest. Patients present with chronic productive sputum and recurrent infection on the same area. Treatment is with postural drainage, antibiotics for exacerbation, and bronchodilators for coexisting airflow obstruction.

Recurrent pneumonia can occur after clinical and radiographic resolution of pneumonia. If it is present, whether it is in the same or a different area as the original infection should be determined. If it is in the same area, an anatomic problem (obstruction by tumor or foreign body) needs to be considered, whereas, if it is at another site, it may be the consequence of general immune impairment. The risk of this problem is higher in the elderly, those with a history of alcoholism, and in smokers. An underlying systemic immune deficiency should be ruled out by measuring quantitative Ig levels.

PREVENTION

A detailed discussion of prevention is beyond the scope of this article. In the IDSA/ATS guidelines, the mainstay of prevention is pneumococcal and influenza vaccination for at-risk individuals, and provision of smoking cessation information to those smoking cigarettes at the time of pneumonia onset.[1] Influenza vaccine is recommended during the appropriate season, for all persons aged 50 years or older, and for those with specific risk factors, including pregnant women and those with chronic heart, lung, metabolic, hematologic, or immune-compromising illnesses. Pneumococcal polysaccharide vaccine should be given to all patients aged 65 years or older, and to younger patients with chronic heart or lung disease, asplenia, diabetes mellitus, and to residents of long-term care facilities. One revaccination after 5 years should be given to those with either a poor immune response or after age 65 years for those first immunized before the age of 65 years. In guidelines, and also in performance measures for hospitalized patients, vaccination should be given before discharge for all patients admitted with CAP.

REFERENCES

1. Mandell LA, Wunderink RG, Anzueto A, et al. Infectious Diseases Society of America/American Thoracic Society consensus guidelines on the management of community-acquired pneumonia in adults. Clin Infect Dis 2007;44:S2–27.
2. Brar NK, Niederman MS. Management of community-acquired pneumonia: a review and update. Ther Adv Respir Dis 2011;5:61–78.
3. Kochanek KD, Xu J, Murphy SL, et al. Deaths: Preliminary data for 2009. National Vital Statistics Reports 59, No. 4.CDC 2011. Available at: http://www.cdc.gov/nchs/data/nvsr/nvsr59/nvsr59_04.pdf. Accessed 30, June 2011.
4. Heron MP, Hoyert DL, Murphy SL, et al. Deaths: Final data for 2006. National Vital Statistics Reports 57. National Center for Health Statistics2009. Available at: http://www.cdc.gov/nchs/fastats/pneumonia.htm. Accessed 10, July 2011.
5. Fine MJ, Smith MA, Carson CA, et al. Prognosis and outcomes of patients with community-acquired pneumonia. A meta-analysis. JAMA 1996;275:134–41.
6. Welte T, Köhnlein T. Global and local epidemiology of community-acquired pneumonia: the experience of the CAPNETZ network. Semin Respir Crit Care Med 2009;30:127–35.
7. Kaplan V, Clermont G, Griffin MF, et al. Pneumonia: still the old man's friend? Arch Intern Med 2003;163:317–23.
8. File TM Jr, Marrie TJ. Burden of community-acquired pneumonia in North American adults. Postgrad Med 2010;122:130–41.
9. Kozma CM, Dickson M, Raut MK, et al. Economic benefit of a 1-day reduction in hospital stay for community-acquired pneumonia (CAP). J Med Econ 2010;13: 719–27.
10. Capelastegui A, Espana PP, Quintana JM, et al. Validation of a predictive rule for the management of community-acquired pneumonia. Eur Respir J 2006;27:151.
11. Aujesky D, Auble TE, Yealy DM, et al. Prospective comparison of three validated prediction rules for prognosis in community-acquired pneumonia. Am J Med 2005;118:384–92.
12. Niederman MS. Biological markers to determine eligibility in trials for community-acquired pneumonia: a focus on procalcitonin. Clin Infect Dis 2008;47:S127–32.

13. Wunderink RG, Waterer GW. Community-acquired pneumonia: pathophysiology and host factors with focus on possible new approaches to management of lower respiratory tract infections. Infect Dis Clin North Am 2004;18:743–59.

14. Sarkar M, Hennessy S, Yang YX. Proton-pump inhibitor use and the risk for community-acquired pneumonia. Ann Intern Med 2008;149:391–8.

15. Waterer GW, Bruns AH. Genetic risk of acute pulmonary infections and sepsis. Expert Rev Respir Med 2010;4:229–38.

16. Niederman MS, Ahmed QA. Inflammation in severe pneumonia: act locally, not globally. Crit Care Med 1999;27:2030–2.

17. Lieberman D. Atypical pathogens in community-acquired pneumonia. Clin Chest Med 1999;20:489–97.

18. Paganin F, Lilienthal F, Bourdin A, et al. Severe community-acquired pneumonia: assessment of microbial aetiology as mortality factor. Eur Respir J 2004;24:779–85.

19. Kang CI, Song JH, Oh WS, et al. Asian Network for Surveillance of Resistant Pathogens (ANSORP) Study Group. Clinical outcomes and risk factors of community-acquired pneumonia caused by gram-negative bacilli. Eur J Clin Microbiol Infect Dis 2008;27:657–61.

20. Boyer A, Amadeo B, Vargas F, et al. Severe community-acquired *Enterobacter* pneumonia: a plea for greater awareness of the concept of health-care-associated pneumonia. BMC Infect Dis 2011;11:120.

21. Arancibia F, Bauer TT, Ewig S, et al. Community-acquired pneumonia due to gram-negative bacteria and *Pseudomonas aeruginosa*: incidence, risk, and prognosis. Arch Intern Med 2002;162:1849–58.

22. de Roux A, Marcos MA, Garcia E, et al. Viral community-acquired pneumonia in non immunocompromised adults. Chest 2004;125:1343–51.

23. Niederman MS. In the clinic - community-acquired pneumonia. Ann Intern Med 2009;151:ITC1–14.

24. Lobo LJ, Reed KD, Wunderink RG. Expanded clinical presentation of community-acquired methicillin-resistant *Staphylococcus aureus* pneumonia. Chest 2010; 138:130–6.

25. Francis JS, Doherty MC, Lopatin U, et al. Severe community-onset pneumonia in healthy adults caused by methicillin-resistant *Staphylococcus aureus* carrying the Panton-Valentine leukocidin genes. Clin Infect Dis 2005;40:100–7.

26. Diep BA, Chambers HF, Graber CJ, et al. Emergence of multidrug-resistant, community associated, methicillin-resistant *Staphylococcus aureus* clone USA300 in men who have sex with men. Ann Intern Med 2008;148:249–57.

27. Torres A, Menendez R, Wunderink R. Infectious disease of lung. In: Mason RJ, Their SO, editors. Murray and Nadel's Textbook of Respiratory Medicine. [Chapter: Pyogenic Bacterial Pneumonia and Lung Abscess] vol. 1. 5th edition. Philadelphia: Saunders; 2010. p. 699–740.

28. Metlay JP, Kapoor WN, Fine MJ. Does this patient have community-acquired pneumonia? Diagnosing pneumonia by history and physical examination. JAMA 1997;278:1440–5.

29. Mandell LA, Marrie TJ, Grossman RF, et al. Canadian guidelines for the initial management of community-acquired pneumonia: an evidence-based update by the Canadian Infectious Diseases Society and the Canadian Thoracic Society. Clin Infect Dis 2000;31:383–421.

30. van der Eerden MM, Vlaspolder F, de Graaff CS, et al. Comparison between pathogen directed antibiotic treatment and empirical broad spectrum antibiotic treatment in patients with community acquired pneumonia: a prospective randomised study. Thorax 2005;60:672–8.

31. van der Eerden MM, Vlaspolder F, de Graaff CS, et al. Value of intensive diagnostic microbiological investigation in low- and high-risk patients with community-acquired pneumonia. Eur J Clin Microbiol Infect Dis 2005;24:241–9.

32. Mirsaeidi M, Peyrani P, Aliberti S, et al. Thrombocytopenia and thrombocytosis at time of hospitalization predict mortality in patients with community-acquired pneumonia. Chest 2010;137:416–20.

33. Nair V, Niederman MS, Masani N, et al. Hyponatremia in community-acquired pneumonia. Am J Nephrol 2007;27:184–90.

34. Hopstaken RM, Witbraad T, van Engelshoven JM, et al. Inter-observer variation in the interpretation of chest radiographs for pneumonia in community-acquired lower respiratory tract infections. Clin Radiol 2004;59:743–52.

35. Syrjälä H, Broas M, Suramo I, et al. High-resolution computed tomography for the diagnosis of community-acquired pneumonia. Clin Infect Dis 1998;27:358–63.

36. Metersky ML, Ma A, Bratzler DW, et al. Predicting bacteremia in patients with community-acquired pneumonia. Am J Respir Crit Care Med 2004;169:342–7.

37. Smith MD, Derrington P, Evans R, et al. Rapid diagnosis of bacteremic pneumococcal infections in adults by using the Binax NOW *Streptococcus pneumoniae* urinary antigen test: a prospective, controlled clinical evaluation. J Clin Microbiol 2003;41:2810–3.

38. Ortega L, Sierra M, Domínguez J, et al. Utility of a pneumonia severity index in the optimization of the diagnostic and therapeutic effort for community-acquired pneumonia. Scand J Infect Dis 2005;37:657–63.

39. Benin AL, Benson RF, Besser RE. Trends in legionnaire's disease, 1980-1998: declining mortality and new patterns of diagnosis. Clin Infect Dis 2002;35: 1039–46.

40. Sordé R, Falcó V, Lowak M, et al. Current and potential usefulness of pneumococcal urinary antigen detection in hospitalized patients with community-acquired pneumonia to guide antimicrobial therapy. Arch Intern Med 2011;171:166–72.

41. Krüger S, Ewig S, Giersdorf S, et al. Cardiovascular and inflammatory biomarkers to predict short- and long-term survival in community-acquired pneumonia: results from the German Competence Network, CAPNETZ. Am J Respir Crit Care Med 2010;182:1426–34.

42. Ramírez P, Ferrer M, Martí V, et al. Inflammatory biomarkers and prediction for intensive care unit admission in severe community-acquired pneumonia. Crit Care Med 2011. [Epub ahead of print]. PMID:21705887.

43. Almirall J, Bolíbar I, Toran P, et al. Contribution of C-reactive protein to the diagnosis and assessment of severity of community-acquired pneumonia. Chest 2004;125:1335–42.

44. Schuetz P, Suter-Widmer I, Chaudri A, et al. Procalcitonin-Guided Antibiotic Therapy and Hospitalisation in Patients with Lower Respiratory Tract Infections (ProHOSP) Study Group. Prognostic value of procalcitonin in community-acquired pneumonia. Eur Respir J 2011;37:384–92.

45. Müller F, Christ-Crain M, Bregenzer T, et al. Procalcitonin levels predict bacteremia in patients with community-acquired pneumonia: a prospective cohort trial. Chest 2010;138:121–9.

46. Christ-Crain M, Stolz D, Bingisser R, et al. Procalcitonin guidance of antibiotic therapy in community- acquired pneumonia: a randomized trial. Am J Respir Crit Care Med 2006;174:84–93.

47. Renaud B, Santin A, Coma E, et al. Association between timing of intensive care unit admission and outcomes for emergency department patients with community acquired pneumonia. Crit Care Med 2009;37:2867–74.

48. Restrepo MI, Mortensen EM, Rello J, et al. Late admission to the ICU in patients with community-acquired pneumonia is associated with higher mortality. Chest 2010;137:552–7.

49. Aujesky D, McCausland JB, Whittle J, et al. Reasons why emergency department providers do not rely on the Pneumonia Severity Index to determine the initial site of treatment for patients with pneumonia. Clin Infect Dis 2009;49: 100–8.

50. Fine MJ, Auble TE, Yealy DM, et al. A prediction rule to identify low-risk patients with community-acquired pneumonia. N Engl J Med 1997;336:243–50.

51. Valencia M, Badia JR, Cavalcanti M, et al. Pneumonia severity index class V patients with community-acquired pneumonia: characteristics, outcomes, and value of severity. Chest 2007;132:515–22.

52. Brito V, Niederman MS. Predicting mortality in the elderly with community-acquired pneumonia: should we design a new car or set a new 'speed limit'? Thorax 2010;65:944–5.

53. Bauer TT, Ewig S, Marre R, et al. CRB-65 predicts death from community-acquired pneumonia. J Intern Med 2006;260:93–101.

54. Blot SI, Rodriguez A, Solé-Violán J, et al. Effects of delayed oxygenation assessment on time to antibiotic delivery and mortality in patients with severe community-acquired pneumonia. Crit Care Med 2007;35:2509–14.

55. Huang DT, Weissfeld LA, Kellum JA, et al. Risk prediction with procalcitonin and clinical rules in community-acquired pneumonia. Ann Emerg Med 2008;52: 48–58.

56. Kruger S, Ewig S, Marre R, et al. Procalcitonin predicts patients at low risk of death from community acquired pneumonia across all CRB-65 classes. Eur Respir J 2008;31:349–55.

57. Liapikou A, Ferrer M, Polverino E, et al. Severe community-acquired pneumonia: validation of the Infectious Diseases Society of America/American Thoracic Society guidelines to predict an intensive care unit admission. Clin Infect Dis 2009;48:377–85.

58. Brown SM, Jones BE, Jephson AR, et al. Validation of the Infectious Disease Society of America/American Thoracic Society 2007 guidelines for severe community-acquired pneumonia. Crit Care Med 2009;37:3010–6.

59. Rello J, Rodriguez A, Lisboa T, et al. PIRO score for community-acquired pneumonia: a new prediction rule for assessment of severity in intensive care unit patients with community-acquired pneumonia. Crit Care Med 2009; 37:456–62.

60. Charles PG, Wolfe R, Whitby M, et al. SMART-COP: a tool for predicting the need for intensive respiratory or vasopressor support in community-acquired pneumonia. Clin Infect Dis 2008;47:375–84.

61. Houck PM, Bratzler DW, Nsa W, et al. Timing of antibiotic administration and outcomes for Medicare patients hospitalized with community-acquired pneumonia. Arch Intern Med 2004;164:637–44.

62. Meehan TP, Fine MJ, Krumholz HM, et al. Quality of care, process, and outcomes in elderly patients with pneumonia. JAMA 1997;278:2080–4.

63. Metersky ML, Ma A, Houck PM, et al. Antibiotics for bacteremic pneumonia: improved outcomes with macrolides but not fluoroquinolones. Chest 2007;131: 466–73.

64. Baddour LM, Yu VL, Klugman KP, et al. Combination antibiotic therapy lowers mortality among severely ill patients with pneumococcal bacteremia. Am J Respir Crit Care Med 2004;170:440–4.

65. Leroy O, Saux P, Bédos JP, et al. Comparison of levofloxacin and cefotaxime combined with ofloxacin for ICU patients with community-acquired pneumonia who do not require vasopressors. Chest 2005;128:172–83.
66. Rodríguez A, Mendia A, Sirvent JM, et al. Combination antibiotic therapy improves survival in patients with community-acquired pneumonia and shock. Crit Care Med 2007;35:1493–8.
67. Ramirez JA, Bordon J. Early switch from intravenous to oral antibiotics in hospitalized patients with bacteremic community-acquired *Streptococcus pneumoniae* pneumonia. Arch Intern Med 2001;161:848–50.

Eosinophilic Lung Diseases

Evans R. Fernández Pérez, MD, MS[a,*],
Amy L. Olson, MD, MSPH[b,d], Stephen K. Frankel, MD[c,d]

KEYWORDS

- Eosinophilic pneumonia • Eosinophils
- Eosinophilic lung disease • Churg-Strauss syndrome
- Allergic bronchopulmonary aspergillosis
- Hypereosinophilic syndrome

The eosinophilic lung diseases consist of a heterogeneous group of disorders characterized by an increased numbers of eosinophils in 1 or more compartments of the lung, radiographic abnormalities, or impaired pulmonary function, and commonly, but not universally, peripheral blood eosinophilia. These disorders may be idiopathic in nature, or the result of a well-defined disease process. Disease severity in these entities can vary from clinically silent disease noted incidentally on radiologic imaging to life-threatening disease. Accurate diagnosis is essential to optimizing patient outcomes but remains challenging. Signs and symptoms frequently overlap among the disorders, and because these disorders are infrequent, expertise is difficult to acquire. Still, these disorders are not rare, and most clinicians periodically encounter patients with one or more of the eosinophilic lung diseases and need to understand how to recognize, diagnose, and manage these diseases. This review focuses on the clinical features, general diagnostic workup, and management of the eosinophilic lung diseases.

CLASSIFICATION OF EOSINOPHILIC LUNG DISEASES

Eosinophilic lung diseases may be divided into primary disorders and secondary disorders (**Fig. 1**). The secondary disorders include those conditions in which the

Financial Disclosure: the authors have no relevant financial disclosures.
[a] Interstitial Lung Disease Program, Autoimmune Lung Center, National Jewish Health, G-010, 1400 Jackson Street, Denver, CO 80206, USA
[b] Interstitial Lung Disease Program, Autoimmune Lung Center, National Jewish Health, F-107, 1400 Jackson Street, Denver, CO 80206, USA
[c] Interstitial Lung Disease Program, Autoimmune Lung Center, National Jewish Health, G-012, 1400 Jackson Street, Denver, CO 80206, USA
[d] Division of Pulmonary Sciences & Critical Care Medicine, University of Colorado Denver, 12700 East, 19th Avenue, Aurora, CO 80045, USA
* Corresponding author.
E-mail address: fernandezevans@njhealth.org

Med Clin N Am 95 (2011) 1163–1187
doi:10.1016/j.mcna.2011.08.006
0025-7125/11/$ – see front matter © 2011 Elsevier Inc. All rights reserved.

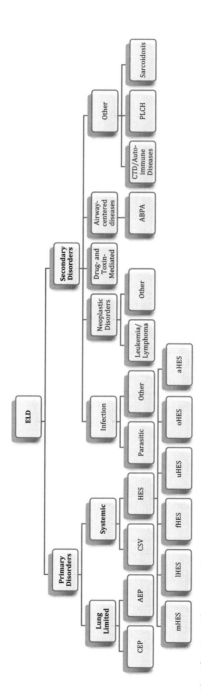

Fig. 1. Classification of eosinophilic lung diseases. aHES, associated variant hypereosinophilic syndrome; CSV, Churg-Strauss vasculitis; CTD, connective tissue disease; ELD, eosinophilic lung disease; fHES, familial variant hypereosinophilic syndrome; IHES, lymphocytic variant hypereosinophilic syndrome; mHES, myeloproliferative variant hypereosinophilic syndrome; oHES, overlap variant hypereosinophilic syndrome; PLCH, pulmonary Langerhans cell histiocytosis. uHES, undefined variant hypereosinophilic syndrome (benign and complex subtypes).

eosinophilia is believed to result from an identifiable, well-defined underlying cause or predisposition.[1] Secondary disorders are more common than primary disorders, and need to be definitively excluded before a primary disorder diagnosis is settled on. Examples of secondary disorders include infections (parasitic, fungal, mycobacterial, bacterial, and viral), drug/medication reactions, inhalant exposure (eg, crack cocaine), allergic bronchopulmonary aspergillosis (ABPA), primary connective tissue disease (eg, rheumatoid arthritis-related eosinophilic pneumonia), and primary malignancy (leukemias, lymphomas, myelodysplastic disorders, and lung carcinoma).

The primary eosinophilic diseases are commonly subdivided into organ-specific disorders and systemic disorders. Lung-limited entities include idiopathic chronic eosinophilic pneumonia (CEP) and idiopathic acute eosinophilic pneumonia (AEP), whereas systemic disorders include Churg-Strauss syndrome (CSS) and the hypereosinophilic syndromes (HES).[1]

DIAGNOSTIC EVALUATION
Clinical Assessment

Once clinical suspicion for an eosinophilic lung disease is aroused, generally by the concurrent findings of pulmonary impairment or radiographic abnormalities plus increased numbers of eosinophils in the peripheral blood or lung tissue, the clinician embarks on a diagnostic evaluation directed toward making a more specific diagnosis (**Fig. 2**).[1] An in-depth medical history should include a detailed characterization of the clinical course, extent, and severity of the presenting disease course; a complete medication history (including not only current medications but previous medication history as well as supplement and nutraceutical use and illicit drug use); complete occupational and travel histories; and a detailed history of the patient's preexisting chronic medical conditions and immune status. In addition, a comprehensive review of systems is required to investigate all extrapulmonary signs and symptoms. Similarly, a comprehensive physical examination is crucial to identify all the potential manifestations (pulmonary and extrapulmonary) of the underlying disorder. For example, the identification of peripheral nervous system deficits consistent with mononeuritis multiplex may lead one toward a diagnosis of CSS, whereas findings of erythema nodosum and arthritis (Löfgren syndrome) argue for sarcoidosis.

Review of previous medical records may be of vital importance in uncovering the cause of the eosinophilic lung disease, particularly in those cases in which there is a protracted clinical course. In addition, previous documentation helps to provide objective baseline data, such as pulmonary physiology and imaging results, as well as highlighting the temporal relationships between potential exposures and the development of the eosinophilic lung disease.

The search for causation can be challenging. The diagnosis may remain elusive, particularly in the earlier stages of the disease. Signs and symptoms tend to be nonspecific and overlap among the various eosinophilic lung diseases. For example, if the clinician confirms a constellation of findings consisting of asthma, peripheral eosinophilia, constitutional symptoms (fatigue, malaise), chronic rhinosinusitis, and parenchymal pulmonary infiltrates on imaging, the differential diagnosis still includes CSS, idiopathic CEP (ICEP), ABPA, infectious causes of eosinophilic lung disease, drug/medication-induced eosinophilic lung disease, and undefined HES, because these findings are common to all of these disease states. Another common confounder to diagnosis is the use of empiric corticosteroids that nonspecifically ameliorates many of the signs and symptoms of eosinophilic lung disease and improves or resolves the peripheral or pulmonary eosinophilia before a definitive diagnosis being made.

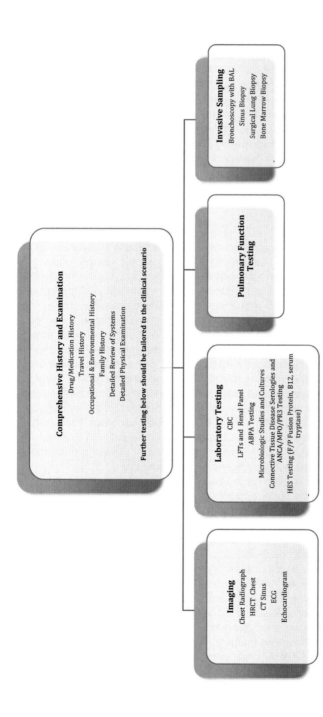

Fig. 2. Diagnostic approach to suspected eosinophilic lung disease. A multidisciplinary approach (eg, radiology, pathology) and appropriate subspecialty consultation as indicated by clinical presentation (eg, rheumatology, infectious disease, hematology-oncology) is recommended. ANCA, antineutrophilic cytoplasmic antibody; BAL, bronchoalveolar lavage; CBC, complete blood count; ECG, electrocardiogram; LFT, liver function test; MPO, myeloperoxidase; PR3, proteinase 3.

Recognizing the challenges surrounding the diagnosis and management of the eosinophilic lung disorders, the benefits of close collaboration among providers, and the importance of a multidisciplinary team approach cannot be overemphasized. Such an approach significantly facilitates the evaluation, diagnosis, and treatment of these conditions.

Laboratory Testing

The laboratory evaluation begins with a complete blood count and circulating eosinophil level count. A circulating eosinophil count greater than 400 cells/mm is abnormal and qualifies as eosinophilia. The terms high-grade eosinophilia or hypereosinophilia indicate a circulating eosinophil count exceeding 1500 cells/mm.[1] It is this finding of peripheral eosinophilia or hypereosinophilia that prompts further diagnostic evaluation.

Additional laboratory assessment, like the clinical evaluation, should be targeted toward assisting with the diagnosis and documenting the full extent of end-organ involvement and injury. Hence, screening for anemia, renal dysfunction, microscopic hematuria, and abnormal liver function tests is appropriate. Hypergammaglobulinemia, an increased erythrocyte sedimentation rate and an increased C-reactive protein level are all common abnormalities, but nonspecific. An increased total IgE level (>100 units/mL) is also common to many of the eosinophilic lung diseases; however, an IgE level greater than 1000 units/mL is more specific for entities such as ABPA, tropical pulmonary eosinophilia (TPE), and hyperimmunoglobulin E syndromes.

Microbiologic testing should be pursued based on clinical suspicion, taking into account the clinical presentation and the environmental and travel histories. Components of the evaluation may include sputum, urine, stool or blood cultures, stool sample for ova and parasites evaluation, and serologic assessments for evidence of parasitic infection (eg, strongyloidiasis, schistosomiasis.) Consultation with an infectious disease specialist is frequently beneficial in addressing potential infectious causes, especially in those patients with significant travel-related exposures.

Eosinophilic pneumonias in association with a primary rheumatologic condition commonly present once other clinical features of the rheumatologic disorder are established. However, in rare cases, pulmonary disease may occur before extrathoracic manifestations become apparent. Thus, the presence of autoantibodies may indicate an underlying collagen vascular disease or autoimmune disease. The choice of serologic testing must be driven by the clinical presentation, but in general terms, antineutrophilic cytoplasmic antibodies (ANCAs) along with antimyeloperoxidase antibodies and antiproteinase 3 antibodies as measured by enzyme-linked immunosorbent assay testing are often obtained to assess for serologic evidence of Churg-Strauss vasculitis. Similarly, antinuclear antibodies (titer, pattern, and profile), anti-dsDNA, anticyclic citrulinated peptide antibodies, rheumatoid factor, anti-Scl-70 (topoisomerase), anti-Ro/SS-A, and anti-La/SS-B antibodies may also be obtained in those cases in which there is a clinical suspicion for a primary connective tissue disease.

Laboratory testing for primary hypereosinophilic syndromes generally includes a serum mast cell tryptase level test to evaluate for systemic mastocytosis and myeloproliferative HES (mHES), along with a serum vitamin B_{12} concentration test for possible mHES.[2,3] FIP1-like protein (FIP1L1) and the platelet-derived growth factor receptor α (PDGFR&alpha) fusion protein (F/P) analysis by fluorescence in situ hybridization (FISH) or reverses transciptase-polymerase chain reaction (RT-PCR) is used to evaluate for F/P-positive mHES (see later discussion) and may be performed on a peripheral blood sample or bone marrow biopsy.[1]

An electrocardiogram and echocardiogram should be used to evaluate for cardiac involvement, which contributes heavily to the morbidity and mortality of CSS and HES. Pulmonary function testing rarely leads to a specific diagnosis but is useful in quantifying pulmonary impairment, in addition to monitoring disease progression and response to therapy.

Radiologic Evaluation

Imaging plays an integral role in the evaluation of the eosinophilic lung diseases. If the chest radiograph is abnormal, this may be the only modality required; however, high-resolution computed tomography (HRCT) of the chest is more sensitive than plain radiograph and provides valuable diagnostic insight in that it permits a more detailed characterization of the parenchymal abnormalities. Additional benefits of HRCT imaging may include the detection of nonparenchymal abnormalities (mediastinal lymphadenopathy, airways disease, or pleural or esophageal disease), prognostic information (eg, fibrotic changes as opposed to pure ground-glass attenuation), and the identification of an optimal location for bronchoalveolar lavage (BAL) or biopsy. Examples of characteristic HRCT patterns include middle and upper lobe predominant peripheral consolidation, also known as the photographic negative pulmonary edema seen in some patients with CEP,[4] or the concomitant findings of bronchiectasis, mucous plugging, atelectasis, and areas of airspace consolidation/ground-glass attenuation in an upper and central lung zone predominant pattern characteristic of ABPA. If one identifies these findings on HRCT it is possible to distinguish these entities from other eosinophilic lung diseases in about 80% of cases.[5]

Imaging of other potential target organs, including sinuses, heart, and upper abdomen, may be helpful in specific cases. Sinus CT is commonly performed in patients with clinical evidence of sinus disease to characterize the pattern and extent of disease. Plain radiographs of the hands may be obtained to evaluate for the presence of an erosive arthropathy in those patients in whom a primary rheumatologic diagnosis is entertained. Abdominal ultrasonography or CT should be obtained when considering infectious causes of eosinophilia such as amebic liver abscess or echinococcal cysts, and also when screening for hepatosplenomegaly in patients with clinical HES. Cardiac magnetic resonance imaging (cMRI) for myocardial disease in CSS remains investigational, but may be performed in some centers with cMRI expertise.[6] Similarly, positron emission tomography using [^{18}F]fluoro-2-deoxy-D-glucose may be used in the evaluation of pulmonary and extrathoracic organ involvement in a subset of patients in whom malignancy is suspected.

Invasive Testing and Histopathology

Bronchoscopy with BAL is often a critical element of the evaluation of eosinophilic lung disease. Specifically, (1) differential cell counts on a formal BAL permit an accurate assessment as to whether or not there is an eosinophilic alveolitis consistent with histopathologic eosinophilic pneumonia, and (2) BAL fluid evaluation permits a more thorough evaluation for infectious processes. In normal individuals, the BAL differential cell count shows only a few lymphocytes, neutrophils, and eosinophils (<1%). If the BAL has more than 25% eosinophils (and even more convincingly >40% eosinophils), then the patient by definition has pulmonary eosinophilia or eosinophilic alveolitis, which in turn correlates with the histopathologic finding of eosinophilic pneumonia. There are 2 major caveats to this statement. First, normal airways have large numbers of eosinophils such that small volume lavages or bronchial washings commonly show eosinophilia. In our experience, for the differential cell count to be informative, the bronchoscope must remain in wedge position as serial lavage is performed, and the lavage must use 3 to 4 instillations of 40 to 60 mL aliquots of saline (for a total volume of at least 120 mL, but no more than 240 mL), and achieve at least a 50% return volume.[7] Second, the finding of an eosinophilic alveolitis or the histo-pathologic finding of eosinophilic pneumonia may be seen with several of the eosino-philic lung diseases and represents a pathologic finding, not a clinical diagnosis. It is still up to the clinician to integrate this important finding with the larger clinical picture to achieve a final clinical diagnosis.

Transbronchial biopsy is useful in the diagnosis of peribronchovascular disease such as that found in sarcoidosis, lymphangitic carcinomatosis, and lymphoma, and in processes with airspace consolidation. However, small specimen size and sampling error are significant limitations, and in general, transbronchial biopsy tends to confirm the findings (or lack thereof) identified on lavage. Endobronchial biopsies are helpful if ulcerative or exophytic tracheobronchial lesions are identified during bronchoscopy, such as those found in sarcoidosis, malignancy, or granulomatosis with polyangitiis (Wegener granulomatosis).

Video-assisted thoracoscopic surgery remains the surgical procedure of choice when a diagnosis cannot be obtained by less invasive tests and procedures. In our experience this surgery is required in only a few patients.[1]

If a secondary cause for persistent high-grade eosinophilia cannot be found, and the patient does not meet criteria for reactive processes such as vasculitis, then evidence for a clonal expansion of eosinophils should be sought. Hematology-oncology consul-tation should be obtained and a bone marrow biopsy performed to exclude leukemia, lymphoma, myelodysplastic syndromes, and HES. An assessment for blasts, mast cells, and lymphocyte subpopulations should be performed, and conventional cytoge-netic, clonality, and flow cytometry studies are often required.[8,9]

PATHOLOGIC PATTERNS

Eosinophil longevity and survival are greater in peripheral tissues than in the circula-tion, and as a result, many eosinophils can be found in the lung even when the periph-eral blood count is low or normal, and this is the case in AEP.[10] In other cases, eosinophils are not a prominent component of the pulmonary cell infiltrate despite an increased blood eosinophil count. This scenario is frequently seen with malignan-cies. Any inflammatory eosinophilic reaction unrelated to host defense (ie, parasitic infection) is abnormal.[11] Although patients who smoke may have modest increases in pulmonary eosinophils, large numbers of eosinophils are unusual.[12,13]

The key histopathologic feature of eosinophilic pneumonia is the presence of eosin-ophils within the alveolar airspace (**Fig. 3**). Its appearance ranges from the simple presence of modest numbers of eosinophils in an otherwise normal lung to dense collections of eosinophils admixed with fibrin and macrophages and associated with architectural distortion. In addition, there may be significant infiltration and expan-sion of the alveolar septa by a mixture of eosinophils and other inflammatory cells. Focal collections of eosinophils and areas of organizing pneumonia may also be seen. The recognition of associated histopathologic features in the proper clinical scenario of eosinophilic pneumonia may have diagnostic significance. Examples include the finding of diffuse alveolar damage in a patient with acute onset disease (ie, idiopathic AEP), extensive intra-alveolar hemorrhage (Goodpasture syndrome),[14] or vasculitis with endothelial cell injury, eosinophilic abscess formation, and granulo-matous inflammation (CSS).[1,15] Still, it is worth reiterating that the finding of a histo-pathologic pattern of eosinophilic pneumonia frequently does not differentiate between eosinophilic lung disease considerations. Therefore, the clinical, physiologic,

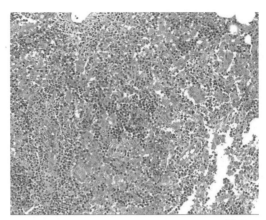

Fig. 3. Eosinophilic pneumonia. Histopathologic section of eosinophilic pneumonia showing airspaces filled with eosinophils, fibrin exudates, and macrophages. The adjacent septa are expanded by inflammation and show reactive pneumocyte hypertrophy.

radiographic, and laboratory findings must be integrated with the pathologic findings to make a specific diagnosis. A final caveat is that patients who received corticosteroid therapy before biopsy may have a paucity of eosinophils within the airspaces, thus producing patterns more similar to acute lung injury (ALI)/diffuse alveolar damage or organizing pneumonia, greatly complicating diagnosis.

SPECIFIC EOSINOPHILIC LUNG DISEASES
Secondary Disorders

ABPA

Aspergillus sp pulmonary infections can manifest with (1) a chronic necrotizing process, (2) aggressive angioinvasive disease (most notably in immunocompromised hosts), or (3) a more indolent, saprophytic process (aspergilloma). However, *Aspergillus* colonization of the airways can also result in ABPA, a hypersensitivity immune response to *Aspergillus* conidial or mycelial antigens.

Approximately 1% to 2% of patients with asthma and 2% to 15% of patients with cystic fibrosis develop ABPA.[16] More than 200 species of *Aspergillus* have been identified, and although ABPA is most commonly caused by *A fumigatus*, this identical hypersensitivity reaction has been described with other *Aspergillus* species as well as other fungal colonizers (and is then termed allergic bronchopulmonary mycosis). In susceptible hosts, the inhalation, colonization, and proliferation of *Aspergillus* in the airway leads to antigenic exposure within the tracheobronchial tree, and results in an intense CD4+ Th2-mediated eosinophilic inflammatory response, IgE, IgA, and IgG synthesis, and interleukin 8 (IL-8) mediated neutrophilic inflammation.[17] The clinical ABPA phenotype is influenced by host genetic susceptibility factors (eg, CFTR gene mutations, class II HLA-DR2/5 antigens),[18,19] host defense function, and underlying medical comorbidities, and organism virulence factors[20] such as the frequency and quantity of inhaled spores.[16]

Clinically, ABPA presents with severe, persistent asthma that is often steroid-dependent, chronic cough with expectoration of brown mucus plugs, constitutional symptoms (fatigue, malaise, weight loss, fever), recurrent, migratory pulmonary infiltrates, and cystic/varicoid bronchiectasis. ABPA preferentially affects persons in their third to fifth decades, but may be seen at any age. Chest CT frequently shows characteristic abnormalities in ABPA, with bronchiectasis being found in about 90% of cases (typically proximal in location, and varicose or cystic in type).[21,22] Peribronchial thickening, mucous plugging and impaction, migratory ground-glass opacities/consolidation, and bronchiolitis are common associated findings.[5,23,24]

In terms of confirming a diagnosis of ABPA, the Rosenberg-Patterson criteria[24,25] remain widely accepted (**Box 1**). Major diagnostic criteria include: (1) asthma, (2) radiographic infiltrates, (3) skin test positivity for *Aspergillus*, (4) peripheral eosinophilia, (5) positive serum precipitating antibodies to *Aspergillus*, (6) increased serum total IgE level (>1000 IU/mL), (7) increased *Aspergillus*-specific IgG and IgE, and (8) central bronchiectasis.[24,25] Minor criteria include: (1) *Aspergillus* in the sputum, (2) the expectoration of brown mucus plugs, and (3) a positive delayed skin test reaction to *Aspergillus*. A confident diagnosis of ABPA may be made when at least 6 of the major Rosenberg-Patterson criteria are present.

Early diagnosis and treatment of ABPA is critical to preventing progressive and debilitating lung disease. Whereas systemic corticosteroid therapy clearly represents the primary treatment of ABPA, the dose and duration of optimal corticosteroid therapy remain unknown. One large cohort study using high dosages for a prolonged period appeared to be associated with higher rates of sustained disease remission compared with other historic case series.[26] On the other hand, the risk of adverse side effects increases with higher dosages administered for longer durations. Therefore, efforts should be made to minimize the total cumulative dose to the necessary dose required to control the disease, and the prescribed doses of corticosteroids must be carefully tailored to clinical, physiologic, and radiographic response.[1] In addition, both high-dose inhaled corticosteroids and oral itraconazole have been

---

Box 1
Rosenberg-Patterson criteria for diagnosis of allergic bronchopulmonary *Aspergillus*

Major criteria

1. History of asthma

2. Radiographic pulmonary opacities

3. Immediate skin reactivity (positive skin testing) to *Aspergillus* antigen

4. Peripheral blood eosinophilia

5. Precipitating antibodies to *Aspergillus* antigen

6. Increased serum total IgE level

7. Increased *A fumigatus*-specific IgE and IgG antibodies

8. Central bronchiectasis

Minor criteria

1. *A fumigatus* in sputum

2. History of expectorating brown plugs

3. Delayed skin reactivity to *Aspergillus* antigen

The presence of 6 of 8 major criteria makes the diagnosis of ABPA nearly certain.

Data from Patterson R, Greenberger PA, Halwig JM, et al. Allergic bronchopulmonary aspergillosis. Natural history and classification of early disease by serologic and roentgenographic studies. Arch Intern Med 1986;146(5):916–8; and Agarwal R, Gupta D, Aggarwal AN, et al. Allergic bronchopulmonary aspergillosis: lessons from 126 patients attending a chest clinic in north India. Chest 2006;130(2):442–8.

associated with reduced oral corticosteroid requirements.[27–32] A systematic review reported that the use of itraconazole, in addition to reducing corticosteroid dose, modifies the immunologic activation associated with ABPA and improves clinical outcomes.[33] Thus, itraconazole and high-dose inhaled corticosteroids should be strongly considered when treating corticosteroid-dependent ABPA patients and those with frequent exacerbations.

Anti-IgE monoclonal antibody therapy has been considered as a potential therapy for ABPA based on biologic plausibility, but no controlled studies of anti-IgE monoclonal antibody therapy have been reported in children or adults with ABPA. Although anti-IgE has been shown to improve respiratory function and reduce glucocorticoid administration in pediatric patients with ABPA with cystic fibrosis at the case report level, this therapy warrants further evaluation in a randomized, controlled trial.[32,34,35]

The nonpharmacologic management of ABPA centers on close patient follow-up with regular monitoring of the total serum IgE level, blood eosinophil count, pulmonary function tests, and imaging studies; airway clearance techniques; pulmonary rehabilitation/regular exercise program to achieve and maintain musculoskeletal conditioning; appropriate vaccination; and the treatment of comorbid conditions. Moreover, given the frequent requirement for prolonged or repeated therapy with oral corticosteroids, screening (eg, periodic electrolytes and bone mineral density testing), prevention (eg, bone mineral preserving therapies), and treatment of glucocorticoid side effects (eg, diabetes) is recommended.

Infectious diseases

Infections, and especially parasitic infections, represent a major cause of eosinophilic lung disease. Infectious causes are often suggested by travel history, but not necessarily so, because the travel history may be remote to the onset of illness (eg, TPE). Fungi may cause pulmonary eosinophilia through direct infection of pulmonary tissue (eg, *Coccidioides*, *Blastomyces*, *Histoplasma*, *Paracoccidioides*) or by triggering an immunologic reaction when fungal antigens are inhaled (eg, ABPA). Also, yeastlike fungal infections (*Pneumocystiis jiroveci*)[36] and viral infections (respiratory syncytial virus)[37] have been associated with eosinophilic pneumonia. Pulmonary disease associated with peripheral eosinophilia may be seen with a wide variety of infectious agents including bacteria, viral infections, mycobacterial pulmonary infections, and fungi.

Parasitic infections are common worldwide, especially in the tropical and subtropical regions. Parasitic pulmonary infections may be divided into those caused by protozoans and those cause by helminths. *Entamoeba histolytica* is spread by the fecal-oral route and is more common in areas with poor sanitation. Pulmonary involvement by *E histolytica* occurs mainly by extension from an amebic liver abscess (hepatopulmonary amebiasis).[38] Metronidazole is the mainstay of treatment.

In its broadest sense, simple pulmonary eosinophilia (also known as Löffler syndrome) is an acute, transient, and often mild hypersensitivity response to parasitic infections or medications/drugs characterized by migratory pulmonary infiltrates and eosinophilia (PIE syndrome). More narrowly, Löffler syndrome has generally been associated with intestinal (*Ascaris*, *Strongyloides*, *Trichinella*, *Ancylostoma*, and *Necator*) and tissue (*Toxocara*) roundworm infections, especially *Ascaris*, because *Ascaris* is the most prevalent roundworm infection worldwide, and hence, the most common parasitic cause of simple pulmonary eosinophilia. Infection is spread by ingestion of eggs from contaminated soil or food. Patients may be asymptomatic, or may present with a constellation of constitutional symptoms (fatigue, fever, night sweats, weight loss), dyspnea, or wheezing. Stool ova and parasite evaluation often confirms the diagnosis, albeit 6 to 12 weeks after the initial infection. At the time of pulmonary symptoms, larvae may be identified in the sputum or on gastric aspirate. Mebendazole is the treatment of choice.

TPE is caused by the host response to the mosquito-borne filarial parasites *Wuchereria bancrofti* and *Brugia malayi*.[39] In contrast to simple pulmonary eosinophilia, most patients are symptomatic with fever, fatigue, malaise, anorexia, weight loss, paroxysmal nocturnal cough, and breathlessness. However, clinical disease may not develop until months or years after the initial infection, greatly complicating diagnosis. Hypereosinophilia and markedly increased IgE levels (>1000 U/mL) are common in TPE. Chest imaging may show reticulonodular, interstitial infiltrates, but is variable, and may even be normal. TPE is commonly treated with diethylcarbamazine.

Drug-induced and toxin-induced eosinophilic lung disease

Illicit,[40] over-the-counter, and prescribed drugs as well as herbal remedies,[41] radiation,[42] environmental, and occupational inhalational exposures[43] have been associated with eosinophilic lung diseases. As the number of available drugs and medications expands, so does the incidence of drug-induced lung diseases. More than 120 medications have been associated with eosinophilic lung disease. An updated list can be found at http://www.pneumotox.com, a Web site database maintained by the Groupe d'Etudes de la Pathologie Pulmonaire Iatrogêne, which regularly updates thousands of bibliographical references of drug-induced lung diseases. Antibiotics and nonsteroidal antiinflammatory drugs are the most common causative agents.[44] Other classes of drugs implicated in eosinophilic lung disease are outlined in **Table 1**.[45]

Drug-induced lung disease findings on histopathology and on high-resolution CT can resemble essentially any of the patterns described in the interstitial lung diseases,

Table 1
Drugs and medications associated with eosinophilic lung disease

Antibiotics	Anticonvulsants	Illicit drug
β-Lactams	Carbamazepine	Cocaine
Tetracyclines	Phenytoin	Heroin
Sulfa agents		
Nitrofurantoin		
Isoniazid		
Ethambutol		
Pentamidine		
Sulfonamides		
Nonsteroidal antiinflammatory	Antidepressants	Chemotherapeutics
drugs	Amitriptyline	Bleomycin
Ibuprofen	Trazadone	Camptothecin
Indomethacine	Venlafaxine	
Naproxen		
Diclofenac		
Sulindac		
Piroxicam		
Cardiovascular	Biologics	Nutraceuticals
Angiotensin-converting	Infliximab	L-Tryptophan
enzyme inhibitors	Interferon alpha	
Amiodarone	Granulocyte-macrophage	
β-blockers	colony stimulating factor	

Data from Solomon J, Schwarz M. Drug-, toxin-, and radiation therapy-induced eosinophilic pneumonia. Semin Respir Crit Care Med. 2006;27(2):192–7; and Frankel SK. Drug-induced lung disease. In: Hanley M, Welsh C, editors. Current diagnosis and treatment in pulmonary medicine. New York: Lange Medical Bools/McGraw-Hill; 2003. p. 337–47.

including desquamative interstitial pneumonia, diffuse alveolar damage, alveolar hemorrhage, hypersensitivity pneumonitis, nonspecific interstitial pneumonia, organizing pneumonia, and eosinophilic pneumonia. Drug-related eosinophilic lung manifestations are remarkably common and varied, and may range from subclinical transient fleeting infiltrates (Löffler syndrome, the most common clinical presentation) to more pronounced presentations characterized by nonspecific constitutional symptoms, cough, dyspnea, and ground-glass infiltrates, and histopathologic findings of CEP. Drug-induced AEP may occur and present with life-threatening respiratory failure.[46–49]

The diagnosis of drug-induced eosinophilic lung disease rests on the temporal association with a potential candidate agent or toxin and the development of disease. This relationship may be confirmed when prompt cessation of the offending agent leads to rapid improvement. In patients with significant symptoms or pulmonary impairment, systemic corticosteroids are often required, especially in those cases that do not resolve quickly and spontaneously, and in those patients who present with fulminant disease, especially those with respiratory distress/failure.

Neoplastic disorders

Eosinophilic lung diseases with or without peripheral blood eosinophilia may occur in the setting of malignancy as a result of opportunistic infections, as a side effect from chemotherapy or radiation therapy, as a host response to the neoplasm, or as a paraneoplastic manifestation. Peripheral blood eosinophilia results from the production of cytokines such as IL-3, IL-5, and granulocyte-macrophage colony stimulating factor that promote eosinophil differentiation and survival. An eosinophilic response may be seen with leukemia, lymphoma, acute graft versus host disease,[50] myelodysplastic disorders, systemic mastocytosis, and solid organ neoplasms including lung cancer.[50–53] In contrast to primary lung neoplasms or thoracic metastases of solid tumors, peripheral blood eosinophilia in blood and bone marrow malignancies is generally considered to be an ominous sign and important factor for determining disease-free survival.[54,55]

Primary Disorders

Lung-limited

ICEP ICEP is an uncommon interstitial lung disease. The true incidence and prevalence are unknown, but based on 2 registry studies, ICEP seems to represent approximately 1% to 2.5% of interstitial lung disease cases.[56,57] The gender distribution favors a female predominance in most series. No clear genetic predisposition exists, but patients frequently have a previous history of asthma or other atopic disease. The relationship between asthma and ICEP is not well understood. Although both entities share similar inflammatory responses and cytokine/chemokine profiles, the precise mechanisms that produce pulmonary parenchymal eosinophilic inflammation in ICEP compared with those associated with asthma alone await further research.[58,59]

Clinical manifestations of ICEP include cough, dyspnea on exertion, exercise intolerance, and systemic symptoms such as fever, chills, night sweats, anorexia, and malaise that evolve insidiously over weeks to months. Chest auscultation may reveal wheeze, consolidative findings, or crackles, but the remainder of the physical examination is largely unremarkable. Signs of pulmonary hypertension as a result of pulmonary fibrosis may be present in advanced cases.

Frequent laboratory findings include peripheral blood eosinophilia or hypereosinophilia, increased inflammatory markers, and increased total IgE levels.[60] Chest films commonly reveal migratory, patchy, bilateral, peripheral-predominant, ground-glass, or consolidative infiltrates. Shadows parallel to the pleural surface (ie, the photoneg-ative pulmonary edema) are virtually pathognomonic[61]; however, this imaging pattern is found in fewer than 25% of patients with CEP.[62] Progressive interstitial changes, including reticular infiltrates and honeycombing, consistent with pulmonary fibrosis have been described.[63] Pulmonary function testing is nonspecific and may show obstructive, restrictive, or mixed patterns of disease, or may be normal. BAL eosino-philia greater than 25% is characteristic in treatment-naive patients. This finding in the correct clinical scenario, and in the absence of alternative diagnostic considerations (ie, drug-induced and infectious causes have been excluded) can obviate a surgical lung biopsy. If a biopsy is performed, histopathologic specimens show an inflamma-tory and eosinophilic cellular infiltrate involving the interstitium and filling the alveolar space. Occasionally, areas of organizing pneumonia can be seen.[62]

The natural history of ICEP is unpredictable at the time of the diagnosis. Some patients may resolve their disease after an initial course of corticosteroid therapy without further recurrence of the disease, whereas others may experience one or more episodes of disease relapse. Still others may have progressive disease despite therapy. It is unclear if these different natural histories represent distinct phenotypes of ICEP or if the natural history is influenced by other factors such as asthma. Among patients with ICEP, asthmatics may have a lower frequency of relapse than nonasth-matics, whereas the occurrence of ICEP in asthmatics is often associated with the development of more severe asthma.[64]

ICEP is typically exquisitely responsive to systemic corticosteroids. Rapid improve-ment in symptoms and radiographic infiltrates is often noted within days after the initi-ation of therapy. However, the disease commonly recurs after corticosteroid therapy is discontinued, and this is especially true for those patients for whom the steroid therapy is quickly tapered.[60–62,65] Steroid-resistant cases should raise the question of a competing diagnostic entity (eg, CSS). No randomized controlled trials have been conducted with corticosteroid monotherapy in ICEP. As with ABPA, the dose and duration of systemic corticosteroids need to be tailored to the severity of disease and individual circumstances. In general, we initiate therapy with 0.5 to 1 mg/kg/d of prednisone or equivalent followed by a gradual tapering over a period of 6 to 12 months. The duration of therapy can be extended beyond 12 months if the disease course is marked by relapses.[62] Screening for and prevention of corticosteroid-related adverse side effects is highly recommended (eg, osteoporosis, diabetes, elec-trolyte abnormalities, ophthalmologic complications). In addition, *Pneumocystis* prophylaxis should be consider for patients who are on high-dose corticosteroids (eg, $\geq$20 mg/d of prednisone or equivalent) for 1 month or longer or if used in combi-nation with another immunosuppressive drug. Steroid-sparing agents may be consid-ered on a case-by-case basis for remission maintenance in patients requiring chronic moderate-dose to high-dose oral corticosteroids (>15 mg/d of prednisone) in an attempt to limit steroid-related toxicity and in patients who develop unacceptable side effects with the doses necessary to control ICEP.[1] The addition of high-dose inhaled corticosteroids, especially in those with concomitant asthma, may reduce ICEP recurrence or total oral corticosteroid requirements.[1,64,66,67]

AEP AEP is a severe and acute illness that clinically resembles ALI/acute respiratory distress syndrome (ALI/ARDS). AEP is often indistinguishable from ALI/ARDS or severe community-acquired pneumonia at the time of initial presentation. However, unlike ALI/ARDS, AEP is rare, making diagnosis challenging. The predominant histologic feature of AEP is eosinophilic pneumonia, although elements of diffuse alveolar damage may also be seen in conjunction with the dominant eosinophilic process.

However, the most telling difference between AEP and ALI/ARDS is that AEP improves dramatically within hours of corticosteroid administration. Thus, the ability to make a prompt diagnosis has important implications for the management and outcome of this disease: AEP may be fatal if not recognized, but has excellent outcomes in most cases that are promptly diagnosed and treated. Therefore, early BAL showing an increased percentage in the total number of eosinophils (>25%) is of paramount importance in the early diagnosis of this disorder. In contrast to patients with ICEP, peripheral blood eosinophilia is usually not a prominent feature. Moreover, a history of asthma or atopy is unusual, and relapses of the idiopathic form of this disease are rare.[68,69]

A temporal relation has been reported between the development of AEP and several inciting factors such as heavy dust exposure,[43] drugs,[46,70] and several occupational exposures.[68,71] However, cigarette smoke is the most frequently implicated trigger in susceptible individuals.[68,69,72]

Patients with AEP typically present with the abrupt onset ($\leq$7 days) of cough, dyspnea, fatigue, malaise, myalgias, fever, chest discomfort, and ultimately hypoxemic respiratory failure, hence the difficulty distinguishing AEP from ALI/ARDS or severe community-acquired pneumonia. On auscultation, crackles are frequently audible although clear lungs have been reported.[1,68,71] Radiographically, the findings are indistinguishable from those of cardiogenic pulmonary edema or ARDS and include bilateral infiltrates (which may be patchy or asymmetric) and in some cases pleural effusions. In the absence of features to suggest cardiovascular dysfunction or other causes of ALI/ARDS, AEP should be suspected.[73]

Significant eosinophilia in BAL fluid is essential for the diagnosis. In the absence of alternative explanations, BAL eosinophilia can help provide a presumptive diagnosis on which to base treatment.[69] Biopsy is usually not necessary, but when obtained, reveals eosinophilic pneumonia with or without a component of acute or organizing diffuse alveolar damage.[1,74]

High-dose, intravenous corticosteroids (1 g/d in divided doses) typically produce rapid and dramatic improvement in clinical symptoms and radiographic abnormalities. Once disease activity is controlled, the corticosteroids may be transitioned to oral therapy. Corticosteroid taper may be performed over approximately a 3-month period, and resolution without recurrence after treatment is characteristic for this disorder.[1]

Primary Disorders, Systemic

CSS

CSS, first described by J. Churg and L. Strauss in 1951,[75] is a distinct clinicopathologic entity characterized by necrotizing vasculitis affecting small to medium-sized vessels, granulomatous inflammation, and eosinophilic tissue infiltration associated with asthma and peripheral eosinophilia.[76,77] CSS is one of the ANCA-associated small-vessel vasculitides, a category that also includes granulomatosis with polyangiitis (Wegener granulomatosis) and microscopic polyangiitis.

Although the pathogenesis of CSS is unknown, several environmental, drugs, and putative triggering factors have been identified.[78,79] Familial clustering of CSS suggests that genetic factors may confer susceptibility to this disease.[80,81] CSS is rare, with an estimated annual incidence of 2.7 cases per million of total population.[82] The disease occurs almost exclusively in asthmatics, with an estimated incidence in this subpopulation of 35 to 67 cases per million person-years.[83,84] The incidence of CSS increases with age until the sixth to seventh decades of life and is more common in men than women.

Given the overlapping signs and symptoms common to both the other ANCA-associated vasculitides and the other eosinophilic lung disorders, careful exclusion of alternative causes through multidisciplinary collaboration is of the utmost importance for a correct diagnosis. Although multiple classification schemes have been proposed, none of the diagnostic schemes identifies all patients with CSS.[85] The diagnosis is usually made or excluded when a preponderance of data derived from the clinical, radiographic, laboratory, and histopathologic findings support or refute a diagnosis of CSS.

CSS has classically been characterized as evolving through 3 distinct phases with different clinical, histopathologic, and radiographic manifestations; and although a useful paradigm, the phases are not necessarily progressive and may overlap. The first stage described is a prodromal allergic/atopic phase and consists of atopic disease, rhinitis, and asthma. Asthma is near universal in patients with CSS, and although the asthma may vary in severity from patient to patient, it is more commonly severe and progressive. Similarly, sinus involvement is present in most patients, but unlike granulomatosis with polyangiitis, lacks destructive features and is more similar to the eosinophilic/allergic rhinosinusitis that is seen in the other eosinophilic lung disorders.[1,79,85] The second phase is described as the eosinophilic phase, which consists of peripheral blood eosinophilia or end-organ eosinophilic infiltration, particularly of the lung, heart, and gastrointestinal tract. Migratory infiltrates consistent with eosinophilic pneumonia may be noted on imaging studies. On the other hand, cardiac and gastroenterologic involvement may present with life-threatening complications.[79,85–87] The third phase is the vasculitic phase and presents with manifestations commonly seen in the other ANCA-associated vasculitides and is often life threatening. At any point throughout the disease process, nonspecific constitutional symptoms may develop, and most patients ultimately complain of fatigue, malaise, anorexia, fever, myalgias, and arthralgias during their disease course.[1]

Recent studies evaluating clinical phenotypes in CSS have suggested that ANCA status may distinguish between 2 different clinical phenotypes of CSS.[88] Patients who are ANCA or myeloperoxidase (MPO)-positive seem to preferentially present with features of small-vessel vasculitis, whereas ANCA-negative patients typically have a clinical presentation dominated by eosinophilic tissue infiltration. The latter population clinically shares more commonality with the HES (see later discussion) and other eosinophilic lung diseases. Whereas the vasculitic phenotype has an increased frequency of neurologic (eg, mononeuritis multiplex), renal (necrotizing glomerulonephritis), and cutaneous (eg, leukocytoclastic vasculitis) manifestations, those with an eosinophilic phenotype typically have more frequent cardiac and pulmonary involvement. Cardiac involvement may be seen in 10% to 50% of patients with CSS and carries an attributable mortality of 33% to 83% of CSS-related deaths.[79,89,90] Common cardiac manifestations include conduction abnormalities, cardiomyopathy, coronary arteritis, heart failure, and pericardial disease.[91–95]

Approximately one-half to two-thirds of patients have a positive ANCA, and there is compelling evidence that ANCA are important in the pathogenesis of the vasculitis. Most CSS patients who are ANCA positive show a perinuclear pattern, called p-ANCA, which in turn corresponds most commonly to autoantibodies directed against MPO. In ANCA-positive patients with CSS, ANCA titers are poor markers of therapeutic response.[79] Furthermore, patient survival and relapse are independent of ANCA status.[96,97]

As with other eosinophilic lung diseases, the radiological findings are nonspecific and most commonly include bilateral, patchy, ground-glass opacities or airspace consolidations. Associated findings may include airway wall thickening, nodules, or pleural effusions.[1] Serial imaging frequently shows migratory infiltrates.[1,98–100] In those patients who undergo biopsy, the classic pathologic findings in the lung include a combination of eosinophilic pneumonia, granulomatous inflammation, and the presence of a small or medium-sized vessel necrotizing vasculitis.[77,101] However, all, some, or none of the 3 findings may be present.

Clinical management in CSS is based on disease extent, severity, and response to treatment. The recently revised French Vasculitis Study Group 5-factor score system (FFS) may be used to grade disease activity and predict the need for cytotoxic agents when poor prognostic factors are present.[102] Of the 5-FSS, 4 of the elements are associated with a poor prognosis (age ≥65 years, renal insufficiency, cardiac involvement, and gastrointestinal manifestations) and the presence of each of these elements is assigned a weight of +1 point, whereas the fifth factor (ear nose and throat involvement) is associated with a better prognosis, and the absence of upper airway manifestations is scored as +1 point. The 5-year mortality for scores of 0, 1, and 2 or more were 9%, 21%, and 40%, respectively.[102]

With regard to treatment, patients with CSS with FFS of 0 may successfully be treated with corticosteroid monotherapy (0.5–1 mg/kg per day of oral prednisone or equivalent) as first-line treatment. Intermittent intravenous cyclophosphamide (CYC) is used in combination with corticosteroids for those patients with an FFS of 1 or more or who present with life-threatening disease manifestations (eg, central nervous system disease or diffuse alveolar hemorrhage). Intravenous CYC is preferable to daily oral CYC in terms of reducing drug-specific toxicity. Unlike the other ANCA-associated vasculitides, a shorter CYC pulse regimen may be less effective in controlling CSS than a longer regimen. A prospective multicenter trial comparing 6 versus 12 CYC pulses (given in conjunction with corticosteroids) in 48 patients with CSS showed that those receiving 6 pulses had significantly more disease relapses than those receiving 12 pulses of therapy (94% vs 41%).[103] Nevertheless, once disease remission is achieved, corticosteroid therapy is slowly tapered. Similarly, once CYC therapy is complete, patients are transitioned to a less toxic agent of moderate potency such as azathioprine or methotrexate for maintenance of disease remission. The recommended duration of moderate potency immunosuppressive therapy for the maintenance of disease remission remains controversial, but most experts seem to favor between 1 and 4 years, barring evidence of disease relapse.

Rituximab, an anti-CD20 monoclonal antibody, may represent an attractive alternative in CSS ANCA-positive patients intolerant or refractory to CYC, and this agent is currently the subject of a phase II/III clinical trial for the treatment of CSS. A recent randomized, controlled, multicenter trial of rituximab versus CYC for the induction of disease remission in patients with granulomatosis with polyangiitis (Wegener granulomatosis) and microscopic polyangiitis showed that the rituximab-based regimen was not inferior to CYC for induction of remission at 6 months in severe ANCA-associated vasculitis and was more efficacious than the CYC-based regimen for inducing remission of relapsing disease.[104] However, further studies are needed to establish whether or not there is a role for rituximab in CSS.

Other agents that may be considered for refractory disease to conventional therapy include α-interferon,[105] intravenous immune globulin,[106] anti–tumor necrosis factor agents,[107] and anti-IgE therapy,[108] although the quality of evidence informing the use of these agents is limited and based on observational uncontrolled data. Anti–IL-5 monoclonal antibodies are under investigation as a potentially novel therapy for the treatment of CSS in both the United States and Europe.[109]

When addressing the total disease management of the patient with CSS, the clinician must also recall that the disease is characterized by severe, steroid-dependent asthma, chronic rhinosinusitis, and oral corticosteroid use, and additional therapies should be directed toward each of these elements. Specifically, most patients require additional therapy directed toward their severe persistent/steroid-dependent asthma including high-potency inhaled corticosteroids, a long-acting β-agonist, and a rescue inhaler. Although leukotriene antagonists were suspected of potentially facilitating a biologic conversation of severe asthma toward Churg-Strauss vasculitis, more recent studies seem to support the notion that the use of leukotriene antagonists permits reductions in oral corticosteroid doses such that incidentally treated, underlying CSS is unmasked and no causal link between leukotriene antagonists and CSS has been reported.[110] The addition of a leukotriene antagonist is often appropriate for patients with CSS whose asthma continues to require oral corticosteroids as per National Heart, Lung, and Blood Institute/National Asthma Education and Prevention Program Asthma Guidelines.[111] Similarly, if patients meet criteria for omalizumab use for management of their severe asthma, are taking no other biologic agents, and there is no other contraindication to their use, then the presence of CSS does not by itself mitigate against their use, and the agent may be used for the management of the severe asthma. Moreover, aggressive therapies directed toward the management of concomitant sinus disease (nasal saline irrigation and topical corticosteroids) and gastroesophageal reflux disease (eg, proton pump inhibitor therapy) may improve asthma control. Up to 10% of the attributable mortality in CSS is caused by asthma/status asthmaticus.

As with ICEP and ABPA, screening for, prevention of, and treatment of steroid-related side effects cannot be overemphasized. Patients should routinely be evaluated for complications of corticosteroid use, including but not limited to osteoporosis/avascular necrosis, diabetes, electrolyte abnormalities, cataract formation, hypertension, and opportunistic infections. Bone mineral–preserving therapies and *Pneumocystis carinii* pneumonia prophylaxis should be strongly considered. Vaccination against pneumococcal disease and influenza is appropriate, as is a regular exercise program, efforts to achieve and maintain optimal body weight, good nutrition, and regular medical follow-up that includes assessments for disease activity, complications of the medications used to manage the disease, opportunistic infections, and the development of comorbid conditions.

HES

HES are a group of rare and heterogeneous disorders characterized by the presence of hypereosinophilia and end-organ damage.[112] The diagnostic criteria for HES have historically included: (1) persistent eosinophilia of 1500 cells/mm^3 or more for longer than 6 months; (2) the absence of known causes of eosinophilia; and (3) signs and symptoms of end-organ damage.[113] Despite the seemingly straightforward nature of these criteria, the diagnosis of HES is complicated by several issues.[114] For example, the first criterion may exclude recognized variants of HES, even those with recognized molecular abnormalities, that present without peripheral blood hypereosinophilia. Second, it is unlikely that a patient with symptomatic HES would remain untreated for 6 months.[114] Likewise, the third criterion would exclude patients with evolving HES who do not yet have documented end-organ injury.[112,114] As a result, the definition of HES was refined in a recent National Institutes of Health workshop summary report to include those disorders in which (1) eosinophils are markedly increased in the peripheral blood ($\geq$1500 mm^3), (2) this degree of eosinophilia is documented on more than 1 occasion, and (3) a secondary cause cannot be identified.[112] The new classification scheme subdivides HES into the following subtypes (see **Fig. 1**): myeloproliferative, lymphocytic, familial, undefined (benign if asymptomatic and without evidence of end-organ involvement, complex if symptomatic or with end-organ damage), overlap (hypereosinophilia in the setting of single organ involvement), and associated (hypereosinophilia associated with another distinct cause, such as CSS) HES.[112] However, the diagnostic classification scheme will likely continue to evolve with increasing knowledge regarding the pathogenesis of disease variants and the identification of specific clinical phenotypes.

The 2 most well-characterized pathogenic HES variants (mHES and lymphocytic HES [lHES]) are associated with dramatic differences in clinical profiles, prognosis, and responses to therapy.[115] The mHES variant is a male-predominant disease subdivided into FIP1L1-PDGFRa F/P-positive mHES, F/P-negative mHES, and chronic eosinophilic leukemia.[112] In F/P-positive patients, a deletion on chromosome 4q12 results in fusion of the FIP1L1 and PDGFRα genes.[116] RT-PCR or FISH testing commonly detects the FIP1L1-PDGFRα F/P. Because the CHIC2 gene is located in this deleted genetic segment, a FISH probe for the CHIC2 deletion is also available. The F/P has constitutive tyrosine kinase activity, and F/P-positive patients are amenable to therapy with the tyrosine kinase inhibitor imatinib mesylate (Gleevec).[116–119] Although additional cytogenetic abnormalities/constitutively active kinase activities have been identified[114,120] not all patients with a clinical phenotype of mHES can be explained at the molecular level. In the absence of the F/P protein, a presumptive diagnosis of mHES is based on a patient having 4 or more of the following criteria: (1) an increased serum tryptase level; (2) an increased serum B_{12} level; (3) splenomegaly; (4) anemia; (5) thrombocytopenia; (6) increased circulating myeloid precursors; (7) bone marrow hypercellularity with reticulin or collagen fibrosis; or (8) increased numbers of atypical (CD25+) mast cells.[119,121]

The lHES is characterized by the expansion of CD3-CD4+ T cells that elaborate IL-3 and IL-5, which in turn drive the polyclonal expansion and survival of eosinophils.[122] In some cases, the aberrant T-cell population is clonal.[1,123] In these cases, malignant transformation into T-cell lymphoma may occur. However, other cases of lHES do not have an identifiable clonal T-cell population. Clinically, patients with lHES present with cutaneous atopic disease such as urticaria or angioedema, increased IgE levels, and increased serum thymus and activation-regulated chemokine (a marker of T-cell eosinophil hematopoietin expression). In contrast to those with mHES, lHES affects men and women equally, rarely results in cardiac involvement, and is typically more steroid responsive.[124]

Virtually any organ system may be involved in HES. Of 188 patients evaluated in a multicenter, retrospective study,[115] the most common presenting manifestations of HES were dermatologic (37%), pulmonary (25%), and gastrointestinal (14%) in nature. Six percent of patients in this series presented with clinically asymptomatic eosinophilia. Less than 5% of patients had cardiac manifestations at the time of diagnosis; however, as with CSS, cardiac involvement in patients with HES (especially mHES) represents a major cause of morbidity and mortality. Pulmonary manifestations of HES include chronic eosinophilia pneumonia, AEP, and ARDS.[125]

Systemic corticosteroids are the first-line therapy for most HES subtypes. Imatinib is indicated for mHES F/P-positive patients, and may result in dramatic improvement, but is not useful in lHES. Second-line modalities include hydroxyurea and interferon-α. One notable concern regarding interferon-α is that it may inhibit clonal CD3-CD4+ T-cell apoptosis, potentially promoting T-cell survival, and therefore it is not used as monotherapy for lHES.[126] Use of monoclonal anti–IL-5 antibody, mepolizumab, and anti-CD52 antibody, alemtuzumab,[127] are under investigation for potential use in refractory disease. A recently completed trial of mepolizumab found that patients who received the agent had clinically significant reductions in corticosteroid dosage, and in some cases, corticosteroid discontinuation.[128] The JAK (janus kinase) signaling pathway has been shown to promote eosinophil activation and survival in human eosinophils and may represent a novel target for future HES therapies.[129–131]

SUMMARY

Eosinophilic lung diseases encompass a heterogeneous group of disorders unified by the presence of peripheral and/or tissue eosinophilia combined with pulmonary impairment and/or radiographic abnormalities. Because their course and prognosis are highly variable, an accurate diagnosis is essential to optimizing outcomes. Therefore, a thorough clinical evaluation using a multidisciplinary care model is recommended to achieve accurate diagnosis and optimize patient outcomes. Although much progress has been made over the last decade, resulting in more accurate diagnosis and decreased morbidity and mortality for these disorders, much remains to be done.

REFERENCES

1. Li H, Groshong SD, Lynch D, et al. Eosinophilic lung disease. Clin Pulm Med 2010;17(2):66–74.
2. Chang HW, Leong KH, Koh DR, et al. Clonal origin of eosinophils in the hypereosinophilic syndrome detected by PCR analysis of DNA polymorphisms of the X linked human androgen receptor gene. Int J Hematol 1996;64:S43.
3. Chang HW, Leong KH, Koh DR, et al. Clonality of isolated eosinophils in the hypereosinophilic syndrome. Blood 1999;93:1651–7.
4. Kagohashi K, Ohara G, Kurishima K, et al. Chronic eosinophilic pneumonia with subpleural curvilinear shadow. Acta Medica (Hradec Kralove) 2011;54(1):45–8.
5. Johkoh T, Muller NL, Akira M, et al. Eosinophilic lung diseases: diagnostic accuracy of thin-section CT in 111 patients. Radiology 2000;216(3):773–80.
6. Marmursztejn J, Vignaux O, Cohen P, et al. Impact of cardiac magnetic resonance imaging for assessment of Churg-Strauss syndrome: a cross-sectional study in 20 patients. Clin Exp Rheumatol 2009;27(1 Suppl 52):S70–6.
7. Bronchoalveolar lavage constituents in healthy individuals, idiopathic pulmonary fibrosis, and selected comparison groups. The BAL Cooperative Group Steering Committee. Am Rev Respir Dis 1990;141(5 Pt 2):S169–202.
8. Kwong YL, Chan LC. Involvement of eosinophils in acute myeloid leukemia with monosomy 7 demonstrated by fluorescence in situ hybridization. Br J Haematol 1994;88:389–91.
9. Luppi M, Marasca R, Morselli M, et al. Clonal nature of hypereosinophilic syndrome. Blood 1994;84:349–50.
10. Giembycz MA, Lindsay MA. Pharmacology of the eosinophil. Pharmacol Rev 1999;51(2):213–340.
11. Kariyawasam HH, Robinson DS. The eosinophil: the cell and its weapons, the cytokines, its locations. Semin Respir Crit Care Med 2006;27(2):117–27.
12. Lams BE, Sousa AR, Rees PJ, et al. Immunopathology of the small-airway submucosa in smokers with and without chronic obstructive pulmonary disease. Am J Respir Crit Care Med 1998;158(5 Pt 1):1518–23.
13. Dippolito R, Foresi A, Chetta A, et al. Eosinophils in induced sputum from asymptomatic smokers with normal lung function. Respir Med 2001;95(12):969–74.
14. Komadina KH, Houk RW, Vicks SL, et al. Goodpasture's syndrome associated with pulmonary eosinophilic vasculitis. J Rheumatol 1988;15(8):1298–301.
15. Travis WD. Pathology of pulmonary vasculitis. Semin Respir Crit Care Med 2004;25(5):475–82.
16. Agarwal R. Allergic bronchopulmonary aspergillosis. Chest 2009;135(3):805–26.

17. Gibson PG, Wark PA, Simpson JL, et al. Induced sputum IL-8 gene expression, neutrophil influx and MMP-9 in allergic bronchopulmonary aspergillosis. Eur Respir J 2003;21(4):582–8.

18. Chauhan B, Santiago L, Hutcheson PS, et al. Evidence for the involvement of two different MHC class II regions in susceptibility or protection in allergic bronchopulmonary aspergillosis. J Allergy Clin Immunol 2000;106(4):723–9.

19. Eaton TE, Weiner Miller P, Garrett JE, et al. Cystic fibrosis transmembrane conductance regulator gene mutations: do they play a role in the aetiology of allergic bronchopulmonary aspergillosis? Clin Exp Allergy 2002;32(5):756–61.

20. Tomee JF, Kauffman HF. Putative virulence factors of *Aspergillus fumigatus*. Clin Exp Allergy 2000;30(4):476–84.

21. Mitchell TA, Hamilos DL, Lynch DA, et al. Distribution and severity of bronchiectasis in allergic bronchopulmonary aspergillosis (ABPA). J Asthma 2000;37(1):65–72.

22. Ward S, Heyneman L, Lee MJ, et al. Accuracy of CT in the diagnosis of allergic bronchopulmonary aspergillosis in asthmatic patients. AJR Am J Roentgenol 1999;173(4):937–42.

23. Agarwal R, Gupta D, Aggarwal AN, et al. Clinical significance of hyperattenuating mucoid impaction in allergic bronchopulmonary aspergillosis: an analysis of 155 patients. Chest 2007;132(4):1183–90.

24. Rosenberg M, Patterson R, Mintzer R, et al. Clinical and immunologic criteria for the diagnosis of allergic bronchopulmonary aspergillosis. Ann Intern Med 1977;86:405–14.

25. Patterson R, Greenberger PA, Halwig JM, et al. Allergic bronchopulmonary aspergillosis. Natural history and classification of early disease by serologic and roentgenographic studies. Arch Intern Med 1986;146(5):916–8.

26. Agarwal R, Gupta D, Aggarwal AN, et al. Allergic bronchopulmonary aspergillosis: lessons from 126 patients attending a chest clinic in north India. Chest 2006;130(2):442–8.

27. Imbeault B, Cormier Y. Usefulness of inhaled high-dose corticosteroids in allergic bronchopulmonary aspergillosis. Chest 1993;103(5):1614–7.

28. Balter MS, Rebuck AS. Treatment of allergic bronchopulmonary aspergillosis with inhaled corticosteroids. Respir Med 1992;86(5):441–2.

29. Wark PA, Hensley MJ, Saltos N, et al. Anti-inflammatory effect of itraconazole in stable allergic bronchopulmonary aspergillosis: a randomized controlled trial. J Allergy Clin Immunol 2003;111(5):952–7.

30. Stevens DA, Schwartz HJ, Lee JY, et al. A randomized trial of itraconazole in allergic bronchopulmonary aspergillosis. N Engl J Med 2000;342(11):756–62.

31. Skov M, Hoiby N, Koch C. Itraconazole treatment of allergic bronchopulmonary aspergillosis in patients with cystic fibrosis. Allergy 2002;57(8):723–8.

32. Kanu A, Patel K. Treatment of allergic bronchopulmonary aspergillosis (ABPA) in CF with anti-IgE antibody (omalizumab). Pediatr Pulmonol 2008;43(12):1249–51.

33. Wark PA, Gibson PG, Wilson AJ. Azoles for allergic bronchopulmonary aspergillosis associated with asthma. Cochrane Database Syst Rev 2004;3:CD001108.

34. van der Ent CK, Hoekstra H, Rijkers GT. Successful treatment of allergic bronchopulmonary aspergillosis with recombinant anti-IgE antibody. Thorax 2007;62(3):276–7.

35. Zirbes JM, Milla CE. Steroid-sparing effect of omalizumab for allergic bronchopulmonary aspergillosis and cystic fibrosis. Pediatr Pulmonol 2008;43(6):607–10.

36. Acute eosinophilic pneumonia. N Engl J Med 1990;322(9):634–6.
37. Rosenberg HF, Dyer KD, Domachowske JB. Respiratory viruses and eosinophils: exploring the connections. Antiviral Res 2009;83(1):1–9.
38. Shenoy VP, Vishwanath S, Indira B, et al. Hepato-pulmonary amebiasis: a case report. Braz J Infect Dis 2010;14(4):372–3.
39. Ong RK, Doyle RL. Tropical pulmonary eosinophilia. Chest 1998;113(6):1673–9.
40. Forrester JM, Steele AW, Waldron JA, et al. Crack lung: an acute pulmonary syndrome with a spectrum of clinical and histopathologic findings. Am Rev Respir Dis 1990;142(2):462–7.
41. Kobashi Y, Nakajima M, Niki Y, et al. [A case of acute eosinophilic pneumonia due to Sho-saiko-to]. Nihon Kyobu Shikkan Gakkai Zasshi 1997;35(12):1372–7 [in Japanese].
42. Cottin V, Frognier R, Monnot H, et al. Chronic eosinophilic pneumonia after radiation therapy for breast cancer. Eur Respir J 2004;23(1):9–13.
43. Rom WN, Weiden M, Garcia R, et al. Acute eosinophilic pneumonia in a New York City firefighter exposed to World Trade Center dust. Am J Respir Crit Care Med 2002;166(6):797–800.
44. Solomon J, Schwarz M. Drug-, toxin-, and radiation therapy-induced eosinophilic pneumonia. Semin Respir Crit Care Med 2006;27(2):192–7.
45. Frankel SK. Drug-induced lung disease. In: Hanley M, Welsh C, editors. Current diagnosis and treatment in pulmonary medicine. New York: Lange Medical Bools/McGraw-Hill; 2003. p. 337–47.
46. Salerno SM, Strong JS, Roth BJ, et al. Eosinophilic pneumonia and respiratory failure associated with a trazodone overdose. Am J Respir Crit Care Med 1995;152(6 Pt 1):2170–2.
47. Fleisch MC, Blauer F, Gubler JG, et al. Eosinophilic pneumonia and respiratory failure associated with venlafaxine treatment. Eur Respir J 2000;15(1):205–8.
48. Hayes D Jr, Anstead MI, Kuhn RJ. Eosinophilic pneumonia induced by daptomycin. J Infect 2007;54(4):e211–3.
49. Honore I, Nunes H, Groussard O, et al. Acute respiratory failure after interferon-gamma therapy of end-stage pulmonary fibrosis. Am J Respir Crit Care Med 2003;167(7):953–7.
50. Paralkar VR, Goradia A, Luger SM, et al. Severe eosinophilia as a manifestation of acute graft-versus-host disease. Oncology 2008;75(3–4):134–6.
51. Pandit R, Scholnik A, Wulfekuhler L, et al. Non-small-cell lung cancer associated with excessive eosinophilia and secretion of interleukin-5 as a paraneoplastic syndrome. Am J Hematol 2007;82(3):234–7.
52. Wilson F, Tefferi A. Acute lymphocytic leukemia with eosinophilia: two case reports and a literature review. Leuk Lymphoma 2005;46(7):1045–50.
53. Slungaard A, Ascensao J, Zanjani E, et al. Pulmonary carcinoma with eosinophilia. Demonstration of a tumor-derived eosinophilopoietic factor. N Engl J Med 1983;309(13):778–81.
54. Enblad G, Sundstrom C, Glimelius B. Infiltration of eosinophils in Hodgkin's disease involved lymph nodes predicts prognosis. Hematol Oncol 1993;11(4):187–93.
55. Utsunomiya A, Ishida T, Inagaki A, et al. Clinical significance of a blood eosinophilia in adult T-cell leukemia/lymphoma: a blood eosinophilia is a significant unfavorable prognostic factor. Leuk Res 2007;31(7):915–20.
56. Coultas DB, Zumwalt RE, Black WC, et al. The epidemiology of interstitial lung diseases. Am J Respir Crit Care Med 1994;150(4):967–72.
57. Thomeer MJ, Costabe U, Rizzato G, et al. Comparison of registries of interstitial lung diseases in three European countries. Eur Respir J Suppl 2001;32:114s–8s.

58. Tateno H, Nakamura H, Minematsu N, et al. Eotaxin and monocyte chemoattractant protein-1 in chronic eosinophilic pneumonia. Eur Respir J 2001;17(5): 962–8.

59. Alam M, Burki NK. Chronic eosinophilic pneumonia: a review. South Med J 2007; 100(1):49–53.

60. Marchand E, Reynaud-Gaubert M, Lauque D, et al. Idiopathic chronic eosinophilic pneumonia. A clinical and follow-up study of 62 cases. The Groupe d'Etudes et de Recherche sur les Maladies "Orphelines" Pulmonaires (GERM"O"P). Medicine (Baltimore) 1998;77:299–312.

61. Gaensler EA, Carrington CB. Peripheral opacities in chronic eosinophilic pneumonia: the photographic negative of pulmonary edema. AJR Am J Roentgenol 1977;128:1–13.

62. Jederlinic PJ, Sicilian L, Gaensler EA. Chronic eosinophilic pneumonia. A report of 19 cases and a review of the literature. Medicine (Baltimore) 1988;67(3): 154–62.

63. Yoshida K, Shijubo N, Koba H, et al. Chronic eosinophilic pneumonia progressing to lung fibrosis. Eur Respir J 1994;7(8):1541–4.

64. Marchand E, Etienne-Mastroianni B, Chanez P, et al. Idiopathic chronic eosinophilic pneumonia and asthma: how do they influence each other? Eur Respir J 2003;22(1):8–13.

65. Durieu J, Wallaert B, Tonnel AB. Long-term follow-up of pulmonary function in chronic eosinophilic pneumonia. Groupe d'Etude en Pathologie Interstitielle de la Societe de Pathologie Thoracique du Nord. Eur Respir J 1997;10:286–91.

66. Naughton M, Fahy J, FitzGerald MX. Chronic eosinophilic pneumonia. A long-term follow-up of 12 patients. Chest 1993;103(1):162–5.

67. Minakuchi M, Niimi A, Matsumoto H, et al. Chronic eosinophilic pneumonia: treatment with inhaled corticosteroids. Respiration 2003;70(4):362–6.

68. Philit F, Etienne-Mastroianni B, Parrot A, et al. Idiopathic acute eosinophilic pneumonia: a study of 22 patients. Am J Respir Crit Care Med 2002;166(9):1235–9.

69. Allen J. Acute eosinophilic pneumonia. Semin Respir Crit Care Med 2006;27(2): 142–7.

70. Liegeon MN, De Blay F, Jaeger A, et al. A cause of respiratory distress: eosinophilic pneumopathy due to minocycline. Rev Mal Respir 1996;13(5):517–9 [in French].

71. Pope-Harman AL, Davis WB, Christoforidis AJ, et al. Acute eosinophilic pneumonia: a summary of fifteen cases and review of the literature. Medicine (Baltimore) 1996;75:334–42.

72. Shintani H, Fujimura M, Ishiura Y, et al. A case of cigarette smoking-induced acute eosinophilic pneumonia showing tolerance. Chest 2000;117:277–9.

73. King MA, Pope-Harman AL, Allen JN, et al. Acute eosinophilic pneumonia: radiologic and clinical features. Radiology 1997;203:715–9.

74. Tazelaar HD, Linz LJ, Colby TV, et al. Acute eosinophilic pneumonia: histopathologic findings in nine patients. Am J Respir Crit Care Med 1997;155:296–302.

75. Churg J, Strauss L. Allergic granulomatosis, allergic angiitis, and periarteritis nodosa. Am J Pathol 1951;27(2):277–301.

76. Lanham JG, Elkon KB, Pusey CD, et al. Systemic vasculitis with asthma and eosinophilia: a clinical approach to the Churg-Strauss syndrome. Medicine (Baltimore) 1984;63:65–81.

77. Jennette JC, Falk RJ, Andrassy K, et al. Nomenclature of systemic vasculitides. Proposal of an international consensus conference. Arthritis Rheum 1994;37(2): 187–92.

78. Lane SE, Watts RA, Bentham G, et al. Are environmental factors important in primary systemic vasculitis? A case-control study. Arthritis Rheum 2003;48(3): 814–23.

79. Guillevin L, Cohen P, Gayraud M, et al. Churg-Strauss syndrome. Clinical study and long-term follow-up of 96 patients. Medicine (Baltimore) 1999;78(1):26–37.

80. Tsurikisawa N, Morita S, Tsuburai T, et al. Familial Churg-Strauss syndrome in two sisters. Chest 2007;131(2):592–4.

81. Manganelli P, Giacosa R, Fietta P, et al. Familial vasculitides: Churg-Strauss syndrome and Wegener's granulomatosis in 2 first-degree relatives. J Rheumatol 2003;30(3):618–21.

82. Watts RA, Lane SE, Bentham G, et al. Epidemiology of systemic vasculitis: a ten-year study in the United Kingdom. Arthritis Rheum 2000;43(2):414–9.

83. Harrold LR, Andrade SE, Go AS, et al. Incidence of Churg-Strauss syndrome in asthma drug users: a population-based perspective. J Rheumatol 2005;32(6): 1076–80.

84. Loughlin JE, Cole JA, Rothman KJ, et al. Prevalence of serious eosinophilia and incidence of Churg-Strauss syndrome in a cohort of asthma patients. Ann Allergy Asthma Immunol 2002;88(3):319–25.

85. Keogh KA, Specks U. Churg-Strauss syndrome: clinical presentation, antineutrophil cytoplasmic antibodies, and leukotriene receptor antagonists. Am J Med 2003;115(4):284–90.

86. Conron M, Beynon HL. Churg-Strauss syndrome. Thorax 2000;55:870–7.

87. Pagnoux C, Mahr A, Cohen P, et al. Presentation and outcome of gastrointestinal involvement in systemic necrotizing vasculitides: analysis of 62 patients with polyarteritis nodosa, microscopic polyangiitis, Wegener granulomatosis, Churg-Strauss syndrome, or rheumatoid arthritis-associated vasculitis. Medicine (Baltimore) 2005;84:115–28.

88. Kallenberg CG. Churg-Strauss syndrome: just one disease entity? Arthritis Rheum 2005;52(9):2589–93.

89. Solans R, Bosch JA, Perez-Bocanegra C, et al. Churg-Strauss syndrome: outcome and long-term follow-up of 32 patients. Rheumatology (Oxford) 2001; 40(7):763–71.

90. Guillevin L, Lhote F, Gayraud M, et al. Prognostic factors in polyarteritis nodosa and Churg-Strauss syndrome. A prospective study in 342 patients. Medicine (Baltimore) 1996;75(1):17–28.

91. Hasley PB, Follansbee WP, Coulehan JL. Cardiac manifestations of Churg-Strauss syndrome: report of a case and review of the literature. Am Heart J 1990;120:996–9.

92. Morgan JM, Raposo L, Gibson DG. Cardiac involvement in Churg-Strauss syndrome shown by echocardiography. Br Heart J 1989;62:462–6.

93. Ramakrishna G, Connolly HM, Tazelaar HD, et al. Churg-Strauss syndrome complicated by eosinophilic endomyocarditis. Mayo Clin Proc 2000;75:631–5.

94. Stollberger C, Finsterer J, Winkler WB. Eosinophilic pericardial effusion in Churg-Strauss syndrome. Respir Med 2005;99:377–9.

95. Val-Bernal JF, Mayorga M, Garcia-Alberdi E, et al. Churg-Strauss syndrome and sudden cardiac death. Cardiovasc Pathol 2003;12:94–7.

96. Sinico RA, Di Toma L, Maggiore U, et al. Prevalence and clinical significance of antineutrophil cytoplasmic antibodies in Churg-Strauss syndrome. Arthritis Rheum 2005;52(9):2926–35.

97. Sable-Fourtassou R, Cohen P, Mahr A, et al. Antineutrophil cytoplasmic antibodies and the Churg-Strauss syndrome. Ann Intern Med 2005;143(9):632–8.

98. Choi YH, Im JG, Han BK, et al. Thoracic manifestation of Churg-Strauss syndrome: radiologic and clinical findings. Chest 2000;117:117–24.
99. Silva CI, Muller NL, Fujimoto K, et al. Churg-Strauss syndrome: high resolution CT and pathologic findings. J Thorac Imaging 2005;20:74–80.
100. Worthy SA, Muller NL, Hansell DM, et al. Churg-Strauss syndrome: the spectrum of pulmonary CT findings in 17 patients. AJR Am J Roentgenol 1998;170: 297–300.
101. Katzenstein AL. Diagnostic features and differential diagnosis of Churg-Strauss syndrome in the lung. A review. Am J Clin Pathol 2000;114(5):767–72.
102. Guillevin L, Pagnoux C, Seror R, et al. The Five-Factor Score revisited: assessment of prognoses of systemic necrotizing vasculitides based on the French Vasculitis Study Group (FVSG) cohort. Medicine 2011;90(1):19–27.
103. Cohen P, Pagnoux C, Mahr A, et al. Churg-Strauss syndrome with poor-prognosis factors: a prospective multicenter trial comparing glucocorticoids and six or twelve cyclophosphamide pulses in forty-eight patients. Arthritis Rheum 2007;57(4):686–93.
104. Stone JH, Merkel PA, Spiera R, et al. Rituximab versus cyclophosphamide for ANCA-associated vasculitis. N Engl J Med 2010;363(3):221–32.
105. Metzler C, Csernok E, Gross WL, et al. Interferon-alpha for maintenance of remission in Churg-Strauss syndrome: a long-term observational study. Clin Exp Rheumatol 2010;28(1 Suppl 57):24–30.
106. Tsurikisawa N, Taniguchi M, Saito H, et al. Treatment of Churg-Strauss syndrome with high-dose intravenous immunoglobulin. Ann Allergy Asthma Immunol 2004; 92(1):80–7.
107. Arbach O, Gross WL, Gause A. Treatment of refractory Churg-Strauss-Syndrome (CSS) by TNF-alpha blockade. Immunobiology 2002;206(5):496–501.
108. Pabst S, Tiyerili V, Grohe C. Apparent response to anti-IgE therapy in two patients with refractory "forme fruste" of Churg-Strauss syndrome. Thorax 2008;63(8):747–8.
109. Kim S, Marigowda G, Oren E, et al. Mepolizumab as a steroid-sparing treatment option in patients with Churg-Strauss syndrome. J Allergy Clin Immunol 2010; 125(6):1336–43.
110. Bibby S, Healy B, Steele R, et al. Association between leukotriene receptor antagonist therapy and Churg-Strauss syndrome: an analysis of the FDA AERS database. Thorax 2010;65(2):132–8.
111. Weller PF, Plaut M, Taggart V, et al. The relationship of asthma therapy and Churg-Strauss syndrome: NIH workshop summary report. J Allergy Clin Immunol 2001;108(2):175–83.
112. Klion AD, Bochner BS, Gleich GJ, et al. Approaches to the treatment of hypereosinophilic syndromes: a workshop summary report. J Allergy Clin Immunol 2006;117(6):1292–302.
113. Chusid MJ, Dale DC, West BC, et al. The hypereosinophilic syndrome: analysis of fourteen cases with review of the literature. Medicine (Baltimore) 1975;54:1–27.
114. Klion A. Hypereosinophilic syndrome: current approach to diagnosis and treatment. Annu Rev Med 2009;60:293–306.
115. Ogbogu PU, Bochner BS, Butterfield JH, et al. Hypereosinophilic syndrome: a multicenter, retrospective analysis of clinical characteristics and response to therapy. J Allergy Clin Immunol 2009;124(6):1319–25. e1313.
116. Cools J, DeAngelo DJ, Gotlib J, et al. A tyrosine kinase created by the fusion of the PDGFRA and FIP1L1 genes as a therapeutic target of imatinib in idiopathic hypereosinophilic syndrome. N Engl J Med 2003;348:1201–14.

117. Klion AD, Noel P, Akin C, et al. Elevated serum tryptase levels identify a subset of patients with a myeloproliferative variant of idiopathic hypereosinophilic syndrome associated with tissue fibrosis, poor prognosis, and imatinib responsiveness. Blood 2003;101(12):4660–6.
118. Vandenberghe P, Wlodarska I, Michaux L, et al. Clinical and molecular features of FIP1L1-PDFGRA(+) chronic eosinophilic leukemias. Leukemia 2004;18: 734–42.
119. Klion AD, Robyn J, Akin C, et al. Molecular remission and reversal of myelofibrosis in response to imatinib mesylate treatment in patients with the myeloproliferative variant of hypereosinophilic syndrome. Blood 2004;103(2):473–8.
120. Curtis CE, Grand FH, Musto P, et al. Two novel imatinib-responsive PDGFRA fusion genes in chronic eosinophilic leukaemia. Br J Haematol 2007;138(1): 77–81.
121. Sheikh J, Weller PF. Clinical overview of hypereosinophilic syndromes. Immunol Allergy Clin North Am 2007;27(3):333–55.
122. Cogan E, Schandene L, Crusiaux A, et al. Brief report: clonal proliferation of type 2 helper T cells in a man with the hypereosinophilic syndrome. N Engl J Med 1994;330:535–8.
123. Roufosse F, Cogan E, Goldman M. Recent advances in pathogenesis and management of hypereosinophilic syndromes. Allergy 2004;59:673–89.
124. Ogbogu PU, Rosing DR, Horne MK 3rd. Cardiovascular manifestations of hypereosinophilic syndromes. Immunol Allergy Clin North Am 2007;27(3):457–75.
125. Winn RE, Kollef MH, Meyer JI. Pulmonary involvement in the hypereosinophilic syndrome. Chest 1994;105(3):656–60.
126. Schandene L, Roufosse F, de Lavareille A, et al. Interferon alpha prevents spontaneous apoptosis of clonal Th2 cells associated with chronic hypereosinophilia. Blood 2000;96(13):4285–92.
127. Verstovsek S, Tefferi A, Kantarjian H, et al. Alemtuzumab therapy for hypereosinophilic syndrome and chronic eosinophilic leukemia. Clin Cancer Res 2009; 15(1):368–73.
128. Rothenberg ME, Klion AD, Roufosse FE, et al. Treatment of patients with the hypereosinophilic syndrome with mepolizumab. N Engl J Med 2008;358(12): 1215–28.
129. Ochiai K, Tanabe E, Ishihara C, et al. Role of JAK2 signal transductional pathway in activation and survival of human peripheral eosinophils by interferon-gamma (IFN-gamma). Clin Exp Immunol 1999;118(3):340–3.
130. Gotlib J. World health organization-defined eosinophilic disorders: 2011 update on diagnosis, risk stratification, and management. Am J Hematol 2011;86(8): 677–88.
131. Jones AV, Kreil S, Zoi K, et al. Widespread occurrence of the JAK2 V617F mutation in chronic myeloproliferative disorders. Blood 2005;106(6):2162–8.

Hypoventilation Syndromes

Ahmad Chebbo, MD, Amer Tfaili, MD, Shirley F. Jones, MD, FCCP*

KEYWORDS

- Hypoventilation • Noninvasive ventilation • Obesity
- Chest wall disorders • Obstructive lung disease
- Neuromuscular disease

DEFINITION AND PHYSIOLOGY

Hypoventilation exists when the arterial partial pressure of carbon dioxide ($Paco_2$) is 45 mm Hg or greater. $Paco_2$ approximates alveolar pressure of carbon dioxide (Pco_2) and is proportional to CO_2 production divided by alveolar ventilation. Alveolar ventilation is equal to minute ventilation (respiratory rate × tidal volume) minus the dead space ventilation (respiratory rate × dead space). Alveolar ventilation is the product of respiratory rate, tidal volume, and dead space to tidal volume ratio. Increases in dead space can effectively lead to reductions in alveolar ventilation and an increase in Pco_2. Reduced alveolar ventilation can classically be divided into conditions of impaired ventilatory drive or altered respiratory mechanics. Impairments in the ventilatory drive are central in nature and include congenital hypoventilation syndrome and congenital disorders with central nervous system involvement in children. However, impairments in drive also partly contribute to the pathophysiology of obesity hypoventilation syndrome (OHS), along with altered respiratory mechanics. OHSs are more frequently encountered and serve as the focus of this review.

EVALUATION OF HYPOVENTILATION

No single specific test exists that can determine the cause of chronic hypoventilation but rather a detailed history taking and physical examination combined with the appropriate test or imaging enables one to differentiate the underlying cause. Useful tests include arterial blood gas analysis, pulmonary function testing, radiologic evaluation, nocturnal oximetry, and polysomnography.

All authors do not have any financial or conflict of interest disclosures.
Division of Pulmonary, Critical Care and Sleep Medicine, Department of Internal Medicine, Scott and White Healthcare/Texas A&M Health Science Center, 2401 South 31st Street, Temple, TX 76508, USA
* Corresponding author.
E-mail address: shjones@swmail.sw.org

Calculation of the alveolar to arterial pressure of oxygen (Po_2) gradient (A-a gradient) from arterial blood gas analysis is useful in the evaluation of hypoventilation. The A-a gradient can be estimated from the following equation:

$$A - a \text{ gradient } = PAo_2 - Pao_2$$

where PAo_2 is the alveolar pressure of oxygen and Pao_2 is the arterial pressure of oxygen. The PAo_2 can be calculated from the Pao_2, $Paco_2$, and fraction of inspired oxygen:

$$PAo_2 = FiO_2(PB - PH_2O) - Pco_2/0.8$$

where PB is the barometric pressure (760 mm Hg) and PH_2O is the partial pressure of H_2O (47 mm Hg) and for simplification purposes

$$PAo_2 = 150 - Paco_2/0.8$$

The normal gradient is 10 mm Hg but varies with age and can be calculated as 0.27 times age in years.[1,2] An elevated A-a gradient in the settings of hypoventilation usually suggests a parenchymal cause. A normal gradient suggests muscle weakness or abnormal ventilatory control as the cause for hypoventilation, although patients with hypoventilation due to neuromuscular disease may have slight elevations in the A-a gradient because of atelectasis, which creates ventilation and perfusion mismatch.

Several pulmonary function tests prove useful in the evaluation of hypoventilation and include spirometry, lung volumes, diffusion capacity for carbon monoxide (DLCO), maximum inspiratory pressure (MIP), and maximum expiratory pressure (MEP). Classification of defects as either airflow obstruction or restrictive ventilatory defects can be very helpful. Patients with hypoventilation secondary to abnormal ventilatory control have normal lung volumes and spirometry results in contrast to those with hypoventilation secondary to neuromuscular disease who exhibit restrictive ventilatory defects with a decrease in total lung capacity (TLC), MIP, and MEP.[3] In patients with hypoventilation due to restrictive chest wall disorders, a restrictive pattern is more common. Obstructive or mixed patterns are found in patients with hypoventilation from obstructive lung disease. The measurement of DLCO is quite helpful and is relatively normal in diseases affecting the chest wall and reduced in chronic obstructive pulmonary disease (COPD), particularly emphysema. The MIP and MEP are sensitive tests of respiratory muscle strength. Although there is no definite normal range, a value less than 60 cm H_2O is associated with a decrease in the forced vital capacity (FVC) and the ability to cough and clear secretions. Reductions in MIP correlate with reductions in the vital capacity (VC). Furthermore, the reductions in VC are more profound than that expected based on muscle strength testing.[4] In general, patients with hypoventilation due to ventilatory apparatus defects usually demonstrate a normal MIP and MEP because of the preservation of the respiratory muscle strength.[5]

Radiographic evaluations, including chest radiographs, or computed tomographic scan can be helpful in detecting chest wall deformity, parenchymal lung disease, or emphysema. In patients suspicious for diaphragm weakness or paralysis, fluoroscopy can be ordered as a sniff test. During inspiration or sniff, paralysis of the involved portion of the diaphragm demonstrates upward excursion.

Overnight oximetry and polysomnography are important in the assessment of nocturnal hypoventilation particularly because some patients experience CO_2 retention only during sleep and exhibit eucapnia during the day. Coexisting obstructive and central sleep apnea can also be detected during polysomnography.

OHS

Although 33% of adults and 17% of children and adolescents in the United States are obese[6,7] and the incidence of morbid obesity is rising, OHS remains underrecognized and underestimated.[8] OHS is defined as obesity (body mass index >30 kg/m^2 [calculated as weight in kilograms divided by height in meters squared]), daytime hypoventilation with awake Pco_2 greater than 45 mm Hg, and sleep-disordered breathing in the absence of other causes of hypoventilation.[9] OHS is also known as pickwickian syndrome, the name given by Dr Burwell in 1956 to describe his patient with a strong resemblance to the character Joe in the Charles Dickens novel *The Posthumous Papers of the Pickwick Club*, having morbid obesity, excessive somnolence, periodic shallow respirations, and cyanosis. About 90% of patients with OHS have concomitant obstructive sleep apnea (OSA),[10] which is defined by recurrent upper airway obstruction generating partial reduction or complete cessation of airflow despite respiratory effort. The prevalence of OHS in patients with OSA is uncertain but is estimated to be between 4% and 20%.[11] However, recognition and initiation of therapy is less than optimal. In a single study of hospitalized obese patients, the prevalence of OHS approximated 30%, but only 10% of them had been diagnosed and started on therapy by discharge.[8]

Hypercapnia in OHS is due to several mechanisms working collectively, including increased work of breathing, OSA, respiratory muscle impairment, decreased central ventilatory drive, and decreased response to leptin. Obesity itself increases the work of breathing through efforts to move the rib cage and the diaphragm and decreases lung compliance. Fifteen percent of the daily oxygen consumption is spent on work of breathing in morbidly obese patients compared with 3% in normal individuals.[12] OSA contributes to hypoventilation through the development of sleep-related hypercapnia, particularly during apneas and hypopneas. Despite hyperpneas between obstructive events, this ventilatory compensation is inadequate to eliminate enough carbon dioxide to maintain eucapnia.[13] The decrease in pH results in reduced bicarbonate excretion at night and progressive elevation in the serum bicarbonate level[14] and subsequent depression of ventilation during the day.[13] Modest degrees of muscle impairment play a role in the pathogenesis of OHS.[15] The decrease in central ventilatory drive is unlikely to be a primary problem and improves once Pco_2 returns to normal with treatment. There is a growing focus on the mechanism of altered leptin levels and resistance in patients with OHS, with such impairments resulting in reduced minute ventilation and hence hypoventilation.[16]

Obesity with OSA is the usual presentation of OHS. Patients exhibit symptoms of OSA, including excessive daytime sleepiness, loud snoring, and morning headache. Dyspnea on exertion is particularly important and may herald the onset of cor pulmonale. Physical examination findings include plethora, large neck circumference, and rapid shallow respirations. A loud pulmonic component of second heart sound, elevated jugular venous pressure and pedal edema indicate the presence of right heart failure. Usually the diagnosis is established in the fifth or sixth decade after frequent hospitalizations for hypercapnic respiratory failure or during evaluation in sleep or pulmonary clinic. The challenge in the diagnosis of OHS is that other diseases that can cause hypoventilation must be eliminated, which is a difficult task because of the significant number of comorbidities associated with obesity and within an individual patient. Furthermore, differentiation between OHS with OSA and OSA alone is important. A Pco_2 greater than 45 during wakefulness on arterial blood gas testing with compensatory metabolic compensation and hypoxemia (Po_2<70)[15,17] suggests the diagnosis. The A-a gradient is usually normal and eliminates pulmonary parenchymal and airway disease as the cause of hypoventilation, but, because of poor ventilation and perfusion mismatch in the lower lobes of the lungs of obese patients, a modest elevation in A-a gradient is not uncommon.[15] Pulmonary function testing shows low FVC and expiratory reserve volume with normal FVC to forced expiratory volume in 1 second (FEV$_1$) ratio.[17,18] The chest radiograph usually shows small lung volume with a mildly elevated diaphragm bilaterally and cardiomegaly if cor pulmonale has ensued. Polysomnography should be performed in every patient with OHS for diagnosis and therapy. The apnea-hypopnea index (AHI) is elevated in most patients because of coexisting OSA. In a study of 46 morbidly obese patients with moderate to severe OSA with and without OHS, the severity of the OSA did not correlate with the development or severity of OHS. However, subjects with OHS had severe oxygen desaturation at night with a larger percentage of total sleep time with saturation less than 90% (75% vs 15%) compared with those with OSA only.[19]

There are no specific and established guidelines for treatment of OHS. The variety of reported therapies target specific components of OHS and aim to improve the ventilatory drive, reverse sleep-disordered breathing, relieve respiratory muscle fatigue, and decrease work of breathing. Medications are used to alter the ventilatory drive act by either direct stimulation of the respiratory center, that is, progestin[20] or inducing metabolic acidosis, that is, acetazolamide.[21] However, this line of treatment does not address other pathologic problems in OHS, including sleep-disordered breathing and increased work of breathing, with one trial of medroxyprogesterone showing no significant change in abnormal breathing events.[22] A potential risk of inducing severe acidosis with long-term use of acetazolamide is also a concern.

Weight loss, both medical and surgical, is associated with improvements in lung volumes, respiratory muscle function and endurance,[23] a significant reduction in the AHI, and improvements in nocturnal oxygen saturation.[24] Follow-up studies of obese patients with OSA after gastric bypass surgery for weight loss found modest reductions in both AHI and measure of pulmonary hypertension. However, in most subjects, the residual AHI was still consistent with moderate OSA.[25,26] A significant amount of weight must be lost before physiologic improvements are seen, with a recent meta-analysis reporting that a weight loss of 45 kg is associated with an improvement of 10 mm Hg in Po$_2$ and a decrease of 3 mm Hg in Pco$_2$.[27] Although lifestyle modifications with dietary change and exercise can help some patients lose weight, most patients regain this weight after 1 year.[28] Bariatric surgery may be a more effective approach in severely obese patients, with achievements of greater degrees of weight loss and long-term maintenance.[29] In general, weight loss requires a multidisciplinary approach with anticipation of degrees of failure and relapse in some patients.

In patients with OHS, continuous positive airway pressure (CPAP) treats coexisting OSA by relieving upper airway obstruction during sleep and improving hypercapnia, oxygenation, and quality of life.[30–32] However, despite improvements in AHI and rapid eye movement (REM) sleep duration, some patients with OHS continue to show significant nocturnal oxygen desaturation.[19] For these patients, noninvasive positive pressure ventilation (NPPV) via bilevel positive airway pressure (BPAP) has the advantage of augmenting ventilation by providing inspiratory pressure and maintenance of airway patency. Long-term NPPV normalizes hypercapnia, improves hypoxemia, and increases lung volumes in patients with OHS.[18] In a retrospective study, use of NPPV for management of hypoventilation in stable settings lowered mortality when compared with untreated patients with OHS.[33]

There are no specific guidelines or criteria when choosing the initial modality of positive airway pressure for treatment of OHS. In general, CPAP can be started if OHS is associated with OSA and severe nocturnal hypoxemia is lacking.[30] Expiratory pressure should be increased to eliminate airflow obstruction; however, if oxygen saturation is less than 90% in the absence of airflow obstruction, then treatment should be switched to BPAP. The BPAP inspiratory pressure should then be increased until oxygen saturation is more than 90%. In patients with OHS without evidence of OSA, BPAP should be used. BPAP should also be considered the first modality in patients with acute decompensation of OHS because it may prevent intubation and is associated with lower mortality.[33,34] Recently, studies of average volume–assured pressure support (AVAPS), another mode of NPPV, showed improvements in ventilation compared with BPAP but achieved less patient tolerance because of high interface pressure.[35,36] Despite this, AVAPS may be considered in patients who lack response to CPAP or BPAP. Supplemental oxygen should be added if optimal positive airway pressure settings fail to resolve nocturnal hypoxemia, especially in cases of coexistent pulmonary parenchymal disease. Although oxygen therapy alone improves nocturnal oxygenation, it does not correct hypoventilation,[37] with a recent study showing more profound degrees of hypercapnia with use of supplemental oxygen in stable patients with OHS.[38]

HYPOVENTILATION IN OBSTRUCTIVE LUNG DISEASE

Both asthma and COPD are associated with hypoventilation. In patients with asthma, it is important to differentiate 2 distinct presentations: stable asthma and severe asthma exacerbation. In stable asthma, hypoventilation is uncommon; thus, chronic hypercapnia with subsequent renal bicarbonate retention is seldom observed. This feature distinguishes asthma from COPD. When chronic hypoventilation occurs in patients with asthma, it is usually the result of an overlapping disorder such as OHS, COPD, or OSA. On the other hand, acute hypercapnic respiratory failure is a well-known complication of asthma exacerbations. Acute hypoventilation in these patients indicates severe bronchial obstruction and has classically been addressed with endotracheal intubation (ETI) and mechanical ventilation. However, increased experience with noninvasive ventilation (NIV) has reduced this need. In a retrospective cohort study of patients admitted to a single academic hospital for severe asthmatic attacks with evidence of hypercapnia, the need for ETI was decreased after introduction of NIV (post-NIV era). Patients treated during this period had shorter hospital length of stay (12.6 ± 4.2 vs 8.4 ± 2.8 days, $P<.01$) compared with those treated in the pre-NIV era.[39] Use of NIV also improves FEV_1 and respiratory rate and decreases rate of hospitalization in patients treated for severe asthma in the emergency department.[40] Despite the number of positive outcomes associated with early institution of NIV in status asthmaticus, the recognition of patients with progressive and declining respiratory status despite NIV is paramount. A continuous increase in Pco_2 or the development of severe acidosis after 1 hour of NIV suggests that ETI and mechanical ventilation are needed.[41] A decrease in pulse volume, dysrhythmias, pneumothorax, and pneumomediastinum are additional criteria. Proper selection of patients who can tolerate and benefit from NIV is crucial. Obtaining an appropriate mask fit to prevent leaks is very important. Inability to protect the airways from excessive secretions or altered mental status, cardiopulmonary arrest and hemodynamic instability, high risk of aspiration, inability of the patient to cooperate, and facial trauma or surgery are respectable contraindications to NIV.[42] If ETI and mechanical ventilation are pursued, the goals of mechanical ventilation are to improve oxygenation, minimize hyperinflation, and provide adequate ventilation. Aggressive correction of hypercapnia and pH is not necessary and could possibly increase the risk of barotrauma.[43] Permissive hypercapnia in the ventilatory management of status asthmaticus is well tolerated but should be avoided in patients with concurrent intracranial hypertension.[43,44] Prolonging expiratory time (or shortening inspiratory time) minimizes hyperinflation. Selection of positive end-expiratory pressure (PEEP) is controversial because of a paradoxic response, hence lowering lung volumes after application of extrinsic PEEP in some patients, whereas others may experience treatment-neutral or positive responses to PEEP.[45]

In contrast to asthma, airflow obstruction that is not fully reversible is the hallmark of COPD. On pulmonary function testing, a decrease in $FEV_1:FVC$ ratio to less than 70% generally indicates airflow obstruction, whereas the percentage of FEV_1 predicted expresses the severity of disease. Although there is an inverse relationship between FEV_1 and $Paco_2$, severe reductions in FEV_1 are not universally predictive of hypercapnia and are likely explained by individual variations in chemoreceptor sensitivity to CO_2 and inspiratory muscle strength.[46] Despite individual differences, 2 phenotypes that predominate in COPD are chronic bronchitis and emphysema. In chronic bronchitis, chronic small and medium-sized airway inflammation with mucous gland hyperplasia, goblet cell metaplasia, and fibrosis lead to luminal narrowing and subsequent airway obstruction.[47] In emphysema, the prominent pathologic condition is destruction of the lung parenchyma, including respiratory bronchioles, alveolar ducts, and alveoli because of smoking-related inflammation, increased proteolytic injury to the extracellular matrix, and subsequent cell death. The destroyed parenchyma is replaced with nonfunctional bullae leading to a decrease in diffusion capacity, a distinguishing feature of pulmonary function testing in these patients with emphysema. The accompanying loss of elastic recoil leads to loss of tethering of the small bronchioles, which then collapse with increased intrathoracic pressure during exhalation.[48] Despite the differences between these 2 phenotypes, both are capable of hypoventilation.

The 4 clinical scenarios of hypoventilation in patients with COPD are acute hypoventilation due to exacerbations of COPD, chronic hypoventilation in COPD, sleep-related hypoventilation, and hypoventilation precipitated by initiation of long-term oxygen therapy (LTOT). During acute hypoventilation from COPD exacerbation, worsening airflow obstruction accompanied by respiratory muscle fatigue leads to inadequate ventilation and subsequent hypercapnia.[49] NIV reduces the work of breathing. The reduction is directly proportional to the level of the inspiratory pressure assist and by the application to extrinsic PEEP to counter the intrinsic PEEP.[50] In a meta-analysis of 14 randomized controlled trials comparing NIV plus usual medical care versus usual medical care alone, NIV reduced mortality, need for invasive mechanical ventilation, rate of treatment failure, rate of complications, and length of stay.[51] Additional studies indicate that NIV is most efficacious in patients with severe exacerbations of COPD and moderate degrees of acidosis (pH<7.3).[52] Close monitoring is important, with direct observations of improvement in hypercapnia and acidosis predicting treatment success. In COPD exacerbations, supplemental oxygen aimed at correcting hypoxia without concurrent effort to correct hypoventilation can be detrimental.

Despite the positive outcomes associated with the use of NIV during acute exacerbations of COPD, studies examining NIV in patients with chronic hypoventilation in severe COPD have generated mixed results. In a randomized controlled clinical trial of 144 patients with severe COPD and daytime hypercapnia randomized to NIV and LTOT versus LTOT alone, NIV improved sleep quality and sleep-related hypercapnia but without change in FEV_1 and $Paco_2$ at 6 and 12 months. Patients randomized to NIV plus LTOT had improved survival at the expense of worsened general and mental health and vigor.[53] These outcomes are in contrast to other studies.[54] In a 2009 Cochrane library review, Wijkstra and colleagues[55] concluded that the use of nocturnal NIV for at least 3 months was not associated with any significant clinical or lung function improvement; however, the number of studies included was quite small, limiting the generalizability of these findings.

Mild physiologic hypoventilation occurs during sleep. This phenomenon is exaggerated in patients with COPD. The effect is most prominent during REM sleep. This hypoventilation can be attributed to coexisting OSA and is termed the overlap syndrome. OSA occurs in 10% to 15% of patients who have COPD.[56] Marin and colleagues[57] studied the outcomes in 441 patients with overlap syndrome, of whom 223 received treatment with CPAP and 213 did not. Patients who were not treated with CPAP had a higher mortality and were more likely to have a severe COPD exacerbation.

Hypoventilation can also be precipitated by oxygen therapy. Even an increase of 1 L/min in oxygen flow at night, as recommended by the American Thoracic Society/European Respiratory Society guidelines, can worsen hypoventilation in severe COPD. In a prospective, crossover, randomized multicenter trial, Samolski and colleagues[58] enrolled 38 patients with GOLD (Global Obstructive Lung Disease initiative) Stage IV COPD, excluding patients with OSAS. The 1-L/min increase in nocturnal oxygen therapy resulted in a larger increase in Pco_2 (62.90 ± 10.60 vs 59.90 ± 8.33 mm Hg, $P = .053$) and a greater reduction in pH (7.32 ± 0.35 vs 7.34 ± 0.35, $P<.05$). The clinical significance of this worsening hypoventilation is still unknown.

HYPOVENTILATION AND RESTRICTIVE CHEST WALL DISORDERS

Restrictive diseases affect the chest wall by limiting expansion of the thorax and may lead to development of hypoventilation. Patients with hypoventilation secondary to chest wall disorders in general demonstrate a restrictive ventilatory impairment on pulmonary function testing. The shallow and reduced tidal volumes increase the dead space fraction. Increases in respiratory rate initially compensate for lower tidal volumes and maintain adequate minute ventilation; however, with progressive restriction of the chest wall and subsequent reduction in the maximum sustainable minute ventilation, hypercapnia and hypoventilation ensue.[59] Restrictive chest wall disorders include, but are not limited to, ankylosing spondylitis, kyphoscoliosis, fibrothorax, and thoracoplasty.

Ankylosing spondylitis is a chronic inflammatory disease affecting the costovertebral joints leading to fusion and fixation of the chest wall and fibrobullous pulmonary disease of the upper lobe.[60] Patients usually have a mild reduction in TLC and VC. The relative preservation of lung volumes compared with other restrictive chest wall disorders is attributed to diaphragmatic compensation and rib cage fixation at higher volumes.[61] Both MEP and MIP are reduced secondary to intercostal muscle atrophy.[62]

Kyphoscoliosis is a combination of anteroposterior (kyphosis) and lateral (scoliosis) angulations of the spine that when excessive can lead to chest wall deformity and restriction. The severity of the spinal curvature is measured by the Cobb angle, which is formed by the intersection of perpendicular lines drawn superior to the highest vertebrae and inferior to the lowest vertebrae involved. Angles greater than 100° are associated with respiratory failure.[63] Pulmonary function testing reveals a restrictive pattern with a significant reduction in TLC, VC, and functional residual capacity with preserved residual volumes. However, the degree of pulmonary involvement can be out of proportion to the radiographic severity of disease, particularly in cases of rotational vertebral involvement at the T8 and T9 levels.[64,65]

Thoracoplasty is a surgical procedure involving resection of ribs or their replacement with an inward convexity device to decrease the thoracic volume.[63]

Thoracoplasty was done before 1950 as a collapse therapy for tuberculosis. In the modern era, thoracoplasty is still performed in patients in need of closure of the pleural space. Pulmonary function testing reveals a restrictive ventilatory defect with reductions in TLC and VC as a result of thoracic volume reduction, residual pulmonary fibrosis, and chest deformity. A unique feature of patients with thoracoplasty is the concomitant presence of irreversible airflow obstruction, which correlates with the development of hypoventilation and respiratory failure.[66]

Fibrothorax is scarring or fibrosis of the visceral pleura caused by inflammation from pleural disease. Although only the pleura is involved initially, extension to the chest wall can lead to involvement of intercostal muscles, endothoracic fascia, and periosteum of the ribs, leading to limitation of chest wall expansion and restrictive ventilatory defects on pulmonary function testing.[67] This process can be the sequela of diseases producing inflammation but is most commonly seen in inadequately treated pleural effusions from chronic empyema, tuberculous effusion, or hemothorax. However, clinical characteristics or pleural fluid analyses are not predictive of pleural thickening or progression.[68]

Although treatment of restrictive chest wall disorders should be aimed at the underlying disease, nocturnal or long-term use of NPPV has been used for management of hypoventilation secondary to restrictive chest disorders. NPPV reduces the work of breathing, increases lung compliance, and treats coexistent sleep-disordered breathing, if applicable. Studies examining the use of NPPV for hypoventilation are most widely reported in kyphoscoliosis. Patients with severe kyphoscoliosis who use long-term NPPV experience improvements in daily symptoms, quality of life, and both nocturnal and daytime oxygen saturation without significant changes in the sleep architecture or breathing patterns. Respiratory muscle function and lung volumes also significantly improve in these patients.[69] Furthermore, in patients with kyphoscoliosis, use of NPPV added to oxygen therapy resulted in improvement in mortality when compared with LTOT alone.[70]

HYPOVENTILATION AND NEUROMUSCULAR DISEASE

Neuromuscular disease may herald the development of both acute and chronic presentations of hypoventilation and are seen in patients affected by several neuromuscular diseases, including, but not limited to, myasthenia gravis, multiple sclerosis, Guillain-Barré syndrome (GBS), spinal muscular atrophy, spinal cord injury, postpolio syndrome (PPS), Lambert-Eaton myasthenic syndrome, Duchenne muscular dystrophy (DMD), and amyotrophic lateral sclerosis (ALS). Although disease-specific characteristics of presentation, evaluation, and treatment are outside the scope of this review, respiratory similarities in this group include sleep disturbances, nocturnal hypoxemia, and eventually hypercapnia due to the involvement of respiratory muscle weakness and alterations in respiratory mechanics. Despite differences in the diseases themselves, assessment and management of hypoventilation in this group have several commonalities.

Assessment of hypoventilation in the patient with neuromuscular disease includes careful history taking, physical examination, and supportive objective evidence, including pulmonary function tests and arterial blood gas analysis. Useful pulmonary function tests include the VC, MIP, and MEP. The reduction in lung and chest wall compliance and respiratory muscle weakness result in decreased VC[71] and hence a restrictive ventilatory defect. The MIP is a measure of inspiratory muscle strength, whereas the MEP is a measure of expiratory muscle strength. Diaphragmatic weakness (the major inspiratory muscle of respiration) leads to reduced tidal volumes.

Compensation for this deficit includes an increase in respiratory rate and use of accessory muscles of inspiration: sternocleidomastoids, scalene, and external intercostal muscles. However, once disease involvement includes the accessory muscles, adequate ventilation cannot be maintained and hypercapnia ensues. Physical examination findings include rapid shallow breathing and visible use of the accessory muscles. If abdominal muscles and internal intercostals (muscles of expiration) are involved along with failure of the glottis to open and close appropriately; this results in impairment of cough and expectoration of secretions[72] and dyspnea. Orthopnea and paradoxic motion of the thorax and abdomen are worthy of notice.

Manifestations of ventilatory impairment may be most evident during sleep, particularly during REM sleep, hallmarked by muscle atonia, with sparing of the diaphragm and extraocular muscles. Minute ventilation during REM sleep is lower in normal individuals but can be much lower in the patient with hypoventilation secondary to neuromuscular disease, such as ALS, which commonly affects the diaphragm. Collectively, these impairments result in more profound degrees of hypoventilation. In addition to sleep-related hypoventilation, nocturnal hypoxemia, reduced sleep efficiency, increased arousals, and obstructive and central sleep apneas and hypopneas have been reported, particularly in myasthenia gravis, PPS, DMD, and ALS.[73–78] Central sleep apnea may result from brainstem involvement, particularly in PPS and ALS with bulbar involvement. However, fatigue may be the only reported symptom of sleep-disordered breathing.

Pulmonary function testing is useful to corroborate clinical examination. As mentioned, the VC is reduced, particularly in the supine position.[79] A reduction of VC of 10% when measured in supine position compared with that in upright position is supportive of diagnosis. During acute presentation of neuromuscular disease, performance of serial measures of VC may be more beneficial and a useful predictor of respiratory failure. In studies involving GBS, a VC less than 50% from baseline or decline in VC by 30% or more predicted the need for mechanical ventilation.[80,81] Additional factors associated with progression to respiratory failure include VC less than 20 mL/kg, MIP less than 30 cm H_2O, and MEP less than 40 cm H_2O.[81] Bulbar or autonomic dysfunction and facial palsy are also clinical predictors. These thresholds may not be applicable in other neuromuscular diseases outside of GBS. Furthermore, their usefulness in predicting successful extubation is not widely accepted, although general guidelines include a positive predictor of successful extubation in patients with myasthenic crisis with an FVC greater than 15 mL/kg.

In addition to pulmonary function testing, arterial blood gas and oximetry can supply valuable information in the assessment of the patient with hypoventilation due to neuromuscular disease. Although there are notable limitations, primary usefulness of these tests is in the evaluation of chronic hypoventilation. In patients with DMD, arterial blood gas analysis is recommended if FEV_1 is less than 40%. In addition, polysomnography is indicated to evaluate for sleep-related hypoventilation when the arterial blood gas analysis reveals a Pco_2 greater than 45 mm Hg and a base excess of 4 mmol/L or greater.[82] Measurement of nocturnal Pco_2 should be performed if possible during polysomnography. In patients with ALS, duration of nocturnal saturations less than 90% may be a measure of early respiratory insufficiency.[3]

Once assessment has been performed and treatment of hypoventilation is needed, options are available. In the setting of cardiopulmonary arrest, altered mental status, and severe ventilatory and oxygenation derangements, invasive mechanical ventilation is needed. Otherwise, NIV can be used for both acute and chronic forms of hypoventilation. In patients with myasthenic crisis, use of NIV before the onset of hypercapnia may prevent intubation. In a retrospective study examining outcomes among patients with myasthenic crisis, average intensive care unit and hospital lengths of stay were significantly less in patients who received NIV compared with those who were intubated.[83] Use of NIV prevented mechanical ventilation in 14 patients; however, a $Paco_2$ level greater than 45 predicted NIV failure. Use of NIV was suspected to result in less atelectasis and pulmonary complications. It is important to recognize that higher degrees of success are expected in patients who do not exhibit hypercapnia.

Positive outcomes with the use of NIV for management of chronic hypoventilation in patients with DMD and ALS have been reported. In a study comparing morbidity and causes of death in patients with DMD receiving mechanical ventilation via tracheostomy versus NIV, patients who had undergone tracheostomy had more cases of mucous hypersecretion, tracheal injury, and chest infection without any improvement in survival.[84] NIV extends survival at 1 and 5 years in patients with DMD.[85] NIV improves hypercapnia and hypoxemia even in patients with DMD with nocturnal hypercapnia but daytime normocapnia.[86] Similar outcomes of improved survival and quality of life are seen with the use of NIV in ALS.[87,88] Furthermore, in patients with neuromuscular disease, the American College of Chest Physicians recommends muscle strength training, manual cough assist, and mechanical cough assist[89] based on studies demonstrating increases in MIP and MEP[90,91] and increases in peak inspiratory cough flow.[92]

REFERENCES

1. Mallemgaard K. The alveolar-arterial oxygen difference: its size and components in normal man. Acta Physiol Scand 1966;67:10–20.
2. Miller WF, Scacci R, Gast LR. Laboratory evaluation of pulmonary function. Philadelphia: JB Lippincott; 1987. p. 101.
3. Jackson CE, Rosenfeld J, Moore DH, et al. A preliminary evaluation of a prospective study of pulmonary function studies and symptoms of hypoventilation in ALS/MND patients. J Neurol Sci 2001;191:75–8.
4. De Troyer A, Borenstein S, Cordier R. Analysis of lung volume restriction in patients with respiratory muscle weakness. Thorax 1980;35:603–10.
5. Gelb AF, Klein E, Schiffman P, et al. Ventilatory response and drive in acute and chronic obstructive pulmonary disease. Am Rev Respir Dis 1977;116:9–16.
6. Ogden CL, Carroll MD, Curtin LR, et al. Prevalence of high body mass index in US children and adolescents, 2007-2008. JAMA 2010;303:242–9.
7. Flegal KM, Carroll MD, Ogden CL, et al. Prevalence and trends in obesity among US adults, 1999-2008. JAMA 2010;303:235–41.
8. Nowbar S, Burkart KM, Gonzales R, et al. Obesity-associated hypoventilation in hospitalized patients: prevalence, effects, and outcome. Am J Med 2004;116:1–7.
9. Mokhlesi B, Tulaimat A. Recent advances in obesity hypoventilation syndrome. Chest 2007;132:1322–36.
10. Kessler R, Chaouat A, Schinkewitch P, et al. The obesity-hypoventilation syndrome revisited: a prospective study of 34 consecutive cases. Chest 2001;120:369–76.
11. Mokhlesi B, Tulaimat A, Faibussowitsch I, et al. Obesity hypoventilation syndrome: prevalence and predictors in patients with obstructive sleep apnea. Sleep Breath 2007;11:117–24.
12. Kress JP, Pohlman AS, Alverdy J, et al. The impact of morbid obesity on oxygen cost of breathing (VO(2RESP)) at rest. Am J Respir Crit Care Med 1999;160:883–6.

13. Ayappa I, Berger KI, Norman RG, et al. Hypercapnia and ventilatory periodicity in obstructive sleep apnea syndrome. Am J Respir Crit Care Med 2002;166:1112–5.
14. Norman RG, Goldring RM, Clain JM, et al. Transition from acute to chronic hypercapnia in patients with periodic breathing: predictions from a computer model. J Appl Phys 2006;100:1733–41.
15. Rochester DS, Arora NS. Respiratory failure from obesity. In: Mancini M, lewis B, Contaldo F, editors. Medical complications of obesity. London: Academic press; 1980. p. 183.
16. O'donnell CP, Schaub CD, Haines AS, et al. Leptin prevents respiratory depression in obesity. Am J Respir Crit Care Med 1999;159(5 Pt 1):1477–84.
17. Bickelmann AG, Burwell CS, Robin ED, et al. Extreme obesity associated with alveolar hypoventilation: a Pickwickian syndrome. Am J Med 1956;21:811–8.
18. Heinemann F, Budweiser S, Dobroschke J, et al. Non-invasive positive pressure ventilation improves lung volumes in the obesity hypoventilation syndrome. Respir Med 2007;101:1229–35.
19. Banerjee D, Yee BJ, Piper AJ, et al. Obesity hypoventilation syndrome: hypoxemia during continuous positive airway pressure. Chest 2007;131:1678–84.
20. Sutton FD Jr, Zwillich CW, Creagh CE, et al. Progesterone for outpatient treatment of Pickwickian syndrome. Ann Intern Med 1975;83:476–9.
21. Tojima H, Kunitomo F, Kimura H, et al. Effects of acetazolamide in patients with the sleep apnoea syndrome. Thorax 1988;43:113–9.
22. Cook WR, Benich JJ, Wooten SA. Indices of severity of obstructive sleep apnea syndrome do not change during medroxyprogesterone acetate therapy. Chest 1989;96:262–6.
23. Weiner P, Waizman J, Weiner M, et al. Influence of excessive weight loss after gastroplasty for morbid obesity on respiratory muscle performance. Thorax 1998;53:39–42.
24. Harman EM, Wynne JW, Block AJ. The effect of weight loss on sleep-disordered breathing and oxygen desaturation in morbidly obese men. Chest 1982;82:291–4.
25. Greenburg DL, Lettieri CJ, Eliasson AH. Effects of surgical weight loss on measures of obstructive sleep apnea: a meta-analysis. Am J Med 2009;122:535–42.
26. Lettieri CJ, Eliasson AH, Greenburg DL. Persistence of obstructive sleep apnea after surgical weight loss. J Clin Sleep Med 2008;4:333–8.
27. Zavorsky GS, Hoffman SL. Pulmonary gas exchange in the morbidly obese. Obes Rev 2008;9:326–39.
28. NIH Technology Assessment Conference Panel. Methods for voluntary weight loss and control. Ann Intern Med 1993;119(7 Pt 2):764–70.
29. Sjöström L, Lindroos AK, Peltonen M. Lifestyle, diabetes, and cardiovascular risk factors 10 years after bariatric surgery. N Engl J Med 2004;351:2683–93.
30. Piper AJ, Wang D, Yee BJ, et al. Randomized trial of CPAP vs bilevel support in the treatment of obesity hypoventilation syndrome without severe nocturnal desaturation. Thorax 2008;63:395–401.
31. Sullivan CE, Berthon-Jones M, Issa FG. Remission of severe obesity-hypoventilation syndrome after short-term treatment during sleep with nasal continuous positive airway pressure. Am Rev Respir Dis 1983;128:177–81.
32. Hida W, Okabe S, Tatsumi K, et al. Nasal continuous positive airway pressure improves quality of life in obesity hypoventilation syndrome. Sleep Breath 2003; 7:3–12.
33. Priou P, Hamel JF, Person C, et al. Long-term outcome of noninvasive positive pressure ventilation for obesity hypoventilation syndrome. Chest 2010;138:84–90.

34. Pérez de Llano LA, Golpe R, Ortiz Piquer M, et al. Short-term and long-term effects of nasal intermittent positive pressure ventilation in patients with obesity-hypoventilation syndrome. Chest 2005;128:587–94.
35. Janssens JP, Metzger M, Sforza E. Impact of volume targeting efficacy of bi-level non-invasive ventilation and sleep in obesity-hypoventilation. Respir Med 2009; 103:165–72.
36. Storre JH, Seuthe B, Fiechter R, et al. Average volume-assured pressure support in obesity hypoventilation. A randomized crossover trial. Chest 2006; 130:815–21.
37. Masa JF, Celli BR, Riesco JA, et al. Noninvasive positive pressure ventilation and not oxygen may prevent overt ventilatory failure in patients with chest wall diseases. Chest 1997;112:207–13.
38. Wijesinghe M, Williams M, Perrin K, et al. The effect of supplemental oxygen on hypercapnia in subjects with obesity-associated hypoventilation: a randomized, crossover, clinical study. Chest 2011;139:1018–24.
39. Murase K, Tomii K, Chin K, et al. The use of non-invasive ventilation for life-threatening asthma attacks: changes in the need for intubation. Respirology 2010;15:714–20.
40. Soroksky A. A pilot prospective, randomized, placebo-controlled trial of bilevel positive airway pressure in acute asthmatic attack. Chest 2003;123:1018–25.
41. Sydow M. Ventilating the patient with severe asthma: nonconventional therapy. Minerva Anestesiol 2003;69:333–7.
42. Gupta D, Nath A, Agarwal R. A prospective randomized controlled trial on the efficacy of noninvasive ventilation in severe acute asthma. Respir Care 2010;55:536–43.
43. Papiris S, Kotanidou A, Malagari K, et al. Clinical review: severe asthma. Crit Care 2002;6:30–44.
44. Mutlu GM, Factor P, Schwartz DE, et al. Severe status asthmaticus: management with permissive hypercapnia and inhalation anesthesia. Crit Care Med 2002;30:477–80.
45. Caramez MP, Borges JB, Tucci MR, et al. Paradoxical responses to positive end-expiratory pressure in patients with airway obstruction during controlled ventilation. Crit Care Med 2005;33:1519–28.
46. Bégin P, Grassino A. Inspiratory muscle dysfunction and chronic hypercapnia in chronic obstructive pulmonary disease. Am Rev Respir Dis 1991;143:905–12.
47. Wise RA. Chronic obstructive pulmonary disease: clinical course and management. In: Fishman AP, Elias JA, Fishman JA, et al, editors. Fishman's pulmonary disease and disorders, vol. 1. 4th edition. New York: McGraw-Hill; 2008. p. 730.
48. Shapiro SD, Reilly JJ, Rennard SI. Chronic bronchitis and emphysema: pathology. In: Mason RJ, Broaddus VC, Martin TR, et al, editors. Murray & Nadel's textbook of respiratory medicine, vol. 1. 5th edition. Philadelphia: Saunders; 2010. p. 933–5.
49. Calverley PM. Respiratory failure in chronic obstructive pulmonary disease. Eur Respir J 2003;22(Suppl 47):26s–30s.
50. Kallet RH, Diaz JV. The physiologic effects of noninvasive ventilation. Respir Care 2009;54:102–15.
51. Ram FS, Picot J, Lightowler J, et al. Non-invasive positive pressure ventilation for treatment of respiratory failure due to exacerbations of chronic obstructive pulmonary disease. Cochrane Database Syst Rev 2004;1:CD004104.
52. Keenan SP, Sinuff T, Cook DJ, et al. Which patients with acute exacerbation of chronic obstructive pulmonary disease benefit from noninvasive positive-pressure ventilation? A systematic review of the literature. Ann Intern Med 2003;138:861–70.

53. McEvoy RD, Pierce RJ, Hillman D, et al. Nocturnal non-invasive nasal ventilation in stable hypercapnic COPD: a randomized controlled trial. Thorax 2009;64(7): 561–6.

54. Lin CC. Comparison between nocturnal nasal positive pressure ventilation combined with oxygen therapy and oxygen monotherapy in patients with severe COPD. Am J Respir Crit Care Med 1996;154(2 Pt 1):353–8.

55. Wijkstra PJ, Lacasse Y, Guyatt GH, et al. Nocturnal non-invasive positive pressure ventilation for stable chronic obstructive pulmonary disease. Cochrane Database Syst Rev 2002;3:CD002878.

56. Capro JD, Glassroth JL, Karlinsky JB, et al. Diagnosis of chronic obstructive pulmonary disease: sleep and chronic obstructive pulmonary disease. In: Baum's textbook of pulmonary disease. 7th edition. Philadelphia: Lippincott Williams & Wilkins; 2004. p. 229.

57. Marin JM, Soriano JB, Carrizo SJ, et al. Outcomes in patients with chronic obstructive pulmonary disease and obstructive sleep apnea: the overlap syndrome. Am J Respir Crit Care Med 2010;182:325–31.

58. Samolski D, Tárrega J, Antón A, et al. Sleep hypoventilation due to increased nocturnal oxygen flow in hypercapnic COPD patients. Respirology 2010;15:283–8.

59. Bergofsky EH. Respiratory failure in disorders of the thoracic cage. Am Rev Respir Dis 1979;119:643–69.

60. Tanoue LT. Pulmonary involvement in collagen vascular disease: a review of the pulmonary manifestations of the Marfan syndrome, ankylosing spondylitis, Sjögren's syndrome, and relapsing polychondritis. J Thorac Imaging 1992;7:62–77.

61. Romagnoli I, Gigliotti F, Galarducci A, et al. Chest wall kinematics and respiratory muscle action in ankylosing spondylitis patients. Eur Respir J 2004;24:453–60.

62. Vanderschueren D, Decramer M, Van den Daele P, et al. Pulmonary function and maximal transrespiratory pressures in ankylosing spondylitis. Ann Rheum Dis 1989;48:632–5.

63. McCool FD, Rochester DF. The lungs and chest wall disease. In: Murray JF, editor. Textbook of Respiratory Medicine, vol. 2. 3rd edition. Philadelphia: Saunders; 2000. p. 2357–76.

64. Takahashi S, Suzuki N, Asazuma T, et al. Factors of thoracic cage deformity that affect pulmonary function in adolescent idiopathic thoracic scoliosis. Spine 2007; 32:106–12.

65. Newton PO, Faro FD, Gollogly S, et al. Results of preoperative pulmonary function testing of adolescents with idiopathic scoliosis. A study of six hundred and thirty-one patients. J Bone Joint Surg Am 2005;87:1937–46.

66. Phillips MS, Miller MR, Kinnear WJ, et al. Importance of airflow obstruction after thoracoplasty. Thorax 1987;42:348–52.

67. Bolliger CT, de Kock MA. Influence of a fibrothorax on the flow/volume curve. Respiration 1988;54:197–200.

68. Barbas CS, Cukier A, de Varvalho CR, et al. The relationship between pleural fluid findings and the development of pleural thickening in patients with pleural tuberculosis. Chest 1991;100(5):1264–7.

69. Gonzalez C, Ferris G, Diaz J, et al. Kyphoscoliotic ventilatory insufficiency: effects of long-term intermittent positive-pressure ventilation. Chest 2003;124:857–62.

70. Buyse B, Meersseman W, Demedts M. Treatment of chronic respiratory failure in kyphoscoliosis: oxygen or ventilation? Eur Respir J 2003;22:525–8.

71. Criner GJ, Kelsen SG. Effects of neuromuscular diseases on ventilation. In: Fishman JA, Grippi MA, Kaiser LR, et al, editors. Fishman's pulmonary disease and disorders. 3rd edition. New York: McGraw-Hill; 1998. p. 1561–85.

72. Haas CF, Loik PS, Gay SE. Airway clearance applications in the elderly and in patients with neurologic or neuromuscular compromise. Respir Care 2007;52:1362–81.
73. Nicolle MW, Rask S, Koopman WJ, et al. Sleep apnea in patients with myasthenia gravis. Neurology 2006;67:140–2.
74. Hsu AA, Staats BA. "Postpolio" sequelae and sleep-related disordered breathing. Mayo Clin Proc 1998;73:216–24.
75. Steljes DG, Kryger MH, Kirk BW, et al. Sleep in postpolio syndrome. Chest 1990; 98:133–40.
76. Suresh S, Wales P, Dakin C, et al. Sleep-related breathing disorder in Duchenne muscular dystrophy: disease spectrum in the pediatric population. J Paediatr Child Health 2005;41:500–3.
77. Atalaia A, De Carvalho M, Evangelista T, et al. Sleep characteristics of amyotrophic lateral sclerosis in patients with preserved diaphragmatic function. Amyotroph Lateral Scler 2007;8:101–5.
78. Arnulf I, Similowski T, Salachas F, et al. Sleep disorders and diaphragmatic function in patients with amyotrophic lateral sclerosis. Am J Respir Crit Care Med 2000;161(3 Pt 1):849–56.
79. Bach JR, Alba AS. Management of chronic alveolar hypoventilation by nasal ventilation. Chest 1990;97:52–7.
80. Chevrolet JC, Deléamont P. Repeated vital capacity measurements as predictive parameters for mechanical ventilation need and weaning success in the Guillain-Barré syndrome. Am Rev Respir Dis 1991;144:814–8.
81. Lawn ND, Fletcher DD, Henderson RD, et al. Anticipating mechanical ventilation in Guillain-Barré syndrome. Arch Neurol 2001;58:893–8.
82. Hukins CA, Hillman DR. Daytime predictors of sleep hypoventilation in Duchenne muscular dystrophy. Am J Respir Crit Care Med 2000;161:166–70.
83. Seneviratne J, Mandrekar J, Wijdicks EF, et al. Noninvasive ventilation in myasthenic crisis. Arch Neurol 2008;65:54–8.
84. Soudon P, Steens M, Toussaint M. A comparison of invasive versus noninvasive full-time mechanical ventilation in Duchenne muscular dystrophy. Chron Respir Dis 2008;5:87–93.
85. Simonds AK, Muntoni F, Heather S, et al. Impact of nasal ventilation on survival in hypercapnic Duchenne muscular dystrophy. Thorax 1998;53:949–52.
86. Ward S, Chatwin M, Heather S, et al. Randomized controlled trial of non-invasive ventilation (NIV) for nocturnal hypoventilation in neuromuscular and chest wall disease patients with daytime normocapnia. Thorax 2005;60:1019–24.
87. Aboussouan LS, Kahn SU, Meeker DP, et al. Effect of noninvasive positive-pressure ventilation on survival in amyotrophic lateral sclerosis. Ann Intern Med 1997;127:450–3.
88. Bourke SC, Bullock RE, William TL, et al. Noninvasive ventilation in ALS: indication and effect on quality of life. Neurology 2003;61:171–7.
89. McCoo RD, Rosen MJ. Nonpharmacological airway clearance therapies: ACCP evidence-based clinical practice guidelines. Chest 2006;129(Suppl 1):28S–32S.
90. Smeltzer SC, Lavietes MH, Cook SD. Expiratory training in multiple sclerosis. Arch Phys Med Rehabil 1996;77:909–12.
91. Fregonezi GA, Resqueti VR, Güell R, et al. Effects of 8-week, interval-based inspiratory muscle training and breathing retraining in patients with generalized myasthenia gravis. Chest 2005;128:1524–30.
92. Bach Jr. Mechanical insufflation-exsufflation: comparison of peak expiratory flow with manually assisted and unassisted coughing techniques. Chest 1993;104: 1553–62.

Clinical Review of Pulmonary Embolism: Diagnosis, Prognosis, and Treatment

James M. Hunt, MD*, Todd M. Bull, MD

KEYWORDS

- Pulmonary embolism • Venous thromboembolic disease
- Biomarkers • Chronic thromboembolic disease

Venous thromboembolism (VTE) refers to the pathologic formation of a thrombus within the veins, and includes both pulmonary embolism (PE) and deep venous thrombosis (DVT). VTE is a common disease causing significant morbidity, mortality, and substantial socioeconomic costs. Consequently, many resources have been devoted to improving its diagnosis and management; resulting in an increasing number of well-designed clinical trials over the past decades. These trials have significantly advanced our understanding of the optimal approach toward diagnosis and treatment of VTE, and are helping resolve existing controversies. The clinical landscape of VTE management, however, continues to evolve rapidly as novel medications, imaging techniques, procedures, and devices present new exciting options and challenges.

EPIDEMIOLOGY AND RISK FACTORS
Epidemiology

Although the exact incidence and prevalence of VTE is unknown, modeling based on epidemiologic studies estimates more than 900,000 incident or recurrent cases in the United States alone.[1] PE is a substantial subset of these cases, with hospital-based studies estimating it is responsible for 200,000 to 300,000 hospital admissions per year.[2] The majority of deaths secondary to VTE are caused by PE, with a 3-month disease specific mortality rate of 10% causing an estimated 30,000 to 50,000 deaths annually.[3–5] Symptomatic PE carries an 18-fold higher risk of early death when

Financial disclosures: Dr Hunt has no competing financial disclosures. Dr Bull has received grant support from the NIH/NHLBI. He has served as a consultant to Actelion.
Division of Pulmonary Sciences and Critical Care Medicine, University of Colorado Denver, Anschutz Medical Campus, Research 2–9th Floor, Mail Stop C-272, 12700 East 19th Avenue, Aurora, CO 80045, USA
* Corresponding author.
E-mail address: James.hunt@ucdenver.edu

compared with DVT alone, and the initial clinical presentation is sudden death in 20% of all cases[2,6] The epidemiology for Europe and other parts of the world is generally similar.[7]

Although the incidence of VTE and PE has not changed dramatically over the past 25 years,[8] the overall mortality rate from PE has decreased substantially in the past several decades.[2,9,10] This decrease has been attributed to improved detection and treatment of DVT, risk-factor modification including protocolization of VTE prophylaxis, and/or improvements in PE diagnostic tests that have increased the specificity and sensitivity of disease diagnosis. Regardless, the annual hospital mortality has decreased by roughly 30% from 1998 to 2009.[2]

Risk Factors

Rudolph Virchow (1821–1902) first coined the term embolism after observing at autopsy blood clots wedged in the pulmonary arteries.[11] From his extensive writings and descriptions of VTE, later investigators coined the term Virchow's Triad, which consists of vascular endothelial injury, hypercoagulability, and venous stasis as the combination of host factors that predispose to VTE.[12] VTE risk factors are traditionally categorized as either acquired or genetic (inherited thrombophilia).

Inherited thrombophilia

Inherited thrombophilias may result in increased levels or function of coagulation factors (activated protein C resistance, factor V Leiden mutation, prothrombin gene mutation, elevated factor VIII levels), defects of coagulation factor inhibitors (antithrombin, protein C, protein S), and defects in fibrolysis, hyperhomocysteinemia, or altered platelet function. The majority of published data regarding the inherited thrombophilias comes from studies of Caucasian populations with VTE.[13–15] It is generally accepted that patients with a "provoked" VTE, such as those with recent surgery, trauma, immobilization, malignancy, or certain inflammatory disorders such as lupus or inflammatory bowel, do not require screening of the hereditary thrombophilias.[16] Screening patients with unprovoked VTE, however, is still a matter of debate, and it is recommended to consult with a coagulopathy specialist before initiating an evaluation.

Acquired risk factors

Acquired risk factors account for the majority of VTE cases. The most significant acquired risk factor for incident VTE is advancing age, especially as age advances beyond 60 years. The most significant risk factor for recurrent VTE is a previous episode of VTE. Other important acquired risk factors include obesity, malignancy, surgery, trauma, hormone replacement therapy, pregnancy, and heparin-induced thrombocytopenia. Roughly 50% or more of patients with VTE will have multiple risk factors,[17] both acquired and inherited, validating the pathophysiologic and clinical relevance of Virchow's Triad.

DIAGNOSIS AND EVALUATION

The diagnosis of PE often presents a significant challenge. The clinical presentations of pulmonary embolic disease are diverse and often incongruous; many patients will experience only a subset of the characteristic symptoms, may have atypical symptoms, or may even be asymptomatic. The signs and symptoms of PE, such as tachycardia, dyspnea, chest pain, hypoxemia, and shock, overlap considerably with other common diseases such as coronary artery disease, congestive heart failure, pericarditis, pneumonia, and exacerbations of chronic obstructive pulmonary disease. Further confounding diagnosis and treatment is that many patients may have a PE in addition to one of the aforementioned diagnoses. The clinical consequences of PE can be equally as diverse, ranging from incidental to catastrophic hemodynamic collapse and sudden death. Consequently, several clinical prediction tools have been developed which, combined with the history and examination, aid clinicians in the choice of appropriate diagnostic tests and therapeutic interventions. Given the high prevalence, diverse symptoms, and mortality associated with PE, it is essential that a high clinical index of suspicion be maintained while using these clinical tools in an efficient and expeditious fashion.

Medical History

Given the diversity and complexity in the clinical presentation of PE, it is crucial to identify risk factors for VTE by performing a careful history. Specifically, the patient's personal and family history of prior VTE, coexisting medical conditions, functional status, travel history, and current medications are fundamental. Recent immobilization, myocardial infarction, cerebrovascular accident, surgery, and recent (within 30 days) trauma are all major risk factors for VTE. Additional major risk factors include advanced age, malignancy, prior VTE, known thrombophilia (inherited or acquired), and indwelling venous catheter. Moderate risk factors include use of estrogen or hormone replacement therapy, obesity, and family history of VTE. These risk factors are used in clinical prediction tools, such as the Wells criteria and the Geneva score, to assess the patient's pretest probability of PE (see the section Clinical Tools).

Clinical Assessment

As previously mentioned, the typical signs and symptoms of PE are nonspecific and include tachypnea, rales, tachycardia, a fourth heart sound, a loud S2, dyspnea, pleuritic chest pain, cough and, in a minority of patients, hemoptysis. Despite, or perhaps because of the complexity in diagnosing PE, clinical judgment is a critical first step in the evaluation and is heavily weighted in diagnostic algorithms. The 1990 PIOPED (Prospective Investigation of Pulmonary Embolism Diagnosis) study first highlighted the importance of a clinician's suspicion in predicting the probability of PE.[18]

In PIOPED, prior to ventilation/perfusion (V/Q) scan and pulmonary arteriogram, physicians recorded their clinical suspicion (low, intermediate, or high probability) of PE in patients evaluated for the disease. A very important finding of PIOPED was that diagnosis or exclusion of PE required concordance between the clinical impression and radiographic findings by V/Q (normal, low, intermediate, or high). There have been many subsequent attempts to quantify and standardize the definition of "clinical impression," 2 of the most widely known being the Wells and Geneva scores, discussed in the Clinical Tools section.

Electrocardiography and Chest Radiography

Chest radiographs (CXR) and electrocardiograms (ECG) are commonly used in the initial evaluation of patients with chest pain or dyspnea. Both lack adequate sensitivity or specificity for diagnosis or exclusion of PE, and do not figure prominently in diagnostic algorithms. It is nevertheless important to appreciate findings that are suggestive of PE. In the case of ECG, evidence of right heart strain should raise suspicion for PE. Signs of right ventricular (RV) strain include T-wave inversions in the anterior precordial leads, new right bundle branch block, or the S1Q3T3 complex (deep S-wave in lead I, and a Q-wave with T-wave inversions in lead III, **Fig. 1**). Other common ECG abnormalities include sinus tachycardia and atrial fibrillation.

Like ECG, CXR is insensitive for PE, but is helpful by excluding other causes of chest pain such as pneumonia or pneumothorax. Although by itself not sensitive or specific

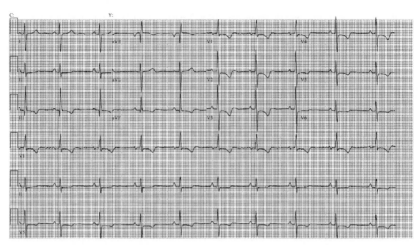

Fig. 1. Electrocardiographic (ECG) findings of right ventricular (RV) strain: This ECG demonstrates many classic findings of right heart strain and hypertrophy. The deep S-wave in lead I, Q-wave in lead III, and inverted T wave in lead III (S1Q3T3 complex) is not sensitive, but is specific for RV strain and should prompt consideration for pulmonary embolism. The inverted T waves in the precordial and inferior leads also suggest RV strain. Of note, there is evidence of RV hypertrophy with tall R waves in the right precordial leads V1-2, and borderline right atrial enlargement. Right bundle branch block can also be seen in patients with acute pulmonary embolism, but is not present in this case. This patient was later diagnosed with chronic thromboembolic pulmonary hypertension.

for PE, ipsilateral elevation of the diaphragm on the affected side can be seen. Other suggestive signs of PE include a wedge-shaped infiltrate (Hampton hump), focal oligemia (Westermark sign), or an enlarged right descending pulmonary artery (Palla sign).

Laboratory Tests

The initial evaluation of patients with dyspnea or chest pain includes several laboratory tests that can aid in the diagnosis and/or prognosis of PE. Common tests include D-dimer, arterial blood gas (ABG), B-type natriuretic peptide (BNP), serum sodium, and troponin. D-dimer is included in many diagnostic algorithms, as a normal level carries a high negative predictive value and is helpful to exclude PE in low to intermediate clinical risk groups. Although not a part of official algorithms at this time, an elevation in either troponin or BNP, or a depression in serum sodium (hyponatremia) has been suggested as a poor prognostic indicator.[16,19,20] Research indicates these markers can differentiate between low and intermediate risk for PE-related complications, including hemodynamic collapse and death.[21,22] Finally, ongoing investigations continue to identify new biomarkers of potential use in the prognosis or diagnosis of PE. One such novel biomarker, growth differentiation factor 15 (GDF-15), is also be discussed herein.[23]

Arterial blood gas

Obtaining an ABG documenting an elevation in alveolar-arterial (A-a) gradient was thought to aid in the diagnosis of PE. It has subsequently been demonstrated, however, that a normal A-a gradient lacks sufficient negative predictive value to exclude PE.[24] Although PE causes increased alveolar dead space and shunt, patients with acute PE will often have hypocapnia and respiratory alkalosis. Also, the partial pressure of oxygen (Po$_2$) may be decreased, normal, or increased. Thus, although an ABG may be indicated for other reasons (dyspnea, hypoxemia, or hypercapnia), its utility in the evaluation of PE is questionable.

D-dimer

D-dimer is a plasmin-derived fibrin degradation product commonly included in the initial evaluation of patients with dyspnea or chest pain. D-dimer represents a direct method to measure endogenous fibrinolysis following a thrombotic event, such as a PE, and is an important screening tool in patients with suspected VTE.[25] Although extremely sensitive, D-dimer lacks specificity for VTE (30%–75%). Many other conditions (eg, trauma, inflammation, surgery) can elevate plasma D-dimer levels; therefore, an abnormal laboratory result has a low positive predictive value for VTE. The strength of the D-dimer is its high sensitivity and ability, with a normal test, to essentially rule out VTE in low-risk and intermediate-risk patients (see Clinical Tools section).

The exact way in which D-dimer is measured has gone through considerable refinement over the past 25 years. Initially several different assays were available, including quantitative enzyme-linked immunosorbent assay (ELISA), quantitative latex agglutination, semiquantitative agglutination latex, and whole blood agglutination. These assays all varied in their sensitivity and specificity, which presented clinicians with a challenge to correctly interpret results. ELISA, however, has now been established as the standard D-dimer test, due to its superior sensitivity and high negative predictive value.[26] Typically a level greater than 500 ng/mL is considered abnormal. When combined with a low clinical probability of VTE, a normal D-dimer level (value <500 ng/mL) has a 99% negative predictive value for PE. This finding was demonstrated in the Christopher study, in which the incidence of PE was on 0.5% at 3 months in patients with a low probability score (by the "modified" Wells criteria) and a D-dimer level less than 500 ng/mL.[27] Other VTE studies looking at outcomes have had similar results, with D-dimer sensitivities ranging between 92% and 99%. In patients with a high clinical suspicion, however, a normal D-dimer cannot adequately rule out VTE, and additional testing is warranted (see Clinical Tools section).[27]

B-type natriuretic peptide

Released by ventricular myocardial cells in response to wall stretch and volume overload, BNP is a prognostic (not diagnostic) biomarker for PE. In the presence of PE, elevated BNP levels generally indicate RV strain due to elevated pulmonary vascular resistance in the clot-burdened lungs. Clinically, BNP levels differentiate between low and intermediate risk of PE-related complications, and alert the clinician to patients at increased risk who are otherwise hemodynamically stable. When measured within 4 hours of admission for PE, elevated BNP levels (>90 pg/mL) have a sensitivity of 85% and specificity of 75% in predicting PE-related clinical outcomes such as need for emergent thrombolysis, mechanical ventilation, vasopressor therapy, emergency surgical embolectomy, cardiopulmonary resuscitation, or death.[28] Conversely, normal BNP values in the setting of acute PE have a 97% to 100% negative predictive value for in-hospital death.[29] Given its short half-life and delay in release, if symptoms have been present for less than 6 hours a repeat test is warranted.

Troponin

Released by damaged myocardial cells, cardiac troponins are extremely sensitive and specific markers of cardiac ischemia and infarction. When elevated in acute PE, troponins are presumed to represent myocyte ischemia and microinfarction due to acute RV strain. Approximately 30% to 50% of patients with large PE will have elevations in troponins I and T that are mild and short-lived when compared with acute coronary syndromes. Similar to BNP, elevated troponin levels correlate with worse RV function and a high incidence of complications while normal troponin T levels have a 97% to 100% negative predictive value for in-hospital death.[19,21] Although BNP and troponins are not a part of diagnostic algorithms at this time, this may change in the future given their usefulness in prognosis and triage of patients.

Growth differentiation factor 15

GDF-15 is a distant member of the transforming growth factor β family of cytokines, and is upregulated in cardiomyocytes in response to stress such as pressure overload or ischemia. GDF-15 levels may also be elevated because of cancer, diabetes, congestive heart failure, or renal failure. A recent prospective cohort study demonstrated GDF-15 to be an independent predictor of PE-related complications including need for vasopressors, mechanical ventilation, cardiopulmonary resuscitation, or death.[23] In this cohort, a cutoff of 4600 ng/L had a positive predictive value of 0.52 and negative predictive value of 0.95 for these PE-related complications. Further studies are needed to validate these findings, but GDF-15 is a promising new prognostic biomarker with potentially superior differentiating power to BNP or troponins.

Hyponatremia

Hyponatremia has been well described as a poor prognostic indicator in a variety of disease processes including congestive heart failure, liver failure, and pulmonary hypertension. Recently, several publications have discussed the prognostic utility of hyponatremia in acute PE. A retrospective analysis of 13,728 patient hospitalizations found serum sodium levels of less than 135 mmol/L in 2907 patients (21.1%).[20] Sodium levels less than 130 mmol/L were independently associated with increased 30-day mortality and readmission. The investigators also found serum sodium levels to improve the accuracy of the pulmonary embolism severity index (PESI) classification of patients into low-risk, intermediate-risk, and high-risk groups (see Clinical Tools section). As with GDF-15, validation of these findings awaits further independent prospective studies.

Advanced Imaging

Venous compression ultrasonography

When initial diagnostic tests are inconclusive, ultrasonography of the deep venous system is a useful adjunctive test in the diagnosis and treatment of PE. Pragmatically the approach to treatment (anticoagulation) of both DVT and submassive PE is the same, and thus a positive ultrasonogram for DVT obviates the immediate need for further diagnostic studies to demonstrate PE. A negative ultrasonogram, however, is a somewhat more complicated result and requires appreciation of several caveats. Ultrasonography of the proximal leg veins detects DVT in roughly 1% to 5% of patients with clinical symptoms consistent with PE but nondiagnostic chest imaging.[30-33] Also, DVT is detectable by ultrasonography in only approximately 50% of patients with an acute PE. Thus, a negative ultrasonogram does not rule out PE. It does, however, slightly reduce the probability of PE and connotes a lower risk of short-term VTE complications should therapeutic anticoagulation be withheld.[34]

Echocardiogram

Transthoracic or transesophageal echocardiography has limited diagnostic value for PE, due to its low sensitivity and specificity. For critically ill patients too unstable for transport, echocardiography can suggest the diagnosis of PE by demonstrating RV dilatation or hypokinesis. Rarely, thrombus within the pulmonary arteries or right ventricle can be visualized on echo. More commonly, acute changes in the RV pressure, size, and function are observed, indicating increased RV strain and pulmonary arterial pressures suggestive of PE in the absence of alternative diagnoses (**Fig. 2**).

Although of limited value in the diagnosis of PE, echocardiography is of great prognostic use in stratifying risk for patients with acute PE. Numerous studies have demonstrated that RV dysfunction or dilatation in acute PE is associated with worse outcomes, including increased mortality.[35–37]

Ventilation/perfusion lung scan

As previously mentioned, the PIOPED study established the role of the V/Q scan in the diagnosis of PE.[18] By correlating the V/Q results (normal, low, high, or indeterminate probability) with a similar clinical impression (low, intermediate, or high probability), the diagnosis or exclusion of PE can be made (**Fig. 3**). It must be noted that a normal V/Q test essentially rules out PE as a diagnosis. Further testing, often by pulmonary or computed tomography (CT) angiogram, is required in patients with discordant or intermediate results. In recent years CT angiography has replaced the V/Q scan as the favored diagnostic test (see CT Angiogram section). V/Q scan remains, however, an important alternative to CT in patients with pregnancy, contrast allergy, or renal insufficiency. V/Q may be the modality of choice to evaluate patients for chronic thromboembolic pulmonary hypertension (CTEPH) (see Chronic Thromboembolic Disease section).

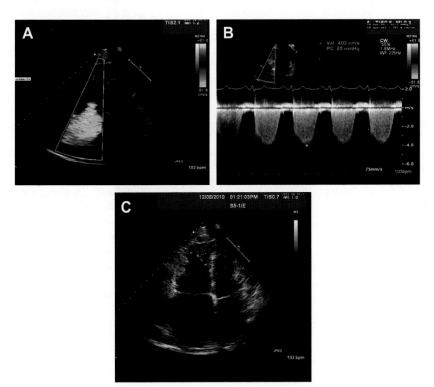

Fig. 2. Echocardiogram of a patient with an RV dysfunction secondary to pulmonary thromboembolic disease. (*A*) Color Doppler of the large tricuspid regurgitant jet. (*B*) M-mode of the tricuspid jet, estimating severely elevated pulmonary arterial pressures. (*C*) Four-chamber view demonstrating enlarged right ventricle and right atria with a flattened septum indicated elevated right-sided ventricular pressures.

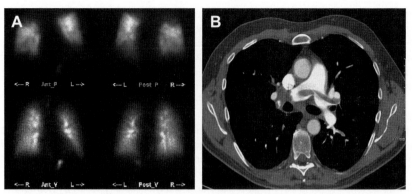

Fig. 3. (*A*) Ventilation/perfusion scan. Ventilation images are below their respective perfusion images. There is significant heterogeneity, especially at the lung apices and bases, consistent with thromboembolic disease. (*B*) Spiral computed tomographic angiogram of the chest, demonstrating a large saddle pulmonary embolism with multiple filling defects of the smaller pulmonary arteries. Modern multidetector computed tomography scanners have the ability to reliably detect pulmonary emboli in the subsegmental branches of the pulmonary artery.

CT angiogram

Over the past 10 years, CT pulmonary angiography (CTA) has become the favored diagnostic study in the evaluation of PE (see **Fig. 3**). There are several practical advantages of CTA, including: (1) common availability, especially after hours; (2) rapid interpretation; (3) direct visualization of the thrombus; (4) evaluation of the chest for alternative or concomitant diagnoses; and (5) simultaneous evaluation for DVT and PE when both the chest and lower extremity deep veins and pelvic veins are imaged. The ability to evaluate the chest for both PE and alternative pathology is not trivial. Up to 75% of patients with suspected PE will actually have an alternative diagnosis, some of which can be just as serious and readily identifiable by CTA, such as thoracic aortic dissection or pneumonia.[27,38]

When evaluating the efficacy of CTA to diagnose PE, it is important to appreciate the improvements in CT technology and the extent these have increased the sensitivity and specificity of CTA over the past 10 years. Early publications of CTA used single-detector scanners that were specific (>90%) but relatively insensitive (~72%), meaning they could not reliably exclude PE.[39,40] Multidetector scanners have significantly improved the sensitivity and specificity as well as the positive and negative predictive value of CTA. Recent outcome studies such as the Christopher study have found the sensitivity and specificity of CTA to be greater than 95%, and a negative CTA carries a 3-month risk of VTE of 1% to 2%, essentially the same as a negative pulmonary arteriogram.[27,30] Current multidetector scanners allow resolution and evaluation of PE down to the sixth-order branches of the pulmonary arteries. In fact, the interobserver agreement for CTA is superior to V/Q scanning, and CTA may be more sensitive than V/Q for subsegmental PE.[41,42] As such, CTA is now the predominant imaging modality used in diagnostic algorithms for the evaluation of PE.

Pulmonary arteriogram

Long considered the gold standard, pulmonary angiography, also known as digital subtraction angiography (DSA), is nowadays rarely performed. The reasons for this are both practical and medical. In practical terms DSA is more expensive than CTA, and is often unavailable in smaller centers. In medical terms outcome studies have found comparable results between DSA and CTA; a negative result with either study confers approximately a 1% VTE rate within 6 months.[18,27,33] Also, because of the invasive nature of DSA, it carries a greater risk of complications and mortality. The mortality from DSA has been estimated at 0.5% while 1% may experience major complications including arrhythmias, hypotension, bleeding, and nephrotoxicity. DSA is also less commonly performed, resulting in fewer clinicians who have experience in both performing and interpreting the test. All these factors have recently made DSA a relatively uncommon test in evaluating acute PE. DSA is still an important test, however, in the evaluation of patients with CTEPH, as discussed later (see Chronic Thromboembolic Disease section).

Magnetic resonance imaging

The Prospective Evaluation Of Pulmonary Embolic Disease—3 (PIOPED 3) trial recently evaluated the efficacy of magnetic resonance angiography (MRA), venography (MRV), or the combination of the two in the diagnosis of acute PE.[43] The gold standard used for comparison was a composite end point of CTA, CTA-CTV, V/Q scan, lower extremity ultrasonography, D-dimer assay, and clinical assessment. Overall, MRA and MRA-MRV were found to be poor tests in the diagnosis of PE. Approximately 25% of the 371 patients enrolled in the study had a technically inadequate MRA, and 48% had either an inadequate MRV or MRA. Considering all patients enrolled, MRA alone identified only 57% of PEs, and had a sensitivity of only 78% when only patients with adequate studies were considered. The combined MRA-MRV studies had a sensitivity of 92%, but only about half of the patients had technically adequate studies. These poor results are generally ascribed to the technical difficulties of MRA in identifying abrupt vessel termination and capturing adequate images of the chest vessels secondary to motion artifact. At this time, MRA-MRV is recommended only in centers with a great deal of experience, and then only when all other imaging modalities are contraindicated.

Clinical Tools

Wells criteria and Geneva score

Two of the most widely known and validated diagnostic scoring systems are the Wells criteria (or modified/dichotomous Wells criteria) and Geneva score.[27,44–46] These tools use a combination of physical examination, history, and vital signs to predict the clinical likelihood of VTE, and thereby inform the appropriate choice of laboratory tests and imaging studies to either diagnose or exclude PE. Notable differences include the use of CXR and ABG in the original Geneva score (subsequent versions do not include these tests), while the Wells criteria use a clinical gestalt in their formula by assigning points to PE if an "alternative diagnosis is less likely." Both scores have been modified and simplified throughout the years, now incorporating many common variables (although scored differently), and have been found to be equally efficacious (**Table 1**).

Pulmonary embolism severity index

Published in 2005 by Aujesky and colleagues,[47] the PESI was originally derived from analysis of 10,354 patients discharged with PE from 186 Pennsylvania hospitals. PESI risk stratifies patients with PE into low (I and II) and high (III, IV, and V) risk groups. In contrast to the Geneva score, which requires an ABG and ultrasonography, PESI only uses data available from a brief history, physical, and vital signs. Low-risk groups have 2% 30-day mortality and are candidates for home-based care, whereas high-risk groups have 14% 30-day mortality and warrant hospitalization and close monitoring.

Table 1
Modified Wells criteria, simplified revised Geneva score, and simplified pulmonary embolism severity index (PESI)

Variable	Clinical Probability Tools		
	Modified Wells (points)	Simplified Revised Geneva (points)	Simplified PESI (points)
Clinical DVT symptoms	3	—	—
Unilateral lower limb pain	—	1	—
Unilateral edema and pain in deep vein	—	1	—
Previous VTE	1.5	1	—
Hemoptysis	1	1	—
Heart rate (bpm)			
75–94	—	1	—
>100	1.5	+1	—
>110	—	—	1
Malignancy	1	1	1
Recent surgery or fracture	—	1	—
Recent surgery or immobilization	1.5	—	—
Age (y)			
>65	—	1	—
>80	—	—	1
Other diagnosis less likely than PE	3	—	—
Heart failure or chronic lung disease	—	—	1
Systolic blood pressure	—	—	1
Arterial oxyhemoglobin saturation <90%	—	—	1

The table lists all the clinical variables considered in the most recent published versions of these 3 algorithms. Both the modified Wells criteria and simplified revised Geneva score are used to predict the likelihood of pulmonary embolism as a diagnosis. In the most recent iteration, the modified Wells criteria is split in a dichotomous fashion with pulmonary embolism (PE) being likely if >4 points are assigned. PE can essentially be ruled out with an unlikely score and a negative D-dimer. The simplified revised Geneva score considers PE likely with >2 points. PE is essentially ruled out with 2 or fewer points and a negative D-dimer. The PESI score assigns a prognostic likelihood of poor clinical outcome once the diagnosis of PE is established. A simplified PESI score of 0 is considered low risk, whereas 1 or greater is high risk. Outpatient treatment of PE can be considered in the low-risk group.

Abbreviations: DVT, deep venous thrombosis; VTE, venous thromboembolism.

The accuracy of PESI has been validated in numerous studies.[48–50] Recently, a simplified version of PESI (sPESI) has been proposed (see **Table 1**).[51] Initial studies indicate PESI and sPESI are very similar in most respects, although PESI classifies more patients as low risk than sPESI (41% vs 37%). Finally, a recent prospective study has reported a high level of PE-related complications in patients classified as low risk by PESI.[52] Further investigation is warranted, but generally this report highlights the potential limitations of PESI and other prognostic algorithms, and serves to remind clinicians to exercise their judgment in conjunction with these clinical prediction tools.

TREATMENT

Prompt anticoagulation has remained the cornerstone of PE treatment for more than 50 years and is life saving. There have been, however, numerous exciting advances in recent decades, which have added new options with nuanced risks and benefits for clinicians to weigh. For example, the number and types of anticoagulant medications available continues to expand; with newer medications providing the ability to treat PE outside the hospital setting and with the potential to change future recommendations for duration of treatment. In addition to medications, widely available minimally invasive interventional techniques placing mechanical barriers in the inferior vena cava can protect patients otherwise ineligible for anticoagulation. Uncertainties remain, however, regarding the extent of indications for their use and their long-term risks and benefits. In addition to these newer therapies, clinical trials continue to refine the use of older treatments such as thrombolysis. Overall, these advances in care can be categorized into one of two categories: (1) treatment of acute PE or (2) prophylaxis against recurrent VTE.

Treatment of Acute Pulmonary Embolism

Anticoagulation

Heparin and vitamin K antagonists Initial treatment with anticoagulation aims at rapidly blocking the clotting cascade, stabilizing existing clot, and allowing the body's endogenous thrombolytic system to dissolve preexisting thrombi. For many years now, the standard of care has been to treat nonmassive pulmonary emboli with at least 5 days of heparin concomitant with commencement of an oral vitamin K antagonist (VKA) for long-term anticoagulation, preferably beginning on the first day of treatment. Intravenous unfractionated heparin (UFH) was the anticoagulant of choice until being recently eclipsed by subcutaneous low molecular weight heparin (LMWH) in many situations. LMWH has many advantages over UFH, including more predictable and reliable anticoagulation, increased patient satisfaction, and the ability to be self-administered, making home-based treatment a possibility. LMWH was first studied and approved for the prevention of DVT.[53] Studies with LMWH have subsequently demonstrated it to have similar morbidity and mortality outcomes to UFH in the treatment of DVT and submassive PE.[54,55] Of interest, a small number of patients in these studies were either discharged early or treated entirely at home, and had similar outcomes to hospitalized patients.[56,57] Combined with risk stratification tools (see Clinical Tools section) such as PESI, LMWH has revolutionized the treatment of low-risk PE by making home-based treatment possible for some patients. Although heparin and VKA continue to play a major role in the treatment of PE, advancements in anticoagulation medications continue to challenge these existing treatment paradigms.

Factor Xa inhibitors Factor Xa is a common factor in both the intrinsic and extrinsic coagulation pathways proximal to fibrin formation, making it ideally positioned as a target for anticoagulation. For many years, the only available factor Xa inhibitor has been subcutaneously administered fondaparinux.[58] With a relatively long half-life (17 hours), fondaparinux can be administered once daily. A newer factor Xa inhibitor with an even longer half-life (80 hours), idraparinux, is currently under evaluation. If approved, idraparinux it could dramatically simplify administration to once a week. Both subcutaneous Xa inhibitors undergo renal clearance, and should be used with caution in patients with renal insufficiency.

Recently, new oral factor Xa inhibitors such as rivaroxaban have undergone evaluation for the treatment of VTE, and appear likely to gain approval. Similar to the subcutaneous LMWH and fondaparinux, these oral preparations have predictable and rapid anticoagulation in addition to excellent bioavailability. The Einstein investigators recently demonstrated "noninferiority" between 3, 6, and 12 months of rivaroxaban compared with 5 days of subcutaneous enoxaparin followed by 3, 6, or 12 months of an oral VKA.[59] Of note, both groups had similar low levels of bleeding complications. Included in this report, the investigators published a long-term continuation study examining patients with VTE who had previously completed 6 to 12 months of treatment with oral VKA and were then randomized to either placebo or rivaroxaban for an additional 6 to 12 months.[59] There was a small increased risk of significant bleeding with rivaroxaban versus placebo, but also a significant decrease in recurrent VTE. Although further study is warranted, the oral Xa inhibitors have the potential to dramatically change the current management of VTE. As with LMWH, the ease of use, efficacy, and predictability of anticoagulation could facilitate outpatient management. For long-term anticoagulation, oral Xa inhibitors would relieve the burden of serial laboratory tests needed with the VKAs. One current point of concern, however, is the lack of an available antidote should rapid reversal of anticoagulation be necessary. The development of a reversal agent, as well as further prospective studies demonstrating efficacy, economy, and safety, will help establish whether outpatient and perhaps prolonged therapy (>6–12 months) with oral Xa inhibitors will become the new treatment of choice.

Direct thrombin inhibitors There are currently several direct thrombin inhibitors (DTIs) approved for use in humans, including hirudin, bivalrudin, dabigatran, and argatroban. There are several potential benefits to these medications. For instance, unlike heparin, which requires antithrombin III, the DTIs do not require cofactors for efficacy. The DTIs are also able to inactivate clot-bound thrombin and are unaffected by activated platelet factors such as heparinase and PF4. These potential benefits are offset, however, by the practical difficulties of using most of these medications, including unpredictable anticoagulation, need for intensive laboratory monitoring, continuous intravenous access, and potential drug-drug interactions. The usefulness of the DTIs currently lies in their lack of interaction with platelets and inability to potentiate or cause heparin-induced thrombocytopenia. It is in the treatment of this dangerous condition that the DTIs are primarily used with respect to VTE, although this may change in the future. Dabigatran is a new DTI with an oral preparation that appears not to have these drawbacks. It produces predictable anticoagulation, does not require monitoring, and is approved for treatment of nonvalvular atrial fibrillation, and may gain approval for treatment of VTE as an alternative to VKAs.[60,61]

Thrombolysis

Thrombolytics represent a potentially life-saving intervention, but have potential complications. Consequently, numerous trials have examined the safety and efficacy of thrombolytics for VTE and PE. Many trials found that thrombolysis improved hemodynamics, imaging studies, and hastened clot resolution but were unable to demonstrate improved mortality. Of concern, increased risk of severe bleeding was observed with thrombolysis. Given these results, investigators have sought to identify subgroups of patients with PE in whom the benefits of thrombolysis outweigh its risks.

Jerjes-Sanchez and colleagues[62] planned to enroll 40 patients into a small prospective, randomized controlled trial comparing streptokinase with placebo in patients with massive PE and cardiogenic shock. The study was terminated early after enrolling only 8 patients, due to a clear benefit of thrombolysis: all 4 patients receiving streptokinase and heparin survived, whereas the 4 patients who received only heparin died within 1 to

3 hours of arrival. It is now widely accepted that the use of thrombolytics in patients with cardiogenic shock and massive PE is critical, barring any absolute contraindications. In the vast majority of patients with PE the use of thrombolytics is more nuanced. As discussed, RV dysfunction in otherwise hemodynamically stable patients is a poor prognostic indicator for both morbidity and mortality. It would stand to reason, then, that this group of patients would benefit from thrombolysis. To date two large prospective trials, the Management Strategies and Prognosis of Pulmonary Embolism (MAPPET) and the Management Strategies and Prognosis of Pulmonary Embolism—3 (MAPPET-3), have investigated this issue and have reported potential benefits.[63,64] Controversy remains, however, because of criticism regarding the design of these studies.

In MAPPET, patients with PE and RV dysfunction received either heparin with thrombolytics (alteplase, streptokinase, or urokinase) or heparin alone as a control group. The use of thrombolytics improved 30-day survival from 11.1% to 4.7%. Recurrent PE was also decreased from 18.7% to 7.7% in the thrombolytic group. The study design, however, was not randomized, and the thrombolytic group was significantly younger and suffered from less cardiovascular and pulmonary disease than controls. These imbalances in patient selection may have inflated the observed benefit of thrombolytics, as age and comorbidities are known risk factors for mortality.

A follow-up study by the same group to address these concerns was the randomized, prospective trial MAPPET-3. Patients with RV dysfunction and PE were randomized to either alteplase and heparin, or a control group receiving only heparin. In contrast to MAPPET whereby the end point was mortality, MAPPET-3 used a combined end point of survival and "escalation in therapy." At its conclusion, MAPPET-3 demonstrated a significant benefit in this combined end point in favor of thrombolysis. On closer analysis, however, critics have pointed out that there was no survival difference between the two groups; the benefit of thrombolytics was almost entirely attributable to attenuation in "escalation of therapy." Furthermore, the primary event leading to escalation of therapy in the control group was the later use of thrombolytics. The results of MAPPET-3 continue to generate controversy; several experts cite them as evidence for the benefit of thrombolytics in patients with PE and RV dysfunction, whereas others are skeptical of these conclusions and the significance of the reported benefits.

Pulmonary embolectomy

Pulmonary embolectomy is the surgical removal of an acute PE. It is generally reserved for specific circumstances due to its high reported mortality (up to 30% in some series), in large part a reflection of the severity of the PE and hemodynamic instability before surgery.[65,66] In general, patients selected for embolectomy have had a large PE resulting in RV dysfunction and shock, and have failed or have contraindications to thrombolytics and anticoagulation.

RECURRENT VTE PROPHYLAXIS
Inferior Vena Cava Filters

Originally conceptualized by Trousseau in 1868, mechanical obstruction of the vena cava is now a safe, reliable procedure with the introduction of inferior vena cava (IVC) filters and minimally invasive placement. More recently, the advent of retrievable IVC filters has broadened the number of patients considered for this procedure. In general, the 2 most common indications for IVC filter placement are (1) contraindications to anticoagulation and (2) inability to adequately anticoagulate patients with VTE. Consideration for IVC filter placement is also given to patients in high-risk situations (despite adequate anticoagulation) such as trauma patients with lower extremity or pelvis fractures, patients at high risk of death from PE, and patients with severe pulmonary hypertension and a known DVT. This being said, there is a remarkable lack of data regarding the use of IVC filters. There is only one published randomized trial of IVC filter use, demonstrating a decrease in PE incidence in the first 12 days after placement (1.1% vs 4.8%). Follow-up of patients at 2 years found, however, that IVC filters increased the incidence of DVT (20% vs 11.6%) with a small decreased incidence of PE (3.4% vs 6.2%).[67] An 8-year follow-up of these same patients found a continuation of the 2-year trends, with an increased incidence of DVT (35.7% vs 27.5%) in patients with IVC filters, but a more dramatic decrease in PE (6.2% vs 15.1%).[68] There were no differences in mortality or postphlebitic syndrome between the two cohorts. Most but not all of the patients in the study were on chronic anticoagulation. Given the high rates of VTE in patients with IVC filters left in place, it is recommended they receive indefinite anticoagulation.

In patients with a transient increased risk of VTE, retrievable IVC filters are an option. Retrievable filters theoretically should protect against PE in the short term while avoiding long-term DVT complications. There are, however, no randomized data demonstrating the outcomes or efficacy of retrievable filters. In general, the retrievable filters are placed to cover the days while a patient is off anticoagulation or is at increased risk of VTE, and should be removed as soon as possible to avoid endothelialization. Current recommendations for duration of deployment vary by filter type and center expertise, but are usually 2 to 6 weeks.[69] Removal after prolonged use is possible, but comes at increasingly greater risk the longer the device has been in place.[70]

Management of Inherited Thrombophilia

The acute management of PE in patients with inherited thrombophilia is no different from that for other patients. Long-term treatment and prophylaxis is somewhat less clear, as there are no randomized controlled trials addressing the inherited thrombophilias. Guidelines suggest permanent anticoagulation in patients with spontaneous VTE and multiple prothrombotic mutations (either homozygous for a single mutation or heterozygous for several), any heritable risk factor and a single idiopathic near-fatal thrombosis such as massive PE or portal, mesenteric, or cerebral thrombosis, or a spontaneous thrombosis and an antithrombin deficiency or antiphospholipid antibody syndrome.[16,71,72] Less consensus exists regarding the treatment length after the first spontaneous VTE and a single heritable mutation. It is recommended that expert consultation be sought to determine the length of anticoagulation.

Treatment of Cancer-Associated VTE

The incidence of VTE in cancer can be remarkably high, and is affected by several factors unique to cancer including tumor type, stage, and total tumor burden. Renal cell carcinoma, for instance, has a 43% incidence of VTE.[73] VTE is also a poor prognostic indicator, with increased 6-month mortality in comparison with similar cancer patients without VTE. The Comparison of LMWH versus Oral anticoagulation Therapy for the prevention of VTE in patients with cancer (CLOT) study randomized patients to receive either 6 months of VKA (warfarin) or LMWH (dalteparin).[74] Patients receiving LMWH had less recurrent VTE (9%) than those receiving VKA (17%). Based on these data, the current recommendation for VTE treatment in patients with cancer is to use LMWH as the first-line agent.

Chronic Thromboembolic Disease

In the majority of patients who suffer PE, resolution of the thrombus and restoration of normal pulmonary artery pressures is complete within 30 days of the event. Pengo and colleagues[75] reported in a prospective incidence study, however, that up to 4% of PE survivors may develop CTEPH. The natural history of CTEPH is unknown, as most patients present late in the clinical course, only after becoming symptomatic with pulmonary artery hypertension (PAH). The predisposing factors to CTEPH are unclear, although an increased incidence of anticardiolipin antibodies and elevated factor VIII levels have been reported. It is thought that CTEPH begins with an acute PE (even an asymptomatic PE) which, instead of undergoing thrombolysis, becomes covered in endothelial cells. Once endothelialization is complete, the thrombus is protected from circulating endogenous or exogenous thrombolytics, and over time obstructs and remodels the pulmonary vasculature, causing PAH.

Overall, untreated severe CTEPH carries a poor prognosis, with 5-year survival estimated at as low as 10%.[76] Chronic anticoagulation is part of the treatment, but will not resolve the organized, endothelialized thrombi. Instead, clot must be physically removed via pulmonary endarterectomy (PEA), a process by which the endothelialized thrombi are carefully dissected from the pulmonary artery wall. PEA is the treatment of choice for CTEPH, but comes with significant morbidity and 5% to 10% postoperative mortality. Given the complexity and magnitude of PEA, it is recommended to be performed only at experienced centers.

Many patients, in some cases up to half, may be ineligible for PEA because of comorbidities or distal clot position. Furthermore, some patients may have persistent or exercise-limiting PAH even after PEA. In such cases, medical therapy is an alternative. Medical therapy can be divided into two categories: general therapies and those specific to PAH. General therapies include correcting hypoxemia with supplementary oxygen, dieresis, indefinite anticoagulation, and digoxin to augment RV contractility. PAH-specific therapies include 3 categories of medications designed for the treatment of idiopathic pulmonary arterial hypertension, and include the phosphodiesterase-5 inhibitors (sildenafil, tadalafil), endothelin receptor antagonists (ambrisentan, bosentan), and the prostacyclin analogues (epoprostenol, treprostinil, and iloprost). The evidence, however, supporting the use of these medications in CTEPH is generally limited to retrospective studies, case series, and prospective cohort series. When subjected to randomized controlled trials, medical therapies such as iloprost,[77] bosentan,[78] and sildenafil[79] have not shown significant clinical benefit.

SUMMARY

VTE is a rapidly evolving field, with advances in biomarkers, imaging, clinical algorithms, devices, and medications improving our ability to diagnose and treat PE. For instance, the development of LMWH, CTA, D-dimer, and clinical scoring tools have all substantially improved diagnostic accuracy and have decreased morbidity and mortality associated with PE. Questions in the diagnosis and management of PE persist, however, such as the significance of heritable thrombophilias or the optimal use of thrombolytics in hemodynamically stable patients with RV dysfunction. In some cases such as CTEPH, medical therapy is inadequate. Ongoing study and advancement in clinical care will attempt to address these deficiencies while continuing to improve clinical care overall.

REFERENCES

1. Heit J, Cohen A, Anderson FJ. Estimated annual number of incident and recurrent, non-fatal and fatal venous thromboembolism (VTE) events in the US. Blood 2005;106:267A.

2. Park B, Messina L, Dargon P, et al. Recent trends in clinical outcomes and resource utilization for pulmonary embolism in the United States: findings from the nationwide inpatient sample. Chest 2009;136:983–90.
3. Goldhaber SZ. Epidemiology of pulmonary embolism. Semin Vasc Med 2001;1: 139–46.
4. Lee CH, Cheng CL, Lin LJ, et al. Epidemiology and predictors of short-term mortality in symptomatic venous thromboembolism. Circ J 2011;75: 1998–2004.
5. Gillum RF. Pulmonary embolism and thrombophlebitis in the United States, 1970-1985. Am Heart J 1987;114:1262–4.
6. Heit JA, Silverstein MD, Mohr DN, et al. Predictors of survival after deep vein thrombosis and pulmonary embolism: a population-based, cohort study. Arch Intern Med 1999;159:445–53.
7. Cohen AT, Agnelli G, Anderson FA, et al. Venous thromboembolism (VTE) in Europe. The number of VTE events and associated morbidity and mortality. Thromb Haemost 2007;98:756–64.
8. Heit J, Petterson T, Farmer S, et al. Trends in incidence of deep vein thrombosis and pulmonary embolism: a 35-year population-based study. Blood 2006;108: 430a.
9. Skaf E, Stein PD, Beemath A, et al. Fatal pulmonary embolism and stroke. Am J Cardiol 2006;97:1776–7.
10. Silverstein MD, Heit JA, Mohr DN, et al. Trends in the incidence of deep vein thrombosis and pulmonary embolism: a 25-year population-based study. Arch Intern Med 1998;158:585–93.
11. Cervantes J, Rojas G. Virchow's legacy: deep vein thrombosis and pulmonary embolism. World J Surg 2005;29(Suppl 1):S30–4.
12. Dickson BC. Venous thrombosis: on the history of Virchow's triad. Univ Toronto Med J 2004;81:166–71.
13. Mateo J, Oliver A, Borrell M, et al. Laboratory evaluation and clinical characteristics of 2,132 consecutive unselected patients with venous thromboembolism—results of the Spanish Multicentric Study on Thrombophilia (EMET-Study). Thromb Haemost 1997;77:444–51.
14. Ridker PM, Hennekens CH, Lindpaintner K, et al. Mutation in the gene coding for coagulation factor V and the risk of myocardial infarction, stroke, and venous thrombosis in apparently healthy men. N Engl J Med 1995;332:912–7.
15. Koster T, Rosendaal FR, de RH, et al. Venous thrombosis due to poor anticoagulant response to activated protein C: Leiden Thrombophilia Study. Lancet 1993; 342:1503–6.
16. Baglin T, Gray E, Greaves M, et al. Clinical guidelines for testing for heritable thrombophilia. Br J Haematol 2010;149:209–20.
17. Spencer FA, Emery C, Lessard D, et al. The Worcester Venous Thromboembolism study: a population-based study of the clinical epidemiology of venous thromboembolism. J Gen Intern Med 2006;21:722–7.
18. Value of the ventilation/perfusion scan in acute pulmonary embolism. Results of the prospective investigation of pulmonary embolism diagnosis (PIOPED). The PIOPED Investigators. JAMA 1990;263:2753–9.
19. Becattini C, Vedovati MC, Agnelli G. Prognostic value of troponins in acute pulmonary embolism: a meta-analysis. Circulation 2007;116:427–33.
20. Scherz N, Labarere J, Mean M, et al. Prognostic importance of hyponatremia in patients with acute pulmonary embolism. Am J Respir Crit Care Med 2010;182: 1178–83.

21. La VL, Ottani F, Favero L, et al. Increased cardiac troponin I on admission predicts in-hospital mortality in acute pulmonary embolism. Heart 2004;90:633–7.

22. Klok FA, Mos IC, Huisman MV. Brain-type natriuretic peptide levels in the prediction of adverse outcome in patients with pulmonary embolism: a systematic review and meta-analysis. Am J Respir Crit Care Med 2008;178:425–30.

23. Lankeit M, Kempf T, Dellas C, et al. Growth differentiation factor-15 for prognostic assessment of patients with acute pulmonary embolism. Am J Respir Crit Care Med 2008;177:1018–25.

24. Stein PD, Goldhaber SZ, Henry JW, et al. Arterial blood gas analysis in the assessment of suspected acute pulmonary embolism. Chest 1996;109:78–81.

25. Righini M, Perrier A, De MP, et al. D-Dimer for venous thromboembolism diagnosis: 20 years later. J Thromb Haemost 2008;6:1059–71.

26. Dempfle CE, Suvajac N, Elmas E, et al. Performance evaluation of a new rapid quantitative assay system for measurement of D-dimer in plasma and whole blood: PATHFAST D-dimer. Thromb Res 2007;120:591–6.

27. van Belle A, Buller HR, Huisman MV, et al. Effectiveness of managing suspected pulmonary embolism using an algorithm combining clinical probability, D-dimer testing, and computed tomography. JAMA 2006;295:172–9.

28. Kucher N, Printzen G, Goldhaber SZ. Prognostic role of brain natriuretic peptide in acute pulmonary embolism. Circulation 2003;107:2545–7.

29. Coutance G, Le PO, Lo T, et al. Prognostic value of brain natriuretic peptide in acute pulmonary embolism. Crit Care 2008;12:R109.

30. Perrier A, Roy PM, Sanchez O, et al. Multidetector-row computed tomography in suspected pulmonary embolism. N Engl J Med 2005;352:1760–8.

31. Righini M, Le GG, Aujesky D, et al. Diagnosis of pulmonary embolism by multidetector CT alone or combined with venous ultrasonography of the leg: a randomised non-inferiority trial. Lancet 2008;371:1343–52.

32. Turkstra F, Kuijer PM, van Beek EJ, et al. Diagnostic utility of ultrasonography of leg veins in patients suspected of having pulmonary embolism. Ann Intern Med 1997;126:775–81.

33. Musset D, Parent F, Meyer G, et al. Diagnostic strategy for patients with suspected pulmonary embolism: a prospective multicentre outcome study. Lancet 2002;360:1914–20.

34. Johnson SA, Stevens SM, Woller SC, et al. Risk of deep vein thrombosis following a single negative whole-leg compression ultrasound: a systematic review and meta-analysis. JAMA 2010;303:438–45.

35. Kucher N, Rossi E, De RM, et al. Prognostic role of echocardiography among patients with acute pulmonary embolism and a systolic arterial pressure of 90 mm Hg or higher. Arch Intern Med 2005;165:1777–81.

36. Kasper W, Konstantinides S, Geibel A, et al. Prognostic significance of right ventricular afterload stress detected by echocardiography in patients with clinically suspected pulmonary embolism. Heart 1997;77:346–9.

37. Kreit JW. The impact of right ventricular dysfunction on the prognosis and therapy of normotensive patients with pulmonary embolism. Chest 2004;125:1539–45.

38. Hall WB, Truitt SG, Scheunemann LP, et al. The prevalence of clinically relevant incidental findings on chest computed tomographic angiograms ordered to diagnose pulmonary embolism. Arch Intern Med 2009;169:1961–5.

39. Van Strijen MJ, De MW, Kieft GJ, et al. Accuracy of single-detector spiral CT in the diagnosis of pulmonary embolism: a prospective multicenter cohort study of consecutive patients with abnormal perfusion scintigraphy. J Thromb Haemost 2005;3:17–25.

40. Perrier A, Howarth N, Didier D, et al. Performance of helical computed tomography in unselected outpatients with suspected pulmonary embolism. Ann Intern Med 2001;135:88–97.
41. Stein PD, Fowler SE, Goodman LR, et al. Multidetector computed tomography for acute pulmonary embolism. N Engl J Med 2006;354:2317–27.
42. Blachere H, Latrabe V, Montaudon M, et al. Pulmonary embolism revealed on helical CT angiography: comparison with ventilation-perfusion radionuclide lung scanning. AJR Am J Roentgenol 2000;174:1041–7.
43. Stein PD, Chenevert TL, Fowler SE, et al. Gadolinium-enhanced magnetic resonance angiography for pulmonary embolism: a multicenter prospective study (PIOPED III). Ann Intern Med 2010;152:434–43.
44. Wells PS, Ginsberg JS, Anderson DR, et al. Use of a clinical model for safe management of patients with suspected pulmonary embolism. Ann Intern Med 1998;129:997–1005.
45. Wells PS, Anderson DR, Rodger M, et al. Derivation of a simple clinical model to categorize patients probability of pulmonary embolism: increasing the models utility with the SimpliRED D-dimer. Thromb Haemost 2000;83:416–20.
46. Wicki J, Perrier A, Perneger TV, et al. Predicting adverse outcome in patients with acute pulmonary embolism: a risk score. Thromb Haemost 2000;84:548–52.
47. Aujesky D, Obrosky DS, Stone RA, et al. Derivation and validation of a prognostic model for pulmonary embolism. Am J Respir Crit Care Med 2005;172:1041–6.
48. Chan CM, Woods C, Shorr AF. The validation and reproducibility of the pulmonary embolism severity index. J Thromb Haemost 2010;8:1509–14.
49. Jimenez D, Yusen RD, Otero R, et al. Prognostic models for selecting patients with acute pulmonary embolism for initial outpatient therapy. Chest 2007;132:24–30.
50. Donze J, Le GG, Fine MJ, et al. Prospective validation of the Pulmonary Embolism Severity Index. A clinical prognostic model for pulmonary embolism. Thromb Haemost 2008;100:943–8.
51. Jimenez D, Aujesky D, Moores L, et al. Simplification of the pulmonary embolism severity index for prognostication in patients with acute symptomatic pulmonary embolism. Arch Intern Med 2010;170:1383–9.
52. Hariharan P, Takayesu JK, Kabrhel C. Association between the Pulmonary Embolism Severity Index (PESI) and short-term clinical deterioration. Thromb Haemost 2011;105:706–11.
53. Nurmohamed MT, Rosendaal FR, Buller HR, et al. Low-molecular-weight heparin versus standard heparin in general and orthopaedic surgery: a meta-analysis. Lancet 1992;340:152–6.
54. Quinlan DJ, McQuillan A, Eikelboom JW. Low-molecular-weight heparin compared with intravenous unfractionated heparin for treatment of pulmonary embolism: a meta-analysis of randomized, controlled trials. Ann Intern Med 2004;140:175–83.
55. Simonneau G, Sors H, Charbonnier B, et al. A comparison of low-molecular-weight heparin with unfractionated heparin for acute pulmonary embolism. The THESEE Study Group. Tinzaparine ou Heparine Standard: evaluations dans l'Embolie Pulmonaire. N Engl J Med 1997;337:663–9.
56. Erkens PM, Gandara E, Wells P, et al. Safety of outpatient treatment in acute pulmonary embolism. J Thromb Haemost 2010;8:2412–7.
57. Kovacs MJ, Hawel JD, Rekman JF, et al. Ambulatory management of pulmonary embolism: a pragmatic evaluation. J Thromb Haemost 2010;8:2406–11.
58. Buller HR, Davidson BL, Decousus H, et al. Subcutaneous fondaparinux versus intravenous unfractionated heparin in the initial treatment of pulmonary embolism. N Engl J Med 2003;349:1695–702.

59. Bauersachs R, Berkowitz SD, Brenner B, et al. Oral rivaroxaban for symptomatic venous thromboembolism. N Engl J Med 2010;363:2499–510.

60. Schulman S, Kearon C, Kakkar AK, et al. Dabigatran versus warfarin in the treatment of acute venous thromboembolism. N Engl J Med 2009;361:2342–52.

61. Ezekowitz MD, Reilly PA, Nehmiz G, et al. Dabigatran with or without concomitant aspirin compared with warfarin alone in patients with nonvalvular atrial fibrillation (PETRO Study). Am J Cardiol 2007;100:1419–26.

62. Jerjes-Sanchez C, Ramirez-Rivera A, de Lourdes GM, et al. Streptokinase and heparin versus heparin alone in massive pulmonary embolism: a randomized controlled trial. J Thromb Thrombolysis 1995;2:227–9.

63. Kasper W, Konstantinides S, Geibel A, et al. Management strategies and determinants of outcome in acute major pulmonary embolism: results of a multicenter registry. J Am Coll Cardiol 1997;30:1165–71.

64. Konstantinides S, Geibel A, Heusel G, et al. Heparin plus alteplase compared with heparin alone in patients with submassive pulmonary embolism. N Engl J Med 2002;347:1143–50.

65. Clarke DB, Abrams LD. Pulmonary embolectomy: a 25 year experience. J Thorac Cardiovasc Surg 1986;92:442–5.

66. Dauphine C, Omari B. Pulmonary embolectomy for acute massive pulmonary embolism. Ann Thorac Surg 2005;79:1240–4.

67. Decousus H, Leizorovicz A, Parent F, et al. A clinical trial of vena caval filters in the prevention of pulmonary embolism in patients with proximal deep-vein thrombosis. Prevention du Risque d'Embolie Pulmonaire par Interruption Cave Study Group. N Engl J Med 1998;338:409–15.

68. PREPIC Study Group. Eight-year follow-up of patients with permanent vena cava filters in the prevention of pulmonary embolism: the PREPIC (Prevention du Risque d'Embolie Pulmonaire par Interruption Cave) randomized study. Circulation 2005;112:416–22.

69. Van Ha TG, Chien AS, Funaki BS, et al. Use of retrievable compared to permanent inferior vena cava filters: a single-institution experience. Cardiovasc Intervent Radiol 2008;31:308–15.

70. Given MF, McDonald BC, Brookfield P, et al. Retrievable Gunther Tulip inferior vena cava filter: experience in 317 patients. J Med Imaging Radiat Oncol 2008;52:452–7.

71. Kearon C, Kahn SR, Agnelli G, et al. Antithrombotic therapy for venous thromboembolic disease: American College of Chest Physicians evidence-based clinical practice guidelines (8th edition). Chest 2008;133:454S–545S.

72. Buller HR, Agnelli G, Hull RD, et al. Antithrombotic therapy for venous thromboembolic disease: the Seventh ACCP Conference on Antithrombotic and Thrombolytic Therapy. Chest 2004;126:401S–28S.

73. Lee AY, Levine MN. Venous thromboembolism and cancer: risks and outcomes. Circulation 2003;107:I17–21.

74. Lee AY, Levine MN, Baker RI, et al. Low-molecular-weight heparin versus a coumarin for the prevention of recurrent venous thromboembolism in patients with cancer. N Engl J Med 2003;349:146–53.

75. Pengo V, Lensing AW, Prins MH, et al. Incidence of chronic thromboembolic pulmonary hypertension after pulmonary embolism. N Engl J Med 2004;350:2257–64.

76. Riedel M, Stanek V, Widimsky J, et al. Longterm follow-up of patients with pulmonary thromboembolism. Late prognosis and evolution of hemodynamic and respiratory data. Chest 1982;81:151–8.

77. Olschewski H, Simonneau G, Galie N, et al. Inhaled iloprost for severe pulmonary hypertension. N Engl J Med 2002;347:322–9.

78. Jais X, D'Armini AM, Jansa P, et al. Bosentan for treatment of inoperable chronic thromboembolic pulmonary hypertension: BENEFiT (Bosentan Effects in iNopErable Forms of chronIc Thromboembolic pulmonary hypertension), a randomized, placebo-controlled trial. J Am Coll Cardiol 2008;52:2127–34.

79. Suntharalingam J, Treacy CM, Doughty NJ, et al. Long-term use of sildenafil in inoperable chronic thromboembolic pulmonary hypertension. Chest 2008;134: 229–36.

Sarcoidosis

Nabeel Hamzeh, MD, FCCP

KEYWORDS

• Sarcoidosis • Management • Pulmonary • Extrapulmonary

Sarcoidosis is a multisystem granulomatous disorder of yet unknown etiology,[1] which predominantly involves the lungs in more than 90% of cases but can also involve any organ in the body, with the lymphatics, skin, eyes, and liver being the most common.[1,2] It was first described in 1877 by Jonathan Hutchinson when he described a patient with raised purple skin lesions, but it was Caesar Boeck who coined the term "sarkoid" when he described the histologic appearance of the skin lesions that he thought resembled sarcoma.[1]

EPIDEMIOLOGY

Sarcoidosis is a worldwide disease but with variable incidences, manifestations, and prognosis.[1] In the United States, the age-adjusted annual incidence rate in Caucasians is 10.9 in 100,000 and in African Americans it is 35.5 in 100,000.[1] In Spain the incidence rate is 1.3 in 100,000,[3] in Eastern Europe 3.7 in 100,000[3] and in Japan 1 in 100,000.[3,4] Sarcoidosis can affect any age group but tends to affect adults 40 years old or younger in the United States.[1] In Japan, it exhibits two peaks in the third and seventh decades of life.[1] Female predominance is common among all regions of the world.[1,4]

Disease manifestation also varies by ethnicity. The Japanese have higher rates of cardiac and ophthalmic involvement whereas Puerto Ricans have a high rate of developing lupus pernio.[1] Lofgren's syndrome is more frequently seen in patients from southern Europe,[3] whereas African Americans tend to have skin involvement other than erythema nodosum, eye, liver, bone marrow, and extrathoracic lymph node involvement.[2]

PATHOPHYSIOLOGY
Environment

The current hypothesis is that sarcoidosis develops when a genetically susceptible host is exposed to a yet unidentified antigen(s) in the environment.[1] Several

Funding support: None.

Financial disclosures/Conflict of interest: The author is a sub-investigator for his institution's site in a multicenter drug study related to sarcoidosis conducted by Centocor.

Division of Environmental and Occupational Health Sciences, National Jewish Health, 1400 Jackson Street, Denver, CO 80206, USA

E-mail address: hamzehn@njhealth.org

Med Clin N Am 95 (2011) 1223–1234

doi:10.1016/j.mcna.2011.08.004

medical.theclinics.com

environmental and infectious agents have been proposed but none have been proven yet. As part of the ACCESS study (A Case Controlled Etiologic Study of Sarcoidosis), which recruited 736 incident cases of sarcoidosis and 706 matched controls, participants completed extensive exposure questionnaires.[5] Five occupations and 5 exposures were more prevalent in the sarcoidosis group. Occupations included agricultural employment, physicians, jobs raising birds, jobs in automotive manufacturing, and middle/secondary school teachers. Exposures included exposure to insecticides and employment in pesticide-using industries, occupational exposure to mold and mildew, occupational exposure to musty odors, and use of home central air-conditioning.[6] A study from Switzerland found a higher frequency of sarcoidosis in regions with metal industry and intense agriculture.[7] In addition, in the aftermath of the 9/11 attacks, sarcoid-like granulomatous pulmonary diseases are being reported at higher rates than in the general population.[8,9] Infectious agents, particularly Mycobacteria, are reemerging as a potential antigen in sarcoidosis, with studies detecting Mycobacteria proteins in tissues from sarcoidosis patients and T cells from sarcoidosis patients responding to stimulation by Mycobacteria antigens.[10–17] Smoking appears to have a protective effect against sarcoidosis.[6,18,19] In the ACCESS study, sarcoidosis subjects were less likely to be smokers or ever-smokers than matched controls.[6] In addition, smoking sarcoidosis patients tended to have less thickening of their bronchovascular bundle on computed tomography (CT) scans.[19]

Chronic beryllium disease is a granulomatous disorder that affects predominantly the lungs, and can be mistaken for sarcoidosis if a history of beryllium exposure is not elicited.[20] Beryllium is a hard metal that is used in several industries including aerospace, automotive parts, computers and electronics, defense, dental, foundries, smelting, recycling, and telecommunications among others.[21] Exposure to beryllium can lead to beryllium sensitization, which can progress to chronic beryllium disease.[21] Beryllium sensitization has also been reported in household members of beryllium workers and from communities downwind from industries using beryllium.[21]

Genetics

The disparity in prevalence and variability of organ involvement between ethnic groups[1] and the familial clustering of sarcoidosis[22] strongly support a genetic basis for sarcoidosis. Several genome-wide association studies have identified potential association of specific genetic loci with sarcoidosis,[23–25] and several studies have also associated various human leukocyte antigen markers and gene-specific single nucleotide polymorphisms[26–28] with the risk, disease course, and organ involvement with sarcoidosis, indicating that sarcoidosis is a multigenetic disease.

Immune Response

Sarcoidosis is a T-helper 1 (Th1) cell biased disease.[1] Antigen presentation in the context of major histocompatibility complex II leads to activation of Th1 cells and subsequent production of various cytokines and chemokines including, but not limited to, interferon-γ, tumor necrosis factor (TNF)-α, transforming growth factor β, interleukin (IL)-2, IL-12, and others.[29] The immune response ultimately leads to the formation of granulomas, which consists of a central core of mononuclear cells surrounded by CD4+ cells and a small number of CD8+ and B cells.[29] A role for regulatory T cells has been proposed, but its exact role in sarcoidosis is yet unknown.[30] Sarcoidosis is also known for its immune paradox with an intense immune response in the organ involved and concomitant peripheral anergy.[29] The peripheral anergy manifests as lack of response to antigen skin testing and relative lymphopenia in the peripheral blood.[29] The exact cause of the peripheral anergy is yet unknown.[29]

Diagnostic Criteria

Sarcoidosis is characterized by the formation of well-formed, nonnecrotizing granulomas in affected organs (**Fig. 1**).[1] There are no formal diagnostic criteria for sarcoidosis, and the presence of noncaseating granulomas does not confirm the diagnosis of sarcoidosis on its own.[1] Sarcoidosis is a diagnosis of exclusion and as such, other causes of granulomas, infectious and noninfectious, need to be evaluated for and ruled out by obtaining a complete medical, occupational, environmental, and medication history as well as physical examination, followed by the appropriate diagnostic testing (**Table 1**).[31]

CLINICAL PRESENTATION

Sarcoidosis is a multisystem disease that can affect any organ.[1] The clinical presentation can vary from asymptomatic organ involvement that is detected incidentally to a slowly progressive disease. An acute form of sarcoidosis, Lofgren syndrome, is defined as an acute onset of fever, erythema nodosum, polyarthritis, and chest radiograph showing bilateral hilar lymphadenopathy with or without parenchymal infiltrates. Lofgren syndrome typically portends an excellent course, with spontaneous resolution.[1,32] The pulmonary system is involved in more than 90% of cases followed by skin, lymph nodes, eyes, and liver.[1,2] In the ACCESS study, half of the sarcoidosis cohort had only one organ involved, 30% had 2 organs involved, 13% had 3 organs involved, and 7% had 4 or more organs involved with sarcoidosis.[2]

Pulmonary

The lungs are the most common organs involved in sarcoidosis.[2] Presenting symptoms are variable. Patients can be asymptomatic with their disease identified on chest imaging obtained for unrelated reasons, but more commonly they have nonspecific symptoms such as cough, fatigue, and dyspnea on exertion. On physical examination, findings can include normal pulmonary examination, dry inspiratory crackles or wheezes from airway involvement with sarcoidosis, or airway distortion from fibrotic changes.[1] Pulmonary function testing can also be variable and may include normal, restrictive, or obstructive patterns with or without bronchodilatory responses, and a normal or reduced diffusion capacity.[33] The Scadding chest radiography staging system is the most common method used to describe chest radiographic findings in sarcoidosis patients, and depends on the presence and absence of hilar lymph

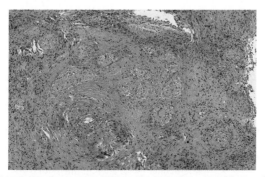

Fig. 1. Noncaseating granuloma. Multiple noncaseating granuloma from lung biopsy (hematoxylin-eosin stain, original magnification ×10). (*Courtesy of* Dr Steve Groshong, National Jewish Health.)

Table 1 Causes of granulomatous diseases	
Causative Agent	**Granulomatous Disease**
Infectious	
Mycobacteria	Tuberculosis
	Atypical mycobacteria infection
Fungi	Histoplasmosis
	Coccidiomycosis
Bacteria	Brucellosis
	Chlamydia infections
	Tularemia
Parasites	Leishmaniasis
	Toxoplasmosis
Occupational and Environmental Exposures	
Organic agents	Hypersensitivity pneumonitis
Heavy metals	Chronic beryllium disease
	Other heavy metals (titanium, aluminum, zirconium)
Drug-induced	Methotrexate-induced pneumonitis
Neoplasia	Lymphoma
	Other tumors—sarcoidlike reactions
Autoimmune disorders	Wegner granulomatosis
	Primary biliary cirrhosis
	Churg-Strauss disease

Data from Newman LS, Rose CS, Maier LA. Sarcoidosis. N Engl J Med 1997;336(17):1224–34.

node enlargement and parenchymal infiltrates on chest radiograph (**Table 2**).[34,35] Chest CT findings include presence or absence of hilar and/or mediastinal lymphadenopathy with or without calcifications, nodular opacities in a perilymphatic distribution, parenchymal opacities, fibrosis with or without traction bronchiectasis, and airway narrowing due to intrinsic airway involvement or extrinsic compression by enlarged lymph nodes.[36] Pleural effusions are rarely seen in sarcoidosis.[37] Workup and follow-up for pulmonary sarcoidosis includes history to determine extent of and changes in dyspnea on exertion, chest radiography, pulmonary function testing, and walk oximetry to assess for oxygen desaturation.[1] Indications for immunosuppressive therapy for pulmonary sarcoidosis depend on the extent of symptoms and evidence of disease progression on follow-up.[1] Therapeutic regimens include corticosteroids and

Table 2 Scadding chest radiograph stages	
Scadding Stage	**Radiographic Description**
0	Normal
I	Bilateral hilar lymphadenopathy *without* parenchymal changes
II	Bilateral hilar lymphadenopathy *with* parenchymal changes
III	Parenchymal changes *without* hilar lymphadenopathy
IV	Pulmonary fibrosis, conglomerate mass formation

steroid-sparing agents such as methotrexate, mycophenolate mofetil, azathioprine, leflunomide, and/or anti–TNF-α agents.[38–41]

Skin

Skin is the second most common organ involved in sarcoidosis, and is seen in 20% to 35% of sarcoidosis patients.[2,42–44] Manifestations of cutaneous sarcoidosis are variable and are categorized as specific and nonspecific lesions. Specific lesions include lupus pernio, maculopapular eruptions, subcutaneous nodules, plaques, and infiltrated scars, and typically show noncaseating granulomas when biopsied. Nonspecific lesions such as erythema nodosum are reactive in nature and do not demonstrate noncaseating granulomas when biopsied.[42–45] Cutaneous sarcoidosis has a predilection for scars and tattoos.[43] Management of cutaneous sarcoidosis is usually accomplished in collaboration with a dermatologist. Depending on the extent and severity of involvement, treatment options include topical steroids, local steroid injections, oral steroids, hydroxychloroquine, methotrexate, and anti–TNF-α agents in cases of recalcitrant lupus pernio.[43,44]

Eyes

Ocular involvement is variable across ethnic groups and can been seen in 10% to 80% of sarcoidosis patients.[1,46–50] Ocular involvement can be the initial manifestation of sarcoidosis.[48] All sarcoidosis patients require an annual ophthalmologic evaluation with a slit lamp, as most patients can be asymptomatic.[1] The most common manifestation is anterior uveitis, but any part of the orbit or adnexa can be involved.[46–50] It can present insidiously or acutely,[46–50] and can lead to visual impairment.[51] Management of ocular sarcoidosis is accomplished in collaboration with an ophthalmologist. Pharmacologic regimens include local topical or injectable steroids, and in refractory or recurrent cases second-line immunosuppressive agents such as methotrexate, leflunomide, mycophenolate mofetil, or anti-TNF agents have been used.[44] In addition to ophthalmic involvement with sarcoidosis, sarcoidosis patients need to be monitored for ophthalmic side effects and toxicities from immunosuppressive agents such as steroids and hydroxychloroquine that are used to manage other organ manifestations of sarcoidosis.[1]

Gastrointestinal

Sarcoidosis of the gastrointestinal system predominantly manifests as liver involvement.[52] The liver is involved in about 30% to 80% of sarcoidosis patients, whereas the gastrointestinal tract is rarely involved.[44,52,53] Hepatic sarcoidosis is twice as common in African Americans than in whites.[44,52] Patients can be asymptomatic or complain of nonspecific abdominal pain, pruritus, and/or jaundice.[44,52] Hepatomegaly is detected clinically in 21% of cases and radiographically in more than 50% of patients.[52] Pathological, findings include noncaseating granulomas mainly in the portal triad in addition to intrahepatic cholestasis and ductopenia with or without fibrosis.[44,52] Differential diagnosis for granulomas on liver biopsy should include primary biliary cirrhosis, tuberculosis, or drug reactions.[44,52,54] Hepatomegaly, lymphadenopathy, and low attenuating lesions of variable size in the liver can be seen on CT. On magnetic resonance imaging (MRI), nodules of various sizes with normal to slightly increased signal intensity can be seen.[44,52] Potential complications from hepatic sarcoidosis include cirrhosis and portal hypertension. Portal hypertension can be present with or without cirrhosis and can also develop from compression of the portal vein by enlarged lymph nodes in the hepatic hilum.[44,52] Most patients with hepatic sarcoidosis do not need therapy, especially if they are asymptomatic.[44,52] For symptomatic patients, low-dose steroids (10–20 mg daily) is usually adequate to control symptoms,[44,52] although hepatic sarcoidosis can progress even with biochemical improvement,[53] and poor responses are usually seen in the setting of established cirrhosis and/or portal hypertension.[44,52] Other agents such as azathioprine, methotrexate, and anti–TNF-α agents have been used to manage hepatic sarcoidosis.[44,52] Ursodeoxycholic acid has been reported to improve symptoms associated with cholestasis in case reports and series.[55] Liver transplant is rarely needed for hepatic sarcoidosis but is successful, with survival rates comparable with those for other indications for liver transplant.[44,52]

Neurologic

Neurosarcoidosis affects 5% to 15% of sarcoidosis patients.[56,57] Any part of the nervous system can be affected but cranial nerves are those most affected, the facial nerve being the most common followed by the optic nerve.[56,57] Parenchymal brain lesions occur in 50% of cases, the meninges are involved in about 20% to 40% of neurosarcoidosis cases, and spinal involvement occurs in fewer than 10% of cases.[56,57]

About 10% of neurosarcoidosis cases are asymptomatic.[56] The signs and symptoms are nonspecific and include cranial neuropathies, meningeal irritation, increased intracranial pressure, peripheral neuropathies, endocrine dysfunction, cognitive dysfunction, and personality changes.[56,57] Fifty percent of patients present within 2 years of diagnosing sarcoidosis.[56]

Diagnosing neurosarcoidosis can be challenging, and other diagnoses with similar manifestations need to be excluded.[56,57] MRI is the imaging modality of choice, but CT can be used in patients who cannot undergo MRI scanning although it has decreased sensitivity compared with MRI.[56,57] Findings on brain MRI include leptomeningeal enhancement, parenchymal lesions, thickening and enhancement of cranial nerves, and hydrocephalus.[56,57] Cerebrospinal fluid (CSF) findings are nonspecific and include lymphocytic pleocytosis, elevated protein level, decreased glucose level, and high opening pressure.[56,57] Although CSF findings are nonspecific, they are important in excluding other causes of the neurologic signs and symptoms.[56,57] The CSF angiotensin-converting enzyme level is nonspecific.[56,57] Electromyography and nerve conduction studies are helpful in assessing peripheral neuropathies.[56]

Diagnosing neurosarcoidosis can pose a challenge. Proposed diagnostic criteria by Zajicek and colleagues[58] include probable neurosarcoidosis, which requires pathologic confirmation of systemic sarcoidosis, clinical presentation suggestive of neurosarcoidosis, and the exclusion of other causes of neurologic dysfunction. If a beneficial response to therapy over a 1-year period is observed in addition to the aforementioned criteria, neurosarcoidosis is characterized as definite. Possible neurosarcoidosis is characterized by a clinical presentation suggestive of neurosarcoidosis but, without pathologic confirmation of systemic sarcoidosis and exclusion of other causes of neurologic dysfunction cannot be confirmed. Small-fiber neuropathy is a newly described entity in sarcoidosis whereby the patient presents with peripheral pain and signs and symptoms of autonomic dysfunction.[56,57] The exact etiology of small-fiber neuropathy in sarcoidosis is yet unknown.

Neurosarcoidosis requires treatment with immunosuppressive therapy to prevent irreversible neurologic deficits.[56,57] Steroids and second-line immunosuppressive agents such as methotrexate, mycophenolate mofetil, azathioprine, cyclophosphamide, and anti–TNF-α agents have all been used with variable success rates.[56,57] The dose and duration of therapy depends on the severity of symptoms and response to therapy.[56,57] Coordinating care with a neurologist who has expertise in neurosarcoidosis is essential.

Hypercalcemia/Hypercalciuria

Hypercalcemia occurs in about 10% of sarcoidosis patients, and hypercalciuria (>300 mg/d) is more common, occurring 3 times more than hypercalcemia.[59] 1α-Hydroxylase, which converts 25-hydroxycholecalciferol to the active form 1,25-dihydroxycholecalciferol, is expressed in the macrophages present in the granulomas and contributes to the abnormal calcium homeostasis seen in sarcoidosis.[59,60] Hypercalcemia and hypercalciuria are usually asymptomatic but could be the initial manifestation of sarcoidosis, with patients presenting with symptoms of hypercalcemia including lethargy, constipation, mental status changes, renal dysfunction, and/or nephrolithiasis. Management of hypercalcemia and/or hypercalciuria includes dietary modifications by avoiding dairy products and other nutrients high in vitamin D and calcium, and avoidance of sun exposure by wearing long sleeves and using sun-blocking products.[61] Other causes of hypercalcemia such as hyperparathyroidism should also be ruled out. Corticosteroids and hydroxychloroquine are the first line of therapy if hypercalcemia and/or hypercalciuria persist in spite of compliance with the aforementioned restrictions.[61]

Cardiac

Cardiac sarcoidosis is detected clinically in about 5% of cases, but on autopsy in about 40% of cases.[62,63] It can be asymptomatic or present with palpitations, dyspnea on exertion out of proportion to pulmonary involvement, syncope or presyncopal episodes or, rarely, sudden cardiac death.[62,63] No official guidelines exist for screening and management of cardiac sarcoidosis.[64] Screening for cardiac sarcoidosis is by history, physical examination, and 12-lead electrocardiogram (ECG).[1] Transthoracic echocardiogram and ambulatory ECG (Holter and event monitors) are helpful in further investigating symptoms that are suspicious of potential cardiac sarcoidosis.[1,63] Cardiac MRI (cMRI) and cardiac [18]fluorodeoxyglucose positron emission tomography (FDG-PET) imaging are new modalities used in the assessment of cardiac sarcoidosis.[65–67] Abnormalities on 12-lead ECG and ambulatory ECG include high-grade conduction blocks and ventricular and atrial arrhythmias.[63] Abnormalities on echocardiogram include unexplained left ventricular dysfunction and wall motion abnormalities.[63] cMRI findings suggestive of cardiac sarcoidosis include delayed hyperenhancement in a noncoronary distribution, suggestive of scar formation, in addition to wall edema.[63] Abnormalities on cardiac FDG-PET include hypermetabolic activity in a patchy or patchy-on-diffuse pattern.[63] Management of cardiac sarcoidosis includes immunosuppressive therapy, arrhythmia management, and management of any underlying left ventricular dysfunction.[68] Electrophysiological studies are important in risk assessment for sudden cardiac death and in determining when an automated implantable cardiac defibrillator is indicated.[69]

Musculoskeletal

Sarcoidosis can involve the articular, skeletal, and muscular systems.[70] Acute arthritis is reactive in nature and commonly manifests as part of Lofgren's syndrome.[70] Chronic arthritis is uncommon (1%–4% of cases), is associated with noncaseating granulomas and lymphocytic infiltration of involved joints, and usually denotes a chronic course.[70] Bone involvement is usually asymptomatic and is detected incidentally. It usually affects the small bones of the hands and feet but can affect any bone.[70] Radiographic findings include osteolysis in the small bones of the hands and feet and osteosclerosis in the long bones and vertebrae.[70] Bone scans and PET can also detect increased activity in the involved bones.[70] Muscle involvement is rare and can present as chronic myopathy, nodules, or masses, and rarely as acute myositis.[70] Management is mainly symptomatic, and includes steroids with or without second-line immunosuppressive agents.[70]

SYNDROMES OF SARCOIDOSIS

Lofgren's syndrome was first described in 1952.[71] Lofgren's syndrome is the acute manifestation of sarcoidosis, typically presenting in the springtime with arthritis, erythema nodosum, uveitis, and enlarged hilar lymph nodes.[72] It usually has an excellent prognosis, with high rates of spontaneous remission.[1] In the United States about 10% of the patients present with manifestations of Lofgren's syndrome, whereas it is rare in Japan but very common in Spain, where about half of the patients present with the syndrome, mostly in the spring.[3] Lofgren's syndrome typically has a benign, self-resolving course. Therapy is usually aimed at symptomatic relief, and includes short courses of nonsteroidal anti-inflammatory agents or corticosteroids.[72]

Heerfordt syndrome, also known as uveoparotid fever, was first described in 1909.[73] Patients present with fever, parotid gland enlargement, anterior uveitis, and facial nerve palsy.[73]

SUMMARY

Sarcoidosis is a multisystem disease with variable presentations, organ manifestations, and disease courses.[1] Histologic confirmation is necessary to confirm sarcoidosis but can be waived in cases of typical Lofgren's syndrome. In assessing a newly diagnosed patient a thorough history, including environmental and occupational history, and physical examination are essential in assessing organ involvement and for exclusion of other disorders that can be mimicked by sarcoidosis.[1] Laboratory and radiographic investigations include chest radiography, pulmonary function testing, annual ophthalmologic examination, 12-lead ECG, comprehensive metabolic panel, and 24-hour urinary calcium level.[1] Other investigations to assess organ involvement are typically guided by the findings of history and physical examination.[1] Sarcoidosis patients need routine follow-up to assess potential organ involvement, disease progression, and response to therapy when instituted.

Management of sarcoidosis patients is best accomplished in collaboration with a sarcoidosis center or expert, and appropriate subspecialists as dictated by organ involvement. Immunosuppressive therapy is indicated when major organs are involved (neurologic, ophthalmologic, or cardiac) or when there is evidence of organ dysfunction or progressive disease in other organs.[1] Immunosuppressive regimens, when indicated, include corticosteroids and steroid-sparing agents, and close monitoring of potential side effects and toxicities of immunosuppressive regimens is necessary.[38,39]

REFERENCES

1. Statement on sarcoidosis. Am J Respir Crit Care Med 1999;160(2):736–55.
2. Baughman RP, Teirstein AS, Judson MA, et al. Clinical characteristics of patients in a case control study of sarcoidosis. Am J Respir Crit Care Med 2001;164: 1885–9.
3. Sharma OP. Sarcoidosis around the world. Clin Chest Med 2008;29(3):357–63.
4. Morimoto T, Azuma A, Abe S, et al. Epidemiology of sarcoidosis in Japan. Eur Respir J 2008;31(2):372–9.

5. Design of a case control etiologic study of sarcoidosis (ACCESS). J Clin Epidemiol 1999;52(12):1173–86.

6. Newman LS, Rose CS, Bresnitz EA, et al. A case control etiologic study of sarcoidosis: environmental and occupational risk factors. Am J Respir Crit Care Med 2004;170(12):1324–30.

7. Deubelbeiss U, Gemperli A, Schindler C, et al. Prevalence of sarcoidosis in Switzerland is associated with environmental factors. Eur Respir J 2010;35(5):1088–97.

8. Crowley LE, Herbert R, Moline JM, et al. "Sarcoid like" granulomatous pulmonary disease in World Trade Center disaster responders. Am J Ind Med 2010;54(3):175–84.

9. Izbicki G, Chavko R, Banauch GI, et al. World trade center "sarcoid-like" granulomatous pulmonary disease in New York City fire department rescue workers. Chest 2007;131(5):1414–23.

10. Song Z, Marzilli L, Greenlee BM, et al. Mycobacterial catalase-peroxidase is a tissue antigen and target of the adaptive immune response in systemic sarcoidosis. J Exp Med 2005;201(5):755–67.

11. Dubaniewicz A, Dubaniewicz-Wybieralska M, Sternau A, et al. *Mycobacterium tuberculosis* complex and mycobacterial heat shock proteins in lymph node tissue from patients with pulmonary sarcoidosis. J Clin Microbiol 2006;44:3448–51.

12. Carlisle J, Evans W, Hajizadeh R, et al. Multiple *Mycobacterium* antigens induce interferon-gamma production from sarcoidosis peripheral blood mononuclear cells. Clin Exp Immunol 2007;150(3):460–8.

13. Carlisle J, Evans W, Hajizadeh R, et al. Immune recognition of multiple mycobacterial antigens by sarcoidosis subjects. J Clin Exp Immunol 2007;150:460–8.

14. Drake WP, Dhason MS, Nadaf M, et al. Cellular recognition of mycobacterium tuberculosis ESAT-6 and KatG peptides in systemic sarcoidosis. Infect Immun 2007;75(1):527–30.

15. Allen S, Evans W, Carlisle J, et al. Superoxide dismutase A antigens derived from molecular analysis of sarcoidosis granulomas elicit systemic Th-1 immune responses. Respir Res 2008;9(1):36.

16. Chen ES, Wahlstrom J, Song Z, et al. T cell responses to mycobacterial catalase-peroxidase profile a pathogenic antigen in systemic sarcoidosis. J Immunol 2008;181(12):8784–96.

17. Oswald-Richter KA, Culver DA, Hawkins C, et al. Cellular responses to mycobacterial antigens are present in bronchoalveolar lavage fluid used in the diagnosis of sarcoidosis. Infect Immun 2009;77(9):3740–8.

18. Douglas JG, Middleton WG, Gaddie J, et al. Sarcoidosis: a disorder commoner in non-smokers? Thorax 1986;41(10):787–91.

19. Gerke AK, van Beek E, Hunninghake GW. Smoking inhibits the frequency of bronchovascular bundle thickening in sarcoidosis. Acad Radiol 2011;18(7):885–91.

20. Muller-Quernheim J, Gaede KI, Fireman E, et al. Diagnoses of chronic beryllium disease within cohorts of sarcoidosis patients. Eur Respir J 2006;27:1190–5.

21. Maier LA. Genetic and exposure risks for chronic beryllium disease. Clin Chest Med 2002;23(4):827–39.

22. Rybicki BA, Iannuzzi MC, Frederick MM, et al. Familial aggregation of sarcoidosis. A case-control etiologic study of sarcoidosis (ACCESS). Am J Respir Crit Care Med 2001;164(11):2085–91.

23. Schurmann M, Reichel P, Muller-Myhsok B, et al. Results from a genome-wide search for predisposing genes in sarcoidosis. Am J Respir Crit Care Med 2001;164(5):840–6.

24. Rybicki BA, Levin AM, McKeigue P, et al. A genome-wide admixture scan for ancestry-linked genes predisposing to sarcoidosis in African-Americans. Genes Immun 2010.

25. Iannuzzi MC, Iyengar SK, Gray-McGuire C, et al. Genome-wide search for sarcoidosis susceptibility genes in African Americans. Genes Immun 2005;6(6):509–18.

26. Muller-Quernheim J, Schurmann M, Hofmann S, et al. Genetics of sarcoidosis. Clin Chest Med 2008;29(3):391–414, viii.

27. Wasfi YS, Silveira LJ, Jonth A, et al. Fas promoter polymorphisms: genetic predisposition to sarcoidosis in African-Americans. Tissue Antigens 2008;72(1):39–48.

28. McDougal KE, Fallin MD, Moller DR, et al. Variation in the lymphotoxin-alpha/tumor necrosis factor locus modifies risk of erythema nodosum in sarcoidosis. J Invest Dermatol 2009;129(8):1921–6.

29. Gerke AK, Hunninghake G. The immunology of sarcoidosis. Clin Chest Med 2008;29(3):379–90, vii.

30. Miyara M, Amoura Z, Parizot C, et al. The immune paradox of sarcoidosis and regulatory T cells. J Exp Med 2006;203(2):359–70.

31. Newman LS, Rose CS, Maier LA. Sarcoidosis. N Engl J Med 1997;336(17):1224–34.

32. Keary PJ, Palmer DG. Benign self-limiting sarcoidosis with skin and joint involvement. N Z Med J 1976;83(560):197–9.

33. Alhamad EH, Lynch JP 3rd, Martinez FJ. Pulmonary function tests in interstitial lung disease: what role do they have? Clin Chest Med 2001;22(4):715–50, ix.

34. Scadding JG. Sarcoidosis, with special reference to lung changes. Br Med J 1950;1(4656):745–53.

35. DeRemee RA. The roentgenographic staging of sarcoidosis. Historic and contemporary perspectives. Chest 1983;83(1):128–33.

36. Nishino M, Lee KS, Itoh H, et al. The spectrum of pulmonary sarcoidosis: variations of high-resolution CT findings and clues for specific diagnosis. Eur J Radiol 2010;73(1):66–73.

37. Huggins JT, Doelken P, Sahn SA, et al. Pleural effusions in a series of 181 outpatients with sarcoidosis. Chest 2006;129(6):1599–604.

38. Paramothayan NS, Lasserson TJ, Jones PW. Corticosteroids for pulmonary sarcoidosis. Cochrane Database Syst Rev 2005;2:CD001114.

39. Paramothayan S, Lasserson TJ, Walters EH. Immunosuppressive and cytotoxic therapy for pulmonary sarcoidosis. Cochrane Database Syst Rev 2006;3:CD003536.

40. Baughman RP, Drent M, Kavuru M, et al. Infliximab therapy in patients with chronic sarcoidosis and pulmonary involvement. Am J Respir Crit Care Med 2006;174(7):795–802.

41. Sahoo DH, Bandyopadhyay D, Xu M, et al. Effectiveness and safety of leflunomide for pulmonary and extrapulmonary sarcoidosis. Eur Respir J 2011. [Epub ahead of print].

42. Collin B, Rajaratnam R, Lim R, et al. A retrospective analysis of 34 patients with cutaneous sarcoidosis assessed in a dermatology department. Clin Exp Dermatol 2008;35(2):131–4.

43. Lodha S, Sanchez M, Prystowsky S. Sarcoidosis of the skin. Chest 2009;136(2):583–96.

44. Rose AS, Tielker MA, Knox KS. Hepatic, ocular, and cutaneous sarcoidosis. Clin Chest Med 2008;29(3):509–24, ix.

45. Ali MM, Atwan AA, Gonzalez ML. Cutaneous sarcoidosis: updates in the pathogenesis. J Eur Acad Dermatol Venereol 2010;24(7):747–55.

46. Baughman RP, Lower EE, Kaufman AH. Ocular sarcoidosis. Semin Respir Crit Care Med 2010;31(04):452–62.
47. Demirci H, Christianson MD. Orbital and adnexal involvement in sarcoidosis: analysis of clinical features and systemic disease in 30 cases. Am J Ophthalmol 2011;151(6):1074–80.
48. Heiligenhaus A, Wefelmeyer D, Wefelmeyer E, et al. The eye as a common site for the early clinical manifestation of sarcoidosis. Ophthalmic Res 2011;46(1):9–12.
49. Miserocchi E, Modorati G, Di Matteo F, et al. Visual outcome in ocular sarcoidosis: retrospective evaluation of risk factors. Eur J Ophthalmol 2011;21(6):802–10.
50. Papadia M, Herbort CP, Mochizuki M. Diagnosis of ocular sarcoidosis. Ocul Immunol Inflamm 2010;18(6):432–41.
51. Edelsten C, Pearson A, Joynes E, et al. The ocular and systemic prognosis of patients presenting with sarcoid uveitis. Eye (Lond) 1999;13(Pt 6):748–53.
52. Ebert EC, Kierson M, Hagspiel KD. Gastrointestinal and hepatic manifestations of sarcoidosis. Am J Gastroenterol 2008;103(12):3184–92 [quiz: 3193].
53. Kennedy PT, Zakaria N, Modawi SB, et al. Natural history of hepatic sarcoidosis and its response to treatment. Eur J Gastroenterol Hepatol 2006;18(7):721–6.
54. Uta D, Hans-Udo K, Judith R, et al. Hepatic granulomas: histological and molecular pathological approach to differential diagnosis—a study of 442 cases. Liver Int 2008;28(6):828–34.
55. Alenezi B, Lamoureux E, Alpert L, et al. Effect of ursodeoxycholic acid on granulomatous liver disease due to sarcoidosis. Dig Dis Sci 2005;50(1):196–200.
56. Terushkin V, Stern BJ, Judson MA, et al. Neurosarcoidosis: presentations and management. Neurologist 2010;16(1):2–15.
57. Hoitsma E, Drent M, Sharma OP. A pragmatic approach to diagnosing and treating neurosarcoidosis in the 21st century. Curr Opin Pulm Med 2010;16(5):472–9.
58. Zajicek JP, Scolding NJ, Foster O, et al. Central nervous system sarcoidosis—diagnosis and management. QJM 1999;92(2):103–17.
59. Sharma OP. Vitamin D, calcium, and sarcoidosis. Chest 1996;109(2):535–9.
60. Sharma OP, Vucinic V. Sarcoidosis of the thyroid and kidneys and calcium metabolism. Semin Respir Crit Care Med 2002;23(6):579–88.
61. Burke RR, Rybicki BA, Rao DS. Calcium and vitamin D in sarcoidosis: how to assess and manage. Semin Respir Crit Care Med 2010;31(4):474–84.
62. Silverman KJ, Hutchins GM, Bulkley BH. Cardiac sarcoid: a clinicopathologic study of 84 unselected patients with systemic sarcoidosis. Circulation 1978; 58(6):1204–11.
63. Mehta D, Lubitz SA, Frankel Z, et al. Cardiac involvement in patients with sarcoidosis: diagnostic and prognostic value of outpatient testing. Chest 2008;133(6): 1426–35.
64. Hamzeh NY, Wamboldt FS, Weinberger HD. Management of cardiac sarcoidosis in the United States: a Delphi study. Chest 2011. [Epub ahead of print].
65. Ohira H, Tsujino I, Ishimaru S, et al. Myocardial imaging with 18-fluoro-2-deoxy-glucose positron emission tomography and magnetic resonance imaging in sarcoidosis. Eur J Nucl Med Mol Imaging 2008;35(5):933–41.
66. Osman F, Foundon A, Leyva P, et al. Early diagnosis of cardiac sarcoidosis using magnetic resonance imaging. Int J Cardiol 2008;125(1):e4–5.
67. Tahara N, Tahara A, Nitta Y, et al. Heterogeneous myocardial FDG uptake and the disease activity in cardiac sarcoidosis. JACC Cardiovasc Imaging 2010;3(12): 1219–28.
68. Ayyala US, Nair AP, Padilla ML. Cardiac sarcoidosis. Clin Chest Med 2008;29(3): 493–508, ix.

69. Writing Committee, Epstein AE, DiMarco JP, et al. ACC/AHA/HRS 2008 Guidelines for Device-Based Therapy of Cardiac Rhythm Abnormalities: executive summary: a report of the American College of Cardiology/American Heart Association Task Force on Practice Guidelines (Writing Committee to Revise the ACC/AHA/NASPE 2002 Guideline Update for Implantation of Cardiac Pacemakers and Antiarrhythmia Devices): developed in collaboration with the American Association for Thoracic Surgery and Society of Thoracic Surgeons. Circulation 2008; 117(21):2820–40.

70. Zisman DA, Shorr AF, Lynch JP 3rd. Sarcoidosis involving the musculoskeletal system. Semin Respir Crit Care Med 2002;23(6):555–70.

71. Lofgren S, Lundback H. The bilateral hilar lymphoma syndrome; a study of the relation to age and sex in 212 cases. Acta Med Scand 1952;142(4):259–64.

72. Mana J, Gomez-Vaquero C, Montero A, et al. Lofgren's syndrome revisited: a study of 186 patients. Am J Med 1999;107(3):240–5.

73. James DG, Sharma OP. Parotid gland sarcoidosis. Sarcoidosis Vasc Diffuse Lung Dis 2000;17(1):27–32.

Index

Note: Page numbers of article titles are in **boldface** type.

A

A Case Controlled Etiologic Study of Sarcoidosis (ACCESS), 1224–1225
Ablation therapies, for airway obstruction, 1104–1106
Abscess, pleural effusion in
    intra-abdominal, 1067
    lung, 1061–1063
ACCESS (A Case Controlled Etiologic Study of Sarcoidosis), 1224–1225
Acetazolamide, for obesity hypoventilation syndrome, 1192
Acute interstitial pneumonia. *See* Interstitial lung disease.
Acute respiratory distress syndrome, versus acute eosinophilic pneumonia, 1175–1176
Airway obstruction
    hypoventilation in, 1193–1195
    interventional pulmonology for, 1101–1106
Alemtuzumab, for hypereosinophilic syndromes, 1180
Allergic bronchopulmonary aspergillosis, 1170–1172
Allergy, asthma with, 1116–1117
Alteplase, for pulmonary embolism, 1215
Amebiasis, eosinophilic lung disease in, 1172
American Cancer Society Cancer Prevention Study, smoking and, 1043
American Thoracic Society, pneumonia guidelines of, 1144
Amyotrophic lateral sclerosis, hypoventilation in, 1196–1198
Angiotensin receptor blockers, for COPD, 1134
Angiotensin-converting enzyme inhibitors, for COPD, 1134
Ankylosing spondylitis, hypoventilation in, 1195
Antibiotics
    eosinophilic lung disease due to, 1173
    for COPD, 1134–1135
    for pleural effusion, 1061–1062
    for pneumonia, 1146–1147, 1153–1156
Anticholinergics
    for COPD, 1132
    for venous thromboembolism, 1216
Anticoagulants, for pulmonary embolism, 1213
Antineutrophilic cytoplasmic antibodies, in eosinophilic lung diseases, 1167, 1177–1178
Antinuclear antibodies, in interstitial lung disease, 1075
Argatroban, for pulmonary embolism, 1214
Argon plasma coagulation, for airway obstruction, 1106
Arterial blood gas measurement
    for pulmonary embolism, 1206–1207
    in hypoventilation syndromes, 1190

Med Clin N Am 95 (2011) 1235–1248
doi:10.1016/S0025-7125(11)00106-4
0025-7125/11/$ – see front matter © 2011 Elsevier Inc. All rights reserved.

medical.theclinics.com